INTERNATIONAL RESEARCH MONOGRAPHS IN THE ADDICTIONS (IRMA)

Series Editor
Professor Griffith Edwards
National Addiction Centre
Institute of Psychiatry, London

A series of volumes presenting important research from major centres around the world on the basic sciences, both biological and behavioural, that have a bearing on the addictions, and also addressing the clinical and public health applications of such research. The series will cover alcohol, illicit drugs, psychotropics and tobacco, and is an important resource for clinicians, researchers and policy makers.

Also in this series:

Alcohol and the Community: A Systems Approach to Prevention
Harold D. Holder

D1336326

CANNABIS AND COGNITIVE FUNCTIONING

NADIA SOLOWIJ

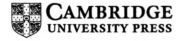

CAMBRIDGE
UNIVERSITY PRESS

CAMBRIDGE UNIVERSITY PRESS
Cambridge, New York, Melbourne, Madrid, Cape Town, Singapore, São Paulo

Cambridge University Press
The Edinburgh Building, Cambridge CB2 2RU, UK

Published in the United States of America by Cambridge University Press, New York

www.cambridge.org
Information on this title: www.cambridge.org/9780521591140

First published 1998
Reprinted 1999
This digitally printed first paperback version 2006

A catalogue record for this publication is available from the British Library

Library of Congress Cataloguing in Publication data
Solowij, Nadia
    Cannabis and cognitive functioning / Nadia Solowij.
  p.   cm. – (International research monographs in the addictions)
    Includes bibliographical references and index.
    ISBN 0 521 59114 7
    1. Cannabis – Physiological effect.   2. Brain – Effect of drugs on.
    3. Cognition.   4. Evoked potentials (Electrophysiology)
    5. Cognition disorders. I. Title II. Series.
    QP801.C27S66   1988
    615'.7827–dc21   97–38655   CIP

ISBN-13 978-0-521-59114-0 hardback
ISBN-10 0-521-59114-7 hardback

ISBN-13 978-0-521-02480-8 paperback
ISBN-10 0-521-02480-3 paperback

Contents

Series editor's preface

This book invites us to examine one single and sharply focused question – can exposure to cannabis result in any kind of long-term cognitive impairment? In considering that question, Dr Nadia Solowij firstly deploys a critical and comprehensive review of the relevant research literature. This part of her writing constitutes a significant contribution in its own right. Second, she reports and integrates the results of a series of experiments which she herself has conducted using event-related potential (ERP) techniques. The background review and her personal research are then together brought to bear on the common and core question. She weighs the evidence and tells us that the long-term use of cannabis may produce "impairment in the higher cognitive functions of memory, attention, and the organisation and integration of complex functions", with that impairment not necessarily recoverable on abstinence.

That is the nub of the matter. Dr Solowij's conclusions are tentative, but if further work confirms her findings there are public health implications of potentially profound importance. Policies on cannabis are at present for the most part, and inevitably, the time warp residuum of positions taken in the absence of knowledge. The present findings should neither be used for scaremongering nor dismissed with easy comfort: in one corner of this complex field Dr Solowij gives us the beginnings of rather worrying knowledge, even though the impairments she describes are subtle in nature.

It has been my privilege to work with Dr Solowij on the preparation of this text for publication. Readers must judge whether the pleasures of that cooperation have made me prejudiced, but my belief is that Dr Solowij provides us here with an exceptionally well-argued and persuasively evidenced analysis of the effects of cannabis on cognitive function. At the same time and beyond the immediate content, I believe she is giving us a disciplined and creative statement which is exemplary of what a scientific monograph, in our day and age, may modestly and with integrity hope to achieve. Readers must judge whether my prejudice is justified.

Griffith Edwards

Author's acknowledgements

A number of people made significant contributions during the course of this research. First and foremost, I thank Associate Professor Patricia Michie, who has been a source of inspiration to me since I first met her some 10 years ago. She introduced me to brain event-related potentials (ERPs) and became my mentor, providing invaluable advice and consultation which enabled this research to come to fruition. Some of the research reported in this monograph was conducted in Dr Michie's laboratory at Macquarie University and I am grateful to Len Glue for his technical expertise and Alan Taylor for statistical guidance.

I wish to express my gratitude to Professor Wayne Hall who has fostered my research at the National Drug and Alcohol Research Centre over the past decade. I have gained a great deal of respect and admiration for him in the course of our professional collaboration. I thank him for his patience in reading, diligently correcting and refining this and other material, and for opening so many opportunities for me in my career.

Most of the research reported here was conducted at the National Drug and Alcohol Research Centre (NDARC), University of New South Wales, funded by the National Campaign Against Drug Abuse (Australia). Portions of the research reported here were funded by the Research Into Drug Abuse Grants Scheme of the Commonwealth Department of Human Services and Health. I thank Heli Wolk for her never ending support, Eva Congreve for library assistance, and Professor Nick Heather for providing the means and facilities to conduct the research. I wish to acknowledge Dr Gregory Chesher and Dr John Prescott for inspiration in formulating some of the early ideas for this research (and Greg for his contributions within our ongoing scholarly deliberations), and Dr Allison Fox for her expertise in setting up the laboratory at NDARC, computer programming and for listening to all my trials and tribulations. I am indebted to all the subjects, cannabis users and nonusers, who participated in the research.

In this monograph I have developed on the text of my previous PhD dissertation while seeking to produce an exposition which is more reader friendly than that academic form. Use has also been made of previously published articles:

Solowij, N., Michie, P.T. & Fox, A.M. (1991). Effects of long-term cannabis use on selective attention: an event-related potential study. *Pharmacology Biochemistry and Behavior*, **40**, 683–8. Portions reprinted by permission of the publisher, copyright 1991 by Elsevier Science Inc.

Solowij, N., Michie, P.T. & Fox, A.M. (1995). Differential impairments of selective attention due to frequency and duration of cannabis use. *Biological Psychiatry*, **37**, 731–9. Portions reprinted by permission of Elsevier Science Inc., copyright 1995 by The Society of Biological Psychiatry.

Solowij, N. (1995). Do cognitive impairments recover following cessation of cannabis use? *Life Sciences*, **56**, 2119–26. Portions reprinted by permission of the publisher, copyright 1995 by Elsevier Science Inc.

Solowij, N., Grenyer, B.F.S., Chesher, G. & Lewis, J. (1995). Biopsychosocial changes associated with cessation of cannabis use: a single case study of acute and chronic cognitive effects, withdrawal and treatment. *Life Sciences*, **56**, 2127–34. Portions reprinted by permission of the publisher, copyright 1995 by Elsevier Science Inc.

Chapters 4 and 5 are updated reviews originally conducted for the World Health Organization project on health implications of cannabis use (reprinted here by permission). These reviews will appear in a forthcoming book, *The Health Effects of Cannabis Use*, to be published by the Addiction Research Foundation, a division of the Addiction and Mental Health Services Corporation.

I thank my family, my parents and my husband, Dr Brin Grenyer, for their encouragement, love and support over all the years. Brin, in particular, has given valuable critical feedback in the course of this research, and contributed his expert clinical skills for the case study reported in Chapter 10. I dedicate this book to Kees, who endured the completion of the thesis while still in the womb, and who played patiently during the endless hours of updating and revision for this monograph.

1

Statement of the problem

What hashish gives with one hand it takes away with the other: that is to say, it gives power of imagination and takes away the ability to profit by it.
Charles Baudelaire (1860) Les Paradis Artificiel, Paris: Poulet-Malassis.

Rarely are the consequences of cannabis use described so eloquently by its users as in this extract from Baudelaire writing in the mid-nineteenth century. After euphoria, the acute cognitive effects of cannabis are among those that are most often sought by those who use the drug. The loosening of associations, the intensification of ordinary experiences, a heightening of humour, pleasant imaginative reverie, are all cognitive effects that provide users with a welcome relief from the tedium of everyday life. Some cannabis users experience these effects daily over a period of many years. It has long been suspected that the price paid for the regular elicitation of these diverting cognitive effects of cannabis may be some type of enduring, and possibly irreversible, cognitive impairment, and thus the loss of ability to profit by its use.

There is a prima facie case to support this suspicion. Some long-term cannabis users who seek help to stop their use complain about various worrying cognitive phenomena. They often report: "I forget what I'm saying in the middle of a sentence", or "I forget why I went from one part of the house to the other" or "I start doing one thing and get distracted into doing something else". Such statements are made by chronic users who perceive there to be a problem but find it difficult to articulate the precise nature of the problem. They may refer to some poorly formulated apprehension of impaired performance: "I can't put my finger on it . . . I'm just not doing as well as I used to . . . I daydream a lot . . . I can't concentrate . . . My memory's not as good as it used to be". While memory has been the cognitive function most often claimed to be affected by long-term use of cannabis, as clinicians and researchers we have not quite been able to put our finger on it either.

Self reports by cannabis users, and those of clinical observers, provide a useful starting point. They suggest a phenomenon worth investigating and provide some clues as to what type of cognitive impairment long-term cannabis use may produce: forgetfulness, distractibility, difficulties in attending and concentrating, and memory problems. It is difficult to be sure that these effects can be unambiguously attributed to cannabis. After all, many people who have not used cannabis complain of similar problems at one time or another, especially as they grow older. It has been difficult enough to discover what changes occur in these cognitive functions with age. Perhaps we should not be surprised that until recently research has not been able to reach consensus on what are the long-term cognitive consequences of cannabis use.

This monograph has several aims. First, it critically reviews the research literature relevant to cannabis use and cognitive functioning. Second, it presents the results of a series of original studies which utilized the most modern and sensitive tools available to assess cognitive functioning, with a view to identifying the specific effects of chronic cannabis use in a more focused way than most previous studies. Third, it is hoped that the integration of evidence from these two approaches will inform not only the research community, but also clinicians and policy makers. For clinicians who deal with long-term cannabis users, a better understanding of the cognitive impairments with which their clients may present might be incorporated to facilitate the treatment process. This might involve tailoring standard clinical interventions to accommodate the difficulties that the client may have with attention, concentration and memory for example, or possibly even designing cognitive rehabilitation programmes (e.g. Sohlberg & Mateer, 1989). As a scholarly work, the aim of this monograph is not to influence policy decision, but inevitably its content may inform debate on the topic.

This monograph is timely. Tremendous advances have been made in recent years in understanding the pharmacology of cannabis. The discovery of a cannabinoid receptor and an endogenous cannabinoid system (Devane *et al.*, 1988, 1992; Matsuda *et al.*, 1990) represented major breakthroughs not only in the cannabis field but also in the field of cognitive neuroscience. The distribution of the receptors throughout the brain and the known pharmacological activity of cannabis suggest roles for the endogenous cannabinoid system in cognition and motor coordination and, thus, provide the potential to enhance our understanding of cognitive processes and executive and motor control in the normal brain. The precise role of the endogenous cannabinoid system and its interaction with other neurotransmitter systems have yet to be elucidated but continued research of the kind presented in this monograph will contribute to our understanding of their dynamics. The knowledge that cannabis acts upon a specific receptor, and that it does not merely nonspecifically perturb cell membranes, for example, has lead to new concerns that prolonged cumulative exposure to cannabis may result in alterations in the functioning of the receptor and its endogenous ligand, which could underly the purported cognitive deficits.

Initiation to cannabis use typically occurs in adolescence and the periods of greatest use coincide with adolescence and young adulthood (Kandel & Logan, 1984). This represents a major concern for society and for the developing individual if there were indeed alterations in brain function and long-term cognitive consequences. These consequences could potentially be compounded by a tendency for more potent strains of cannabis to be developed (Jones, 1987; Adams & Martin, 1996). Despite law enforcement efforts to inhibit its sale and consumption, cannabis remains the most widely used illicit substance in the world with estimates of between 12 and 20 million current users in the USA alone (Kozel & Adams, 1986; Jones, 1987; Goldstein & Kalant, 1990). The prevalence of its use indicates a potentially major public health concern as the costs to society could be high in terms of health risks in general.

There is no reason to believe that cannabis causes gross impairment of cognitive functioning. Given the rates of use worldwide over the past two decades, if chronic cannabis use produced severe cognitive impairments, it is likely that there would be no need to be researching the question in the 1990s: it appears that the question as to whether long-term cannabis use does indeed have any long-term cognitive consequences has never been entirely resolved. While it seems clear that the cognitive consequences are probably not extremely debilitating, there has been sufficient evidence to warrant further investigation of perhaps more subtle impairments.

Clarification of the possible long-term cognitive effects, among other health and psychological consequences, will no doubt contribute to policy considerations regarding the legal status of cannabis. It is not the purpose nor intention of this monograph to influence policy makers in either direction; the reviews were prepared in an attempt to present a balanced appraisal of the scientific literature. In general, this area is one in which opinions have typically been polarized between, on the one hand, a scepticism that is impervious to any evidence of the harmful effects of cannabis and, on the other, a credulous preparedness to take at face value any suggestion that cannabis is harmful to health (Hall & Solowij, 1996). The guidelines adopted here for evaluating the evidence have been clearly set out elsewhere (Hall *et al.*, 1994) and the extent to which the objective of remaining free from bias was achieved is discussed by a number of commentators (see *Addiction* (1996). **91**, 759–73; Hall & Solowij, 1996). Both the reviews and the original research contained within this monograph have previously been published elsewhere and peer reviewed. Their compilation and revision for this monograph provide an update that includes the most recent literature.

Definitions

A number of terms that have been used frequently or interchangeably throughout the literature require definition and clarification at the outset. "Cannabinoids" is the collective term for a variety of compounds which can either be: (1) extracted from the cannabis plant, (2) produced synthetically to mimic the effects of natural cannabis compounds, (3) produced within the body after ingestion and metabolism of cannabis, or (4) found to occur naturally within the body or brain and bind to the recently discovered cannabinoid receptors. Some of these compounds are psychoactive, i.e. they have an effect upon the mind of the users. Others are pharmacologically or biologically active, i.e. they have an effect upon cells or the function of other body tissues and organs, but are not psychoactive. Where the term "cannabis" is used in this monograph, it is used generically to refer only to preparations of the natural plant matter as consumed by illicit drug users. Terms such as "marijuana", "hashish" and others are defined in Chapter 2. Animal and human experimentation indicates that delta-9-tetrahydrocannabinol (THC) is the major psychoactive constituent of cannabis (Gaoni & Mechoulam, 1964).

Terms frequently used to describe the toxicity of a drug are acute, subacute and chronic. These terms strictly apply to the duration of the treatment given to experimental animals in a toxicity study. When applied to human research, they refer to the effects which may follow the acute, subacute or chronic use of the drug. Definitions of these terms may vary according to the substance in question; the definitions below are specific to cannabis.

Acute effects refer to those effects produced by a single dose of cannabis and these include the effects sought by the user, as well as the short lived unwanted side effects that are usually associated with higher doses. The duration of the acute effects depends essentially on the dose and the route of administration, but it may also depend on the specific drug effect measured and on whether the user is experienced or naive. Subacute effects are those that result from repeated administration over several days; each dose itself does not necessarily produce a detrimental effect, but cumulatively may result in an adverse response.

Chronic effects refer to the consequences of repeated administration of cannabis over a prolonged period. Chronic or long-term effects, while not necessarily permanent, persist beyond the phase of elimination of cannabinoids from the body, and hence are not attributable to a direct (acute or subacute) action of cannabinoids. The term "residual" has often been used in the literature to indicate long-term effects, but this term will not be used in this monograph in order to avoid the mistaken implication that these effects may solely be due to drug residues remaining in the body. In this monograph, the hypothesized contribution of drug residues will be clearly differentiated from effects purported to reflect longer lasting changes in brain function. Such changes can be either a result of neuroadaptive mechanisms, such as have been described in the opioid literature (e.g. Cox, 1990), or the result of drug induced neurotoxicity. In the former case, the effects are self limiting if no further drug is taken but may be expressed as a "withdrawal" syndrome. In the latter case, the neurotoxicity may be functional and may or may not be structural and/or irreversible.

Wherever the prevalence, patterns and mode of cannabis use are referred to throughout this monograph, these apply primarily to culturally similar English speaking countries such as Australia, Canada, New Zealand, the UK and the USA, and particularly so because the original research reported here was conducted in Australia. The concepts are also appropriate for many European countries and probably for many other parts of the world as well. While it is acknowledged that the patterns and prevalence of use may vary widely (see Chapter 2), the unifying factor is that cannabis is used primarily for recreational purposes and cannabis is regarded as an illicit drug. This is the framework within which this monograph is written. The use of cannabis for religious or therapeutic purposes is not specifically considered, but the long-term cognitive consequences would be expected to be the same across a variety of cultures, regardless of the purposes for which the drug is used. Nevertheless, the significance of such consequences would vary from culture to culture depending upon the social importance of the cognitive functions affected by cannabis use (see Chapter 5).

Structure of the monograph and overview of the problem

The monograph is divided into two distinct sections. The first presents extensive reviews of the literature which set the scene for the original research presented in part two. The literature review commences in Chapter 2 with a description of the research that led to the discovery of the cannabinoid receptor and endogenous cannabinoid like substances, as this important information must by necessity shape the way all other material is considered. A description of the forms of cannabis the drug, methods of administration, dosage and patterns of use follow, and the metabolism of cannabinoids is discussed together with their detection in body fluids and the issue of passive inhalation.

The acute effects of cannabis on human behaviour and cognition are reasonably well documented. Numerous studies have reported the acute effects of cannabis on psychomotor and cognitive performance, and these are briefly and selectively reviewed in Chapter 3. The most frequently affected cognitive functions are those of memory and attention; the results of many behavioural studies attest that cannabis impairs short-term memory and various kinds of attention while intoxicated, impairing also the ability to perform complex functions requiring attention and mental coordination (Casswell & Marks, 1973a; MacAvoy & Marks, 1975; Miller & Branconnier, 1983; Chait & Pierri, 1992). The long-term consequences of cannabis use on memory and attentional processes are unclear. Memory and attention are inextricably linked: effective memory function is dependent on efficient attentional processes. Impaired attentional processing in the long-term may have serious implications given that such processes are required for successful work performance, learning, memory and everyday tasks such as driving a motor vehicle.

A logical starting point for examining the consequences of long-term exposure to cannabis is to assess precisely those functions most consistently disrupted by acute intoxication. Relatively few studies have investigated cognitive functioning in chronic cannabis users, fewer still in any rigorous way. Many were performed more than a decade ago in response to wide community concern following: (1) the explosion of cannabis use in western societies in the 1970s, (2) the appearance of reports in the clinical literature describing mental deterioration associated with chronic use of cannabis (e.g. Kolansky & Moore, 1971, 1972), (3) the publication of a medical report of cerebral atrophy in young cannabis users (Campbell *et al.*, 1971), and (4) the concurrent sensationalist media reports of cannabis induced "brain damage". Chapter 4 discusses the evidence pertaining to possible neurological damage as a result of exposure to cannabis.

The studies of cognitive functioning in chronic users are reviewed in depth in Chapter 5. The early studies produced essentially contradictory results due in part to the gross measures used and to methodological difficulties. Researchers relied primarily on the use of psychometric tests to assess the presence of dysfunction in fairly broad areas of cognition. While some studies did find significant differences between cannabis users and controls on a number of cognitive tests, these could variously be attributed to acute intoxication (e.g. Stefanis *et al.*, 1977), lack of pre-standardization of test batteries for the subject populations used (e.g. Rubin & Comitas, 1975), or the unrepresentative populations tested (e.g. Soueif, 1971). Many studies were unable to replicate the findings (e.g. Carlin & Trupin, 1977; see also Fehr & Kalant, 1983b). Positive results were often reported nonspecifically as "impairment of cognitive functions associated with long-term heavy cannabis use" (e.g. Mendhiratta *et al.*, 1988). The lack of specificity and sensitivity of assessment techniques led to equivocal results. The long-term effects of cannabis, if they exist, are likely to be subtle rather than grossly debilitating. Following the research efforts of the 1970s and early 1980s, the question as to whether chronic use of cannabis leads to any long-term impairment remained unresolved and there remained considerable controversy over this issue.

The involvement of cannabinoids in the central nervous system was underscored by the discovery and anatomical localization of a specific cannabinoid receptor in the brain (Devane *et al.*, 1988; Bidaut-Russel *et al.*, 1990; Herkenham *et al.*, 1990; Matsuda *et al.*, 1990; Gerard *et al.*, 1991) and by the identification of an endogenous brain molecule, named anandamide, that binds to the receptor and mimics the action of cannabinoids (Devane *et al.*, 1992). Cannabinoid receptors are distributed throughout brain regions known to be involved in attention, with high densities in the cerebral cortex and hippocampus (Bidaut-Russell *et al.*, 1990; Herkenham *et al.*, 1990). The hippocampus plays a role in excluding extraneous stimuli during concentration of attention and it was suggested that cannabinoids may disinhibit septal-hippocampal inputs to the reticular activating system resulting in failure to habituate to irrelevant stimuli (Miller & Branconnier, 1983).

In the original research presented in this monograph, the integrity of attentional processes in long-term cannabis users was assessed using a combination of performance and event-related potential (ERP) measures, which together can provide insight into the nature of cognitive dysfunction (Ward *et al.*, 1991). Event-related potentials are scalp recorded electrical responses of the brain to a particular event or stimulus, usually recorded during the performance of a cognitive task. ERP components are sensitive markers of specific stages of information processing, reflecting the nature, timing and duration of cognitive processes (Hillyard & Kutas, 1983; Näätänen, 1990). In ERP studies of auditory selective attention (reviewed in Chapter 6) directing attention to a particular channel of information results in the onset of a negative shift of the ERP waveform, which is referred to as processing negativity (PN) (Näätänen, 1982; Hansen & Hillyard, 1983). Processing negativity is evident in the auditory system as early as 60 to 80 ms after presentation of a stimulus. It reflects the selection of relevant from irrelevant sources of information. Ongoing negativity beyond 600 ms in the ERP waveform to attended stimuli is referred to as late PN and reflects the maintenance and rehearsal of the attentional trace (Näätänen, 1982). The other component of interest is the P300, a large positive peak which is elicited by infrequent stimuli in the attended channel when a response is required (Donchin, 1981; Pritchard, 1981). The latency of the P300 component reflects the time taken to evaluate a stimulus, while its amplitude reflects the nature of stimulus evaluation processes. It is these two components that are of particular interest in the series of studies reported here.

In the first study, presented in Chapter 7, a small group of cannabis users was compared with a group of nonuser controls in their performance of a complex selective attention task. The results of this study were then replicated with a larger sample which enabled the effects of frequency and duration of cannabis use to be assessed. This study is reported in Chapter 8. The extent of reversibility of the impairments observed was examined in a group of long-term cannabis users who had previously given up, presented in Chapter 9. Finally, a single case study of cessation of cannabis use, which monitored ERPs before and after quitting cannabis use and also during acute intoxication, is reported in Chapter 10. Some descriptive, quantitative and qualitative data over all samples, paying particular attention to psychopathological symptoms and self-reported cognitive dysfunction, are presented in Chapter 11. The monograph concludes with a synthesis of the evidence from the literature reviews and the original research, a discussion of the implications of the findings and recommendations for future research.

The weight of the evidence

The weight of the available evidence suggests that long-term heavy use of cannabis does not produce any severe or grossly debilitating impairment of cognitive function. If it did, research to date should have detected it. Nonetheless, the original ERP studies presented here, together with the results of other research reviewed here, indicate that the long-term use of cannabis may produce more subtle cognitive impairment in the higher cognitive functions of memory, attention and the organization and integration of complex information. While subtle in nature, these impairments could affect everyday functioning, particularly among individuals in occupations that require high levels of cognitive capacity. The evidence suggests there may be different cognitive consequences associated with frequency and duration of cannabis use, but the longer the period that cannabis has been used, the more pronounced is the cognitive impairment. Preliminary work suggests that there may be only partial recovery of function, although it remains to be seen with further research whether the impairment can be fully reversed by an extended period of abstinence from cannabis and what factors may contribute to individual differences in recovery.

Part 1

A review of the literature

2
Cannabis the drug

Cannabis is the material derived from the herbaceous plant *Cannabis sativa* which grows vigorously throughout many regions of the world. It occurs in male and female forms with both sexes having large leaves which consist of 5–11 leaflets with serrated margins. A sticky resin which covers the flowering tops and upper leaves is secreted most abundantly by the female plant and this resin contains the active agents of the plant. While the cannabis plant contains more than 60 cannabinoid compounds, such as cannabidiol and cannabinol, the primary psychoactive constituent is delta-9-tetrahydrocannabinol or THC (Gaoni & Mechoulam, 1964), the concentration of which largely determines the potency of the cannabis preparation. Most of the other cannabinoids are either inactive or only weakly active, although they may increase or decrease potency by interacting with THC (Abood & Martin, 1992).

Previously cannabis had been erroneously classified as a narcotic, as a sedative and most recently as a hallucinogen. While the cannabinoids do possess hallucinogenic properties, together with stimulant and sedative effects (Dewey, 1986; Adams & Martin, 1996), they in fact represent a unique pharmacological class of compounds. Unlike other hallucinogenic drugs, cannabis acts on specific receptors in the brain and periphery. The recent discovery of the receptors and the naturally occurring substances in the brain that bind to these receptors, is of great importance in that it signifies an entirely new pathway system in the brain.

The cannabinoid receptor
The desire to identify a specific biochemical pathway responsible for the expression of the psychoactive effects of cannabis has prompted a prodigious amount of cannabinoid research (Martin, 1986). Early studies

found that radioactively labelled THC would nonspecifically attach to all neural surfaces, which suggested that it produced its effects by perturbing cell membranes (Martin, 1986; Makriyannis & Rapaka, 1990). The work of Howlett and colleagues (Howlett *et al.*, 1986, 1988; Howlett, 1987) however, showed that cannabinoids inhibit the enzyme that synthesizes cyclic AMP in cultured nerve cells, and that the degree of inhibition was correlated with the potency of the cannabinoid. As many receptors relay their signals to the cell interior by changing cellular cyclic AMP, this finding strongly suggested that cannabinoids were not just dissolving nonspecifically in membranes. After eliminating all the known receptors that act by inhibiting adenylate cyclase, it was concluded that cannabinoids acted through their own receptor. The determination and characterization of a specific cannabinoid receptor in brain followed soon after (Devane *et al.*, 1988), paving the way for its distribution in the brain to be mapped (Bidaut-Russell *et al.*, 1990; Herkenham *et al.*, 1990).

It is now accepted that cannabinoids act on specific receptors in the brain and periphery, although probably not all effects are receptor mediated. Conclusive evidence for the receptor was provided by the cloning of the gene for the cannabinoid receptor in rat brain (Matsuda *et al.*, 1990). A cDNA which encodes the human cannabinoid receptor was also cloned (Gerard *et al.*, 1991) and the human receptor was found to exhibit more than 97% identity with the rat receptor. Cannabinoid receptors have also been found in the nervous system of lower vertebrates, including chickens, turtles and trout (Howlett *et al.*, 1990) and there is preliminary evidence that they exist in low concentration in fruit flies (Bonner quoted in Abbott, 1990; Howlett *et al.*, 1992). This phylogenetic distribution suggests that the gene must have been present early in evolution, and its conservation implies that the receptor serves an important biological function.

The localization of cannabinoid receptors in brain has elucidated the pharmacology of the cannabinoids. Herkenham and colleagues (Herkenham, *et al.*, 1990, 1991a, b; Herkenham, 1992) used autoradiography to localize receptors in fresh cut brain sections of a number of species, including human. Dense binding was detected in the cerebral cortex, hippocampus, cerebellum and in outflow nuclei of the basal ganglia, particularly the substantia nigra pars reticulata and globus pallidus. Few receptors were present in the brainstem and spinal cord. Bidaut-Russell, *et al.* (1990) located cannabinoid receptors in greatest abundance in the rat cortex, cerebellum, hippocampus and striatum, with substantially smaller yet significant binding in the hypothalamus, brainstem and spinal cord.

High densities of receptors in the hippocampus and cortex suggest roles for the cannabinoid receptor in cognitive functions. This is consistent with evidence in humans that the dominant effects of cannabis are cognitive: loosening of associations, fragmentation of thought and confusion on attempting to remember recent occurrences (Miller & Branconnier, 1983; Hollister, 1986). High densities of receptors in the basal ganglia and cere-bellum suggested a role for the cannabinoid receptor in movement control, a finding that is also consistent with the ability of cannabinoids to inter-fere with coordinated movements and general motor function (Pertwee, 1992). Recent research has also determined a role for the cerebellum in cognition (e.g. Petersen *et al.*, 1989; Fiez *et al.*, 1992), and particularly in the switching of attention (Akshoomoff & Courchesne, 1992). The globus pallidus, rich in cannabinoid receptors, has also been shown to be acti-vated in positron emission tomography (PET) studies of selective attention (Corbetta *et al.*, 1991).

Cannabis has a mild effect on cardiovascular and respiratory function in humans (Hollister, 1986) which is consistent with the observation that the lower brainstem area has few cannabinoid receptors. The absence of sites in the lower brainstem may in fact explain why high doses of THC are not lethal. Cannabinoid receptors do not appear to reside in the dopaminergic neurons once thought to constitute the reward system of the brain (Herkenham *et al.*, 1991a; Herkenham, 1992). This was at first taken to imply that the euphoric effects of cannabinoids are produced by a different mechanism than the euphoria produced by cocaine and morphine which directly act on the dopamine reward system. Recent conceptualizations of the role of the mesolimbic dopamine neurons in drug taking behaviour have changed from the view that these neurons are a substrate whose activation produces the euphoric or hedonic effects of a drug to one in which the cells are thought to mediate incentive motivational processes or sensitization to drugs (Robinson & Berridge, 1993). The absence of cannabinoid receptors in the mesolimbic dopamine projection is thus of obvious speculative interest in terms of the dependence liability of cannabis. A recent article reports a link between nondrug craving, for chocolate, and the endogenous cannabinoid system (Di Tomaso *et al.*, 1996; see below).

The mappings of cannabinoid receptors have been broadly confirmed by Matsuda *et al.* (1992, 1993) using a histochemistry technique to neuro-anatomically localize cannabinoid receptor mRNA in rats. Labelling intensities were highest in forebrain regions (olfactory areas, caudate nucleus, hippocampus) and in the cerebellar cortex; the role of the cerebellum in cognition has been referred to above. Clear labelling observed in the rat forebrain suggests several potential sites in the human brain that could mediate an impairment of memory function (Miller & Branconnier, 1983), such as the hippocampus, medial septal complex, lateral nucleus of the mamillary body and the amygdaloid complex. Similarly, labelling was detected clearly in rat forebrain regions that correspond to those which could mediate cannabis induced effects on human appetite and mood, namely the hypothalamus, amygdaloid complex and anterior cingulate cortex. Interestingly, the anterior cingulate cortex has been consistently implicated in human PET studies of attention (Posner *et al.*, 1988; Petersen *et al.*, 1989; Pardo *et al.*, 1990; Posner & Petersen, 1990), particularly divided attention (Corbetta *et al.*, 1991) and data on lesions suggest that the anterior cingulate plays an important role in aspects of attention such as neglect (Mesulam, 1981).

Quantitative autoradiographic examinations of the neuroanatomical distribution and density of cannabinoid receptor binding in the human brain at post-mortem have been reported by Westlake *et al.* (1994) and Biegon & Kerman (1995). These studies confirmed a widespread distribution of receptors with high densities in regions consistent with those found in animal research, such as the substantia nigra pars reticulata, basal ganglia (particularly the medial part of the globus pallidus), dentate gyrus, hippocampus, neocortex, amygdala, striatum and cerebellum. In human brain particularly high density bands of receptors were observed in prefrontal cortex, notably around the cingulate and superior frontal gyri (Biegon & Kerman, 1995). These findings reinforce the possible role for the cannabinoid receptor in higher order cognitive functions. It should be borne in mind, however, that the regions where cannabinoid receptors occur may have long projections to other areas, contributing to the multiplicity of effects of the cannabinoids.

The unique psychoactivity of the cannabinoids may be described as a composite of numerous effects which would not arise from a single biochemical alteration, but rather from multiple actions (Martin, 1986). Thus, the diverse pharmacological actions of the various psychoactive and non-psychoactive cannabinoids suggested the existence of receptor subtypes. The cloning of a structurally different receptor in spleen that does not exist in brain and which binds THC and cannabinol (Munro *et al.*, 1993), raises the possibility that other receptor subtypes with entirely unique functional roles may exist (Mechoulam *et al.*, 1994). With the discovery of the cannabinoid receptor in spleen, the cannabinoid receptor in brain came to be known as CB_1 and that in the periphery (spleen) as CB_2.

As THC is not a naturally occurring substance within the brain, the existence of a brain cannabinoid receptor implied the existence of an endogenous cannabinoid like substance. Devane *et al.* (1992) identified a brain molecule that binds to the receptor and mimics the action of cannabinoids. The molecule, arachidonylethanolamide, which is fat soluble like THC, has been named "anandamide" from a Sanskrit word meaning "bliss". Anandamide has been found to act on cells that express the cannabinoid receptor but has no effect on identical cells that lack the receptor. Research has established that anandamide exhibits the essential criteria to be classified as a genuine neurotransmitter for the cannabinoid receptor (Felder *et al.*, 1993; Vogel *et al.*, 1993). A comparison between anandamide and THC showed that anandamide was 4 to 20-fold less potent and had a shorter duration of action than THC in mice (Smith *et al.*, 1994). Mechoulam *et al.* (1994) describe the search for the endogenous ligand that lead to the subsequent discovery of two other endogenous compounds, thus providing evidence for a family of anandamides. They discuss the biochemical and pharmacological properties of the compounds and speculate on their physiological roles. Recent and ongoing research is establishing which neurons are responsible for producing anandamide molecules (e.g. Devane & Axelrod, 1994; Di Marzo *et al.*, 1994) and future research will determine their role. Recently, Di Tomaso *et al.* (1996) reported the detection of three novel constituents of chocolate that were chemically related to anandamide and that may interact with the cannabinoid system in the brain, possibly pointing to a similar mechanism of craving.

Felder *et al.* (1996) have reported the first isolation of anandamide in human brain and other tissues. Significant levels of anandamide were found in hippocampus, parahippocampal cortex, striatum and cerebellum, brain areas known to express high levels of CB_1 cannabinoid receptors, but also in the thalamus which expresses low levels of CB_1 receptors. Anandamide was also found in human spleen which expresses high levels of the CB_2 cannabinoid receptor. Small amounts of anandamide were found in human heart and trace quantities were detected in pooled human serum, plasma and cerebrospinal fluid, which suggests that anandamide is metabolized in tissues where it is synthesized, and that its action is not hormonal in nature (Felder *et al.*, 1996).

The development of potent cannabinoid agonists, such as CP-55,940 and WIN 55,212 (see Adams & Martin, 1996), and recently of at least two different cannabinoid antagonists, SR141716A (Rinaldi-Carmona *et al.*, 1994, 1995) and AM630 (Pertwee *et al.*, 1995), have paved the way for the separation of desired pharmacological effects of cannabinoids from the undesirable or adverse effects. Cannabinoids have great therapeutic potential and have been used for medicinal purposes for many centuries (see Abel, 1980; Mechoulam, 1986). If receptors with the potential for mediating the therapeutic uses of cannabis are different from those responsible for their psychoactive effects, cannabinoid receptor cDNA cloning and new synthetic cannabinoids modelled on anandamide may help to uncover further receptor subtypes and develop drugs to target them, thus fulfilling "the ancient promise of marijuana as medicine" (Snyder, 1990).

Forms of cannabis

The concentration of THC varies with the forms in which cannabis is prepared for ingestion, the most common of which are marijuana, hashish and hash oil. Marijuana is prepared from the dried flowering tops and leaves of the harvested plant. Its potency depends on the growing conditions, the genetic characteristics of the plant and the proportions of plant matter. The flowering tops and bracts, known as "heads", are highest in THC concentration, with potency descending through the upper leaves, lower leaves, stems and seeds. Some varieties of the cannabis plant contain little or no THC, such as the hemp varieties used for making rope, while others have been specifically cultivated for their high THC content, such as "sinsemilla".

Marijuana may range in colour from green to grey or brown, depending on the variety and where it was grown, and in texture from a dry powder or finely divided tea like substance to a dry leafy material. The concentration of THC in a batch of marijuana containing mostly leaves and stems may range from 0.5% to 8% (Fehr & Kalant, 1983a), while the "sinsemilla" variety with "heads" may result in concentrations from 7% to 14% (Jones, 1987). High potency preparations of 17% THC have also been detected (Solowij *et al.*, 1995). Anecdotal evidence abounds for an enhancement of the concentration of Dutch hemp ("Netherweed") to as much as 20% THC through developments in indoor hydroponic cultivation techniques (Adams & Martin, 1996). The potency of marijuana preparations being sold has probably increased in the past decade (Cohen, 1986; Jones, 1987; ElSohly & ElSohly, 1989; American Psychiatric Association, 1994), although the evidence for this has been contested (Mikuriya & Aldrich, 1988).

Hashish or "hash" consists of dried cannabis resin and compressed flowers. It ranges in colour from light blonde/brown to almost black, and is usually sold in the form of hard chunks or cubes. The concentration of THC in hashish generally ranges from 2% to 8%, although it can be as high as 10–20% (Fehr & Kalant, 1983a). Hash oil is a highly potent and viscous substance obtained by using an organic solvent to extract THC from hashish (or marijuana), concentrating the filtered extract and, in some cases, subjecting it to further purification. The colour may range from clear to pale yellow/green, through brown to black. The concentration of the THC in hash oil is generally between 15% and 50%, although samples as high as 60–70% have been detected (Fehr & Kalant, 1983a).

Routes of administration

Almost all possible routes of administration have been used but by far the most common method is smoking (inhaling). Marijuana is most often smoked as a handrolled "joint", the size of a cigarette or larger and often thicker. Tobacco is often added to marijuana to assist burning and "make it go further", and a filter may be inserted. Hashish may be mixed with tobacco and smoked as a joint, but is more often smoked through a pipe, either with or without tobacco. The resin may also be heated in a variety of ways and the fumes inhaled through a funnel or hollow tube. A water pipe known as a "bong" is a popular implement for all cannabis preparations because the water cools the hot smoke before it is inhaled and there is little loss of the drug through sidestream smoke. Hash oil is used sparingly because of its extremely high psychoactive potency; a few drops may be applied to a cigarette or a joint, to the mixture in a pipe, or the oil may be heated and the vapours inhaled. Whatever method is used, smokers inhale deeply and hold their breath for several seconds to ensure maximum absorption of THC by the lungs.

Hashish or marijuana may also be baked in foods and eaten. When ingested orally the onset of the psychoactive effects is delayed by about an hour. In clinical and experimental research, THC has often been prepared in gelatine capsules and administered orally. In India, a popular method of ingestion is in the form of a tea like brew of the leaves and stems, known as "bhang". The "high" is of lesser intensity but the duration of intoxication is longer by several hours. It is easier to titrate the dose and achieve the desired level of intoxication by smoking than ingestion as the effects are more immediate.

Crude aqueous extracts of cannabis have on very rare occasions been injected intravenously. THC is insoluble in water and so little or no drug is actually present in these extracts, and the injection of tiny undissolved particles may cause severe pain and inflammation at the site of injection and a variety of toxic systemic effects. Injection of cannabis is ineffective as a route of cannabis administration, but it has been used for administering THC extract in research to investigate pharmacokinetics.

Different routes of administration give rise to differing pharmacokinetics. For the remainder of this monograph the reader may assume that the method of ingestion is by smoking unless explicitly stated otherwise.

Dosage

A typical joint contains between 0.3 and 1.0 g of cannabis plant matter, which varies in THC content between 2.5 and 150 mg (typically between 1% and 15% THC). Not all of the available THC is ingested; the actual amount of THC delivered in the smoke has been estimated at 20–70% of that in the cigarette (Hawks, 1982), with the rest being lost through combustion or escaping in sidestream smoke. The bioavailability of THC from marijuana cigarettes (the fraction of THC in the cigarette which reaches the bloodstream) has been reported to range between 5% and 24% (mean 18.6%) (Ohlsson *et al.*, 1980). For these reasons, the actual dose of THC that is absorbed when cannabis is smoked is not easily estimated.

In general, only a small amount of smoked cannabis (e.g. 2–3 mg of available THC) is required to produce a brief pleasurable high for the occasional user, and a single joint may be sufficient for two or three individuals. A heavy smoker may consume five or more joints per day, while heavy users in Jamaica, for example, may consume up to 420 mg THC per day (Rubin & Comitas, 1975). In clinical trials designed to assess the therapeutic potential of THC, single doses have ranged up to 20 mg in capsule form. In human experimental research, THC doses of 10, 20 and 25 mg have been administered as low, medium and high doses (e.g. Perez-Reyes *et al.*, 1982; Barnett *et al.*, 1985).

Perez-Reyes *et al.* (1974) determined the amount of THC required to produce the desired effects by slow intravenous administration. They estimated that the threshold for perception of an effect was 1.5 mg (i.e. the dose delivered averaged 21 ng/kg), while a peak social "high" required 2–3 mg THC (an average of 37 ng/kg). These levels did not differ between frequent and infrequent users so Perez-Reyes and colleagues concluded that tolerance or sensitivity to the perceived high does not develop. While tolerance does develop to a wide range of the pharmacological effects of cannabinoids, for tolerance to develop to the subjective effects, high doses must be taken for a prolonged period of time (Adams & Martin, 1996).

Patterns of use

Hall *et al.* (in press) review the epidemiological evidence for patterns of cannabis use in a number of countries throughout the world where survey data were available (e.g. Australia, Canada, the Netherlands, the UK and the USA. Limited data are also compiled for Africa, Central and South America and Asia). Cannabis is the most widely used illicit drug in Australia, having been tried by a third of the adult population and by the majority of young adults between the ages of 18 and 25 years (e.g. for males aged 20–24, up to 84% have used cannabis and 26% currently use it on at least a weekly basis). The USA has probably had the highest prevalence of illicit drug use of any English speaking country, and has also undertaken the longest series of national surveys of drug use, commencing in the 1970s. In 1992, 33% of a national sample reported that they had tried cannabis, 9% had used it in the past year and 4% reported that they were current users, but 21% of those aged 12–17 who had ever used were using weekly (Substance Abuse and Mental Health Services Administration, 1993). The prevalence of cannabis use in Canada is somewhat lower than that of both the USA and Australia. Cannabis use in New Zealand is comparable to that in Australia when adjusted for age: a survey excluding older age groups found that 52% of males and 35% of females aged 15–45 years report ever having tried the drug (Black & Casswell, 1993). In the UK no specific national surveys of illicit drug use comparable in frequency and coverage to the USA household surveys have been regularly undertaken, but some reasonable inferences can be made about trends in drug use from national surveys conducted for other purposes that have also asked about drug use. Data are also available for specific localities where a drug problem is perceived to exist. The data suggest a similar typology but lower rates of use in Britain compared with the other countries examined above (Hall *et al.*, in press). The Netherlands is an interesting case given its policy of de facto decriminalization since 1976. Unfortunately, results of drug use monitoring over time are not readily available in English, nor comparable in methodology to surveys in other countries. The data suggest rates of use that are lower than those in the USA but it is difficult to draw confident conclusions about the prevalence of cannabis use resulting from the Dutch policy (Hall *et al.*, in press). Patterns of use are affected by numerous factors including personal characteristics such as age, sex and socioeconomic status, availability of the drug, perceived risks, social attitudes and criminal sanctions. In many countries, cannabis is merely one drug among many used concurrently or sequentially.

Data regarding the types of cannabis preparations used in different countries are very limited (Hall *et al.*, in press), but there do appear to be culturally specific preferences, probably based to a large degree upon availability. It is probably safe to assume that the most common route of administration in the culturally similar English speaking countries reviewed above is by smoking, and the most widely used form of the drug is marijuana. Anecdotal evidence suggests that hashish is far more prevalent in the UK, while Australia favours heads and New Zealand manufactures substantial quantities of hash oil.

The majority of cannabis use is experimental and recreational, i.e. most users use the drug to experience its euphoric and relaxing effects on a limited number of occasions only. Most of those who have tried cannabis either discontinue their use after a small number of occasions or, if they continue to use, do so intermittently and episodically whenever the drug is available. Only a small proportion of those who ever use cannabis become regular users. The best estimate from the available survey data is that about 10% of those who ever use cannabis become daily users while a further 20–30% use on a weekly basis (Hall *et al.*, in press). Among those who continue to use cannabis, the majority discontinue their use in their mid to late twenties (Kandel & Logan, 1984; Kandel & Raveis, 1989; Kandel & Davies, 1992).

The existence of a cannabis dependence syndrome would have serious implications for cannabis users and for public health (Edwards, 1982). There is clinical and epidemiological evidence that some heavy cannabis users experience problems in controlling their cannabis use and continue to use the drug despite experiencing adverse personal consequences (Hall *et al.*, in press). Cannabis dependence may be the most common form of dependence on illicit drugs in the USA (Anthony & Helzer, 1991) (and probably throughout most "western" countries), but the precise nature of cannabis dependence remains poorly understood. Evidence for a syndrome analogous to the alcohol dependence syndrome is equivocal, but a cannabis dependence syndrome like that defined in DSM-III-R and DSM-IV (Diagnostic and Statistical Manual of Mental Disorders) (American

Psychiatric Association, 1987, 1994) probably occurs in heavy, chronic users (Hall *et al.*, 1994, in press; see Chapter 11 for definitions).

There is no information on the amount of THC ingested by regular cannabis users because of uncertainties about the dose of THC contained in illicit marijuana. "Heavy" cannabis use has typically been defined in the literature in terms of the frequency of use rather than average dose of THC received. Daily or near daily use probably places users at greatest risk of experiencing negative long-term health and psychological consequences (Hall *et al.*, 1994). Such users are more likely to be male and less well educated, and are more likely to regularly consume alcohol and to have experimented with a variety of other illicit drugs, such as amphetamines, hallucinogens, psychostimulants, sedatives and opioids (Kandel, 1984; Newcomb & Bentler, 1988).

Metabolism of cannabinoids

THC is rapidly and extensively metabolized in humans. Different methods of ingesting cannabis give rise to different patterns of absorption, metabolism and excretion of THC. Upon inhalation, THC is absorbed within minutes from the lungs into the bloodstream. Absorption of THC is much slower after oral administration, entering the bloodstream within 1–3 hours and delaying the onset of psychoactive effects (Wall, *et al.*, 1983).

After smoking, the initial metabolism of THC takes place in the lungs, followed by more extensive metabolism by liver enzymes that transform THC to a number of metabolites. The most rapidly produced metabolite is 9-carboxy-THC (or THC-COOH) which is detectable in blood within minutes of smoking cannabis. It is not psychoactive. Another major metabolite of THC is 11-hydroxy-THC (11-OH-THC), which is approximately 20% more potent than THC, and which penetrates the blood–brain barrier more rapidly than THC. 11-OH-THC is only present at very low concentrations in the blood after smoking, but at high concentrations after the oral route (Hawks, 1982). THC and its hydroxylated metabolites account for most of the psychoactive effects of the cannabinoids.

Peak blood levels of THC are reached very rapidly, usually within 10 minutes of smoking and before the joint is fully smoked, and decline rapidly to about 5–10% of their initial level within the first hour (Jones, 1980; Huestis *et al.*, 1992a). This initial rapid decline reflects the rapid conversion of THC to its metabolites, as well as the distribution of THC to lipid rich tissues, including the brain (Jones, 1980; 1987; Fehr Kalant,

1983a). THC and its metabolites are highly fat soluble and may remain for long periods of time in the fatty tissues of the body, including brain, from which they are slowly released back into the bloodstream (Kreuz & Axelrod, 1973). This phenomenon slows the elimination of cannabinoids from the body.

The time required to clear half of the administered dose of THC from the body has been found to be shorter for experienced or daily users (19–27 hours) than for inexperienced users (50–57 hours) (Lemberger *et al.*, 1970; Lemberger & Rubin, 1978; Hunt and Jones, 1980; Ohlsson *et al.*, 1980; Agurell *et al.*, 1986). Recent research using more sensitive detection techniques suggests that the half life in chronic users may be closer to 3–5 days (Johansson *et al.*, 1988). It is the immediate and subsequent metabolism of THC that occurs more rapidly in experienced users (Blum, 1984). Given the slow clearance, repeated administration of cannabis results in the accumulation of THC and its metabolites in the body, and because of its slow release from fatty tissues into the bloodstream, THC and its metabolites may be detectable in blood for several days, and traces may persist for several weeks. The release of stored THC has been suggested as an explanation of "flashback experiences" (e.g. Negrete, 1988; Thomas, 1993).

While blood levels of THC peak within a few minutes, THC-COOH levels peak approximately 20 minutes after commencing smoking and then decline slowly. The elimination curve for THC crosses the THC-COOH curve around the time of the peak of the latter and subjective intoxication also peaks around this time (i.e. 20–30 minutes later than peak THC blood levels), with acute effects persisting for approximately 2–3 hours (Hawks, 1982; Perez-Reyes *et al.*, 1982). Many factors influence the bioavailability of THC (Perez-Reyes, 1990).

Detection of cannabinoids in body fluids

Cannabinoid levels in the body, which depend on both the dose given, the route of administration and the smoking history of the individual, are subject to substantial individual variability. Plasma levels of THC in humans typically range between 0–200 ng/ml, depending on the potency of the cannabis ingested and the time since smoking (e.g. Ohlsson *et al.*, 1980; Agurell *et al.*, 1986). For example, blood levels of THC may decline to 2 ng/ml 1 hour after smoking a low potency cannabis cigarette, a level that may be achieved only 9 hours after smoking a high potency cannabis cigarette (Hawks, 1982; Perez-Reyes *et al.*, 1982). In habitual and chronic users such levels may persist for several days after use because of the slow release of accumulated THC.

The detection of THC in blood above 10–15 ng/ml provides presumptive evidence of "recent" consumption of cannabis but it is not possible to determine how recently it was consumed. A somewhat more precise estimate of the time of consumption may be obtained from the ratio of THC to THC-COOH: similar concentrations of each in blood could be an indication of use within the last 20–40 minutes, and would predict a high probability of the user being intoxicated. When the levels of THC-COOH are substantially higher than those of THC, ingestion can be estimated to have occurred more than half an hour ago (Hawks, 1982; Perez-Reyes *et al.*, 1982). Such an interpretation, however, is probably only applicable to the naive user who has resting levels of 0 ng of THC. Background levels of cannabinoids (particularly THC-COOH) in habitual users make the estimation of time of ingestion almost impossible. As it is very difficult to determine the time of administration from blood concentrations of THC and its metabolites (even if the smoking habits of the individual and the exact dose consumed are known), the results of blood analyses indicate, at best, the "recent" use of cannabis.

Urinary cannabinoid levels provide an even weaker indicator of current cannabis intake. In general, the greater the level of cannabinoid metabolites in urine, the greater the possibility of recent use but again it is impossible to be precise about how recent use has been (Hawks, 1982; Hawks & Chiang, 1986). Only minute traces of THC itself appear in the urine due to its extensive metabolism and most of the administered dose is excreted in the form of metabolites in faeces and urine (Hunt & Jones, 1980). THC-COOH is detectable in urine within 30 minutes of smoking. This and other metabolites may be present for several days in first time or irregular cannabis users while frequent users may continue to excrete metabolites for weeks or months after last use because of the accumulation and slow elimination of these compounds (Dackis *et al.*, 1982; Ellis *et al.*, 1985). As with blood levels, there is substantial human variability in the metabolism of THC and no simple relation exists between urinary levels of THC metabolites and time of consumption. Hence, urinalysis results cannot be used to distinguish between use within the last 24 hours and use more than a month ago.

Several studies have examined measures of cannabinoids in fat and saliva. Analyses of human fat biopsies confirm an accumulation of the drug for at least 28 days (Johansson *et al.*, 1987). Detection of cannabinoids in saliva holds more promise for forensic purposes because it has the capacity to reduce the time frame of "recent" use from days and weeks to hours (Hawks, 1982; Gross *et al.*, 1985; Thompson & Cone, 1987). Salivary THC levels have also been shown to correlate with subjective intoxication and heart rate changes (Menkes *et al.*, 1991).

Intoxication and levels of cannabinoids

Ingestion of cannabis produces a dose related impairment on a wide range of cognitive and behavioural functions. As there is evidence that cannabis intoxication adversely affects skills required to drive a motor vehicle (see Chapter 3), it would be desirable to have a reliable measure of impairment due to cannabis intoxication that was comparable to the breath test of alcohol intoxication.

While the degree of impairment due to alcohol proved possible to determine from a single blood alcohol estimate, a clear relation between blood levels of THC or its metabolites and degree of either impairment or subjective intoxication has not been demonstrated (Mason & McBay, 1985; Agurell *et al.*, 1986). The estimation of the degree of intoxication from a single value of blood THC level is difficult, not only because of the time delay between peak THC blood levels and subjective high, but also because of large individual variations in the effects experienced at the same blood levels (e.g. Hollister *et al.*, 1981; Huestis *et al.*, 1992). The difficulty is compounded by the distribution of THC to body tissues and its metabolism to other psychoactive compounds.

Blood levels of THC metabolites, such as 11-OH-THC, correlate temporally with subjective effects but are not readily detectable in blood after smoking cannabis, while blood levels of THC correlate only modestly with cannabis intoxication, in part because of the lipid solubility of THC (Ohlsson *et al.*, 1980; Barnett *et al.*, 1985; McBay, 1988). The level of intoxication could only realistically be related to the total sum of all the psychoactive cannabinoids present in body fluids and in the brain and various tissues.

No realistic limit of cannabinoid levels in blood has been set which can be related to an undesirable level of intoxication due to large human variability. Tolerance also develops to many of the effects of cannabis. Hence, a given dose consumed by a naive individual may produce greater impairment on a task than the same dose consumed by a chronic heavy user.

THC may also be active in the nervous system long after it is no longer detectable in the blood so there may be long-term subtle effects of cannabis on the cognitive functioning of chronic users even in the unintoxicated state. To date, there is no consistently demonstrated correlation between blood levels of THC and its effect on the human mind and performance. Thus, no practical method has been developed as a forensic tool for determining levels of intoxication based on detectable cannabinoids. A consensus conference of forensic toxicologists has concluded that blood concentrations of THC which cause impairment have not been sufficiently established to provide a basis for legal testimony in cases concerning driving a motor vehicle while under the influence (Consensus Report, 1985).

Passive inhalation

In the USA, urine testing for drug traces and metabolites is increasingly used to identify illicit drug users in the workplace (Hayden, 1991). A technical concern raised by the opponents of this practice has been the possibility of a person having a urine positive for cannabinoids as the result of the passive inhalation of marijuana smoke at a social event immediately prior to the provision of the urine sample. A number of research studies have attempted to determine the relation between passive inhalation of marijuana smoke and consequent production of urinary cannabinoids (Hayden, 1991).

In one of the first studies on passive inhalation, Perez-Reyes *et al.* (1983) found that nonsmokers who had been confined for over an hour in a very small unventilated space containing the smoke of at least eight cannabis cigarettes over 3 consecutive days had insignificant amounts of urinary cannabinoids. Law *et al.* (1984) and Mule *et al.* (1988) also showed that passive inhalation produced urinary cannabinoid concentrations well below the detection limit of 20 ng/ml THC-COOH used in workplace drug screens.

Morland *et al.* (1985) produced urinary cannabinoid levels above 20 ng/ml in nonsmokers but the conditions were extreme, namely confinement in a space the size of a packing box with exposure to the smoke of six cannabis cigarettes. The studies of Cone and colleagues (Cone *et al.*, 1986; Cone & Johnson, 1987a, b) confirmed the necessity to apply extreme experimental conditions to which they claimed nonsmokers were unlikely to submit themselves for the long periods of time required to produce urinary metabolites above 20 ng/ml. They also showed that non-smokers with significant amounts of cannabinoids in their urine experienced the subjective effects of intoxication.

No single mechanism of action can explain the multitude of effects

This overview of the pharmacokinetics and pharmacodynamics of cannabinoids paves the way for considering the effects of cannabis upon the central nervous system and on cognition in the chapters to follow. No single mechanism of action can explain, however, the multitude of effects that cannabis produces and it must be remembered that the endogenous cannabinoid system in the brain has numerous interconnections with a variety of brain structures and interacts with a host of neurochemical systems. Nevertheless, we are clearly substantially more advanced in our understanding of basic cannabinoid pharmacology now than we were ten to 20 years ago when the last surge of cognitive studies were carried out. Based on the premise that consideration of the long-term consequences of cannabis on cognition should commence with an examination of its acute effects, we turn to that literature in the next chapter.

3

Acute effects of cannabis on cognitive functioning

The acute effects of cannabis on cognitive functioning have been reasonably well researched. The literature, though, is so vast that any attempt to summarize the findings will necessarily be an oversimplification. This review will selectively focus on those aspects of cognitive functioning that are of relevance to the research reported in Part 2 of this monograph. The substance of this research concerns the long-term cognitive effects of cannabis and accordingly the review of the literature on chronic effects in Chapter 5 is very thorough. While the premise that a knowledge of the acute effects of a drug may provide the basis for research into possible long-term consequences of use is reasonable, the acute and chronic effects of a drug need not necessarily be the same (Block *et al.*, 1992; Block & Ghoneim, 1993) and can in fact be markedly different (Pomara *et al.*, 1983). Also to be borne in mind is the fact that many factors impinge on the effects experienced by the user when acutely intoxicated. These include the dose, the mode of administration, the user's prior experiences with the drug, any concurrent drug use, the "set and setting", i.e. the complex of user's expectations, attitudes towards drug effects and mood state, and the social environment in which the drug is used (Jaffe, 1990; O'Brien, 1996). Many of the effects of cannabis are also subject to the development of tolerance (Jones, 1983; O'Brien, 1996) and thus naive users may show a greater decrement in performance than experienced users.

Acute intoxication

The major motive for the widespread recreational use of cannabis is the experience of a subjective "high", an altered state of consciousness that is characterized by emotional changes such as mild euphoria and relaxation, and by perceptual alterations, such as time distortion and the intensification of ordinary sensory experiences, such as eating, watching films, listening to music and engaging in sex (Tart, 1970; Jones, 1980; Jaffe, 1990; O'Brien, 1996). When used in a social setting, the high is often accompanied by infectious laughter, talkativeness and increased sociability.

Not all the effects of cannabis intoxication are welcomed by users. Some users report unpleasant psychological reactions, ranging from a feeling of anxiety to frank panic reactions and depressed mood, to a fear of going mad (Smith, 1968; Weil, 1970; Negrete, 1983; Thomas, 1993; O'Brien, 1996). Anxiety, dysphoria, panic and paranoia are most often reported by naive users who are unfamiliar with the effects of cannabis, and by some patients given THC for therapeutic purposes. More experienced users may also report these effects on occasion, especially after the oral ingestion of cannabis when the effects may be more pronounced and of longer duration than those usually experienced after smoking cannabis. If such effects develop they can usually be managed by reassurance and support. Occasionally users may report "flashback experiences" of the intoxicated state. It has been suggested that the release of stored cannabinoids may explain these phenomena (Negrete, 1988; Thomas, 1993). Such experiences, however, have been rarely reported by cannabis users (Edwards, 1983), and even in these cases interpretation of their significance is complicated by the fact that those who have reported such experiences have typically used other hallucinogenic drugs.

There is some evidence that large doses of potent cannabis products can produce a short-term toxic psychotic illness in persons who do not have a personal history of psychotic illness (Negrete, 1983; Ghodse, 1986; Thomas, 1993). Such psychoses are very rare experiences characterized by symptoms of confusion and amnesia, paranoid delusions and auditory and visual hallucinations. They may occur with very high doses of THC, and perhaps in susceptible individuals at lower doses (Smith, 1968; Weil, 1970; Thomas, 1993), and they have a relatively benign course in that they typically remit within a week of abstinence (Thomas, 1993). There is an increased risk of experiencing psychotic symptoms among those who use cannabis and who are vulnerable because of a personal or family history of psychosis (Thornicroft, 1990). There is also evidence of an association between cannabis use and the precipitation of schizophrenia (Andreasson *et al.*, 1987) which is not completely explained by prior psychiatric history, but the causal significance of the association remains unclear (see Hall *et al.*, 1994).

It is not surprising, then, that this state of altered awareness is also marked by a disruption of cognitive functions: cognitive changes are usually marked during acute intoxication. These include impaired concentration and short-term memory, and a loosening of associations, which make it possible for the user to become lost in pleasant reverie and fantasy while making it difficult to sustain goal directed mental activity. Motor skills, reaction time and motor coordination are also affected, so many forms of skilled psychomotor activity are impaired while the user is intoxicated (Hollister, 1986; Jaffe, 1990; O'Brien, 1996). As with most recreational drugs, cannabis is valued for effects which remove the user from mundane concerns, produce relaxation and enhance experiences that would normally interfere with concentration on a skilled task.

Perceptual abilities

A multitude of studies have shown that cannabis disrupts performance on a variety of cognitive and psychomotor tasks. Various mechanisms have been proposed to explain these effects. Alterations in all sensory modalities and the subjective distortion of space and time perception suggest that sensory and perceptual disturbances may underly many of the functions required to successfully perform complex neuropsychological tests and the laboratory tasks used in research. For instance, the perceptual identification of simple geometric figures embedded within complex designs has been shown to be impaired by cannabis (e.g. Carlin *et al.*, 1972). Emrich *et al.* (1991) demonstrated a strong cannabis induced impairment of binocular depth inversion, suggesting that the central nervous system is unable to correct implausible perceptual information during acute intoxication.

The perception of time has been studied using two methods: time production or time estimation. In time production tasks, the subject is asked to indicate when an interval of a duration specified by the experimenter has passed. In time estimation, the subject is asked to estimate the duration of a certain interval of time generated by the experimenter. Both methods have reliably produced significant effects of cannabis on the perception of time, with subjects overestimating the amount of elapsed time in the estimation method (e.g. Jones & Stone, 1970; Cappell & Pliner, 1973), and producing shorter than requested intervals with the production method (e.g. Tinklenberg *et al.*, 1972; Vachon *et al.*, 1974; Chait *et al.*, 1985). This indicates that subjects experience time as passing more quickly relative to real time, i.e. cannabis increases the subjective time rate.

Attention and task accuracy

The subjective effects of cannabis might be expected to decrease performance in situations where both perceptual accuracy and attention are important. The Digit Symbol Substitution Test, a component of the Wechsler Adult Intelligence Scale, is a speed based task of associative ability which requires subjects to copy symbols that correspond to particular digits. This test has been shown to be consistently disrupted by acute cannabis intoxication (e.g. Carlin *et al.*, 1972; Vachon *et al.*, 1974; Heishman *et al.*, 1988, 1989). The results of some studies suggested that heavy users may develop tolerance to the effects of the drug on this task (e.g. Jones & Stone, 1970; Chait *et al.*, 1985).

Few studies have systematically compared the effects of cannabis with other substances such as alcohol. An exception is the study by Heishman *et al.* (1988) who compared performance on the Digit Symbol Substitution Test following placebo, two different doses of smoked THC and two different doses of alcohol. They found stronger dose related impairment following alcohol than THC, but the two doses of THC were both relatively low (1.3% and 2.7%) and would be unlikely to be differentiated. The impairment due to both THC doses was equivalent to the low dose of alcohol (0.6 g/kg).

The administration of the Stroop Colour Word Test, which measures aspects of attention and in particular the ability to inhibit an automatic response, has produced mixed results (e.g. Carlin *et al.*, 1972; Miller *et al.*, 1972; Hooker & Jones, 1987), although various versions of the task were employed and a variety of measures analysed.

Braff *et al.* (1981) reported that cannabis impaired the speed of visual information processing in a backward masking task of letter matching. The interval between the target and mask necessary for the conscious registration of the stimulus was longer following cannabis than placebo, and the authors interpreted this finding as a slowed speed of information processing from labile iconic memory to more permanent registration and processing.

Reaction time and motor control

While early in the phase of intoxication (and at low doses), cannabis produces a mild stimulant effect on the central nervous system, this soon becomes a depression (at moderate to high doses). This general depressant effect might contribute to slowed reaction times, inability to maintain concentration and lapses in attention. This occurs with other central nervous system depressants such as alcohol, but the large and reliable depressant effects of moderate doses of alcohol, and the relatively inconsistent effects obtained with moderate doses of cannabis, suggest that this effect of cannabis is not the primary mediator of performance changes.

Fine motor control and manual dexterity are generally adversely affected, although simple reaction time may or may not be (Chait & Pierri, 1992). Choice or complex reaction time is more likely to be affected, with reaction time consistently (and sometimes error rate) increasing with the difficulty of the task (e.g. Low *et al.*, 1973; Moskowitz *et al.*, 1974; Block & Wittenborn, 1984, 1986).

Sustained and divided attention

Sustained attention, or vigilance, refers to the ability to maintain concentration over an extended period of time, particularly on a task that is relatively simple and boring. Cannabis has been shown to affect sustained attention on simple visual and auditory tasks of particularly long duration (in excess of 50 minutes), impairing accuracy by increasing the number of errors of omission and commission (e.g. Moskowitz *et al.*, 1972; Moskowitz & McGlothlin, 1974; Sharma & Moskowitz, 1974). No drug effects were found in studies using short versions of less than 10 minutes of the Continuous Performance Test (CPT) (e.g. Vachon *et al.*, 1974).

A number of studies have utilized dual or concurrent tasks, where one task requires almost continuous attention, typically tracking, and the other involves the detection of an infrequent stimulus from a variety of sporadically occurring stimuli, often presented on the periphery of vision. These tasks are often referred to as the central and peripheral task, respectively, and the paradigm referred to as a dual task or divided attention paradigm. This paradigm has been one of the most widely studied in the field of research into the acute effects of cannabis, probably because of its presumed relevance to driving related skills. Performance on such tasks is almost always adversely affected by cannabis, although the effects on the component tasks are not consistent. The number or proportion of peripheral targets missed (Moskowitz *et al.*, 1972; Casswell & Marks, 1973a; MacAvoy & Marks, 1975; Marks & MacAvoy, 1989), the proportion of hits (Moskowitz *et al.*, 1972), the number of false alarms (Moskowitz & McGlothlin, 1974; MacAvoy & Marks, 1975), reaction time to peripheral targets (Moskowitz *et al.*, 1976; Perez-Reyes *et al.*, 1988) and tracking errors (Barnett *et al.*, 1985) have all been shown to reflect impaired performance, but no interpretable pattern of decrements has consistently emerged. It seems to be the case that overall performance on divided attention tasks is impaired during cannabis intoxication, and the differences between studies are task dependent. There is no consistency either as to whether it is the performance of the central or peripheral task that is mainly affected by cannabis. Impairments are more likely to be seen in more complex or demanding tasks of divided attention, and complex or choice reaction time tasks.

Driving and flying

A major societal concern about cannabis intoxication is its potential to impair psychomotor performance in ways that may directly affect the well being of nonusers of cannabis. The prototype outcome is a motor accident caused by a cannabis user driving while intoxicated. It is well known that individuals who drive while intoxicated with alcohol are dangerous to others in proportion to their level of intoxication. Is there evidence that intoxication with cannabis produces impaired psychomotor performance of a nature and degree sufficient to warrant restrictions on its use by drivers?

There is considerable evidence, as reviewed above, that cannabis intoxication has some negative effects upon performance which become more pronounced with increasing task difficulty. Motor vehicle driving is a complex task, particularly in conditions of heavy traffic or poor road or weather conditions and, as such, might be expected to be adversely affected by cannabis. Simulated driving tasks require skills that are similar to those involved in driving, which can be performed under controlled laboratory conditions. Smiley (1986) critically reviewed the research on the effects of cannabis intoxication on simulated driving. She reported that early studies found less impairment than more recent studies, but that this was due to the unrealistic car dynamics employed. Later studies demonstrated impairments of lane control after cannabis use, but also showed reductions in risk taking as manifested in slower speeds and the maintenance of a larger distance from the vehicle in front.

Studies of actual on road driving performance have been relatively uncommon due to ethical and safety concerns. Generally, such studies have been carried out on a closed course, although a few have actually been conducted in city traffic (e.g. Klonoff, 1974). The measures in such studies have generally been the number of lane defining markers hit, speed, manoeuvrability, observer ratings and various measures used in actual driving tests. Generally, cannabis has impaired performance more on closed courses than in real traffic, and the mechanism proposed for this phenomenon is an ability of users to compensate for the impairing effects of cannabis in more serious situations (e.g. Robbe & O'Hanlon, 1993). Previous experimental evidence suggested also that cannabis users can voluntarily compensate for some of the impairing effects of the drug (e.g. Cappell & Pliner, 1973).

The effects of cannabis have also been found to be generally less impairing than those due to alcohol intoxication (Smiley, 1986); for example, cannabis users tend to drive more slowly whereas those under the influence of alcohol tend to drive faster and more dangerously than normal. The few studies that have tested the response of cannabis intoxicated drivers in situations that require emergency decision making have found that this is in fact impaired regardless of the ability to compensate under more normal driving circumstances (Smiley, 1986).

The relatively small impairment of driving skills associated with cannabis intoxication appears to be at odds with the predictions from results of laboratory divided attention tasks. While the combination of performance abilities that are tapped by the typical divided attention task, such as concurrent pursuit tracking and visual discrimination, is plausibly related to driving, the tracking task is usually a much more difficult task than driving under normal conditions. Greater attentional resources must be allocated to the central task in most divided attention tests for example, leading to a substantial decrease in performance when drugs such as cannabis are ingested. Thus, the findings of laboratory tasks are difficult to extrapolate to actual driving. An up to date review of the literature is provided by Smiley (in press).

The tasks relevant to flying an aircraft have also been investigated in the laboratory using flight simulators and have generally been found to be impaired by cannabis (Janowsky *et al.*, 1976; Yesavage *et al.*, 1985; Leirer *et al.*, 1989, 1991). The latter two studies found performance to be impaired in experienced pilots for as long as 24 hours after smoking without any subjective awareness of the drug's influence. The impairment in flight simulators appears to be greater than in motor vehicle driving. This may be due to the greater complexity involved in manoeuvring an aircraft, with a greater number of controls to be monitored. It may be that flight simulators are more similar to the laboratory tasks of divided attention.

Memory and higher cognitive functions

"The single, most consistently reported, behavioural effect of cannabinoids in humans is an alteration in memory functioning" (Miller, 1984). Memory is one of the most frequently cited functions to be impaired by cannabis acutely, and numerous studies have investigated the processes of acquisition, storage and retrieval in a variety of tasks. State dependent effects of cannabis on memory have been demonstrated (e.g. Stillman *et al.*, 1974).

One of the simplest measures of short-term memory function is the digit span test, in which subjects are required to reproduce increasingly longer strings of digits in the order presented or reversed. The effects of cannabis on this task have been inconsistent but impairment appears to be highly dose dependent (e.g. Melges *et al.*, 1970; Tinklenberg *et al.*, 1970; Casswell & Marks, 1973b; Hooker & Jones, 1987; Heishman *et al.*, 1989b).

Similarly, the effects on recognition memory have been inconsistent, but generally indicate a greater number of intrusion errors, seen as errors of commission (e.g. Abel, 1971a; b; Dornbush, 1974; Miller *et al.*, 1977a; Miller & Branconnier, 1983). Almost all studies utilizing free recall tasks have demonstrated impairment following cannabis administration. These tasks usually involve the presentation of a list of words (or other items), which the subject must then recall (repeat or write down) either immediately or following some delay. The number of items recalled is invariably fewer, and the next most consistent effect is an increase in the number of intrusion errors (e.g. Dornbush *et al.*, 1971; Cappell & Pliner, 1973; Dornbush, 1974; Miller *et al.*, 1977a, b, 1978; Miller & Branconnier, 1983; Chait *et al.*, 1985). Intrusion errors are items recalled by subjects that were not present in the original list. Miller & Branconnier (1983) suggested that the mechanism behind the large number of intrusion errors generated by subjects acutely intoxicated with cannabis may be due to a failure to habituate to irrelevant stimuli which results in an inability to exclude extraneous information. Similarly, the effects of cannabis on the number of errors and out of sequence distortions in the recall of prose or narrative material were greater than the effects on the number of factual elements recalled (Miller *et al.*, 1972; Hooker & Jones, 1987). Remote memory of previously learned material does not appear to be affected by cannabis (Dornbush, 1974; Hooker & Jones, 1987). The cumulative data from the studies reviewed above, suggest that particularly under conditions of distraction or interference, cannabis may affect the acquisition of information by dysfunction in the processes of focusing attention and maintaining concentration. Furthermore, cannabis may interfere with the transfer from short to long-term memory storage.

A number of other higher cognitive functions are affected by acute cannabis intoxication. Among these is the ability to perform mental arithmetic. This has been examined in a number of studies demonstrating impairment in addition, subtraction, goal directed serial alternation and numerous other variations (Melges *et al.*, 1970; Tinklenberg *et al.*, 1972; Casswell & Marks, 1973b; Chait & Pierri, 1993). Many of these tasks involve holding some information in memory while manipulating other information. A number of studies have attempted to verify empirically the claim that cannabis can promote creative thought processes and enhance artistic creativity but the results have been equivocal (e.g. Carlin *et al.*, 1972). Block & Wittenborn (1984) reported that cannabis decreased the vividness of visual imagery when subjects were instructed to use this in a paired-associate learning task, contrary to previous subjective reports that imagery is enhanced by cannabis. More recently, Block *et al.* (1992) reported that cannabis intoxication altered associative processes, encouraging more uncommon associations. This study also compared the acute effects of cannabis on a test battery which assessed learning and memory, abstraction and psychomotor performance, with the chronic effects of cannabis on the same test battery. The acute effects were far more pervasive, but there were some similarities between acute and chronic impairments (see Chapter 5).

The possibility that cannabis use detrimentally affects planning and organizational strategies and a multitude of frontal lobe functions is becoming increasingly apparent in clinical observations (see Chapter 5), but has not been investigated in any rigorous manner.

Cannabis and alcohol

Cannabis is often used in combination with alcohol. Alcohol and cannabis have a number of effects in common although the mechanisms of these actions appear to be different, with the activity of cannabinoids being receptor mediated (see Chapter 2). Low doses of cannabis and alcohol in combination are perceived to enhance the intoxication (Chesher *et al.*, 1976), while large doses are reported to be aversive (Chesher *et al.*, 1986). Chesher *et al.* (1976, 1977, 1986) studied the effects of orally administered THC and alcohol and their interaction on psychomotor performance on a battery of tests. They found that their combination is approximately additive, but at low doses there is a less than additive effect. After approximately 2 hours, the effects of THC alone were more detrimental than were those of THC plus alcohol, suggesting an antagonism of the effects of THC by alcohol (Chesher *et al.*, 1977). A further study (Belgrave *et al.*, 1979) found no antagonism when cannabis was administered an hour earlier than the alcohol, but demonstrated that performance decrements of THC were slower in onset and lasted longer than those induced by alcohol. Perez-Reyes *et al.* (1988) administered alcohol prior to smoked cannabis and found that the decrements due to alcohol in the performance of skills necessary to drive a motor vehicle were significantly enhanced by cannabis in an additive and possibly synergistic manner. The prior administration of alcohol did not affect subjective ratings of intoxication, heart rate acceleration or THC plasma concentrations.

Strong evidence for adverse cognitive effects but what consequences?

In summary, there is no doubt that cannabis adversely affects the performance of a number of cognitive and psychomotor tasks, and that the effects are dose dependent, and larger, more consistent and persistent in complex and unfamiliar tasks. The acute effects on performance of doses of cannabis which are comparable to those subjects report using recreationally, are similar to, if smaller than, those of intoxicating doses of alcohol.

Most of the studies reviewed above reported that the effects on cognition and psychomotor performance persisted no longer than 4 hours, although many did not measure performance beyond this period. At least two studies have reported dysfunction to persist for longer: up to 24 hours after smoking in one instance (Barnett *et al.*, 1985; Yesavage *et al.*, 1985). Maximal impairment was generally reported to coincide with the peak level of intoxication, approximately 40 minutes after smoking (longer after oral administration of THC). Memory impairment is the most consistently reported effect associated with acute cannabis intoxication; however, the most robust explanation for the mechanism of memory impairment is in reduced attention because of increased competition by the intrusion of irrelevant associations (Miller & Branconnier, 1983).

In recent years, there has been a shift away from further research into the acute effects of cannabis on cognitive functioning because it is now reasonably well established that cannabis affects a wide range of psychomotor and cognitive tasks at doses that produce moderate levels of intoxication. It has been considered of greater importance to investigate the possible long-term effects of chronic cannabis use. Nevertheless, the acute effects of cannabis do have practical significance in terms of impaired learning, driving and operating complex machinery while intoxicated. Further research might aim to elucidate the mechanisms of impairment with greater specificity, investigate individual differences in response to cannabis, and develop test batteries that might reliably detect impairments associated with recent use of cannabis for purposes of ensuring safety in the workplace and on the roads. It is beyond the scope of this monograph to consider the possible mechanisms of cognitive impairment associated with acute cannabis intoxication, particularly as the acute and chronic effects may be quite different. As reviewed in the next chapter, however, there is a growing body of evidence from animal research that the cognitive effects are receptor mediated.

4

Evidence for brain damage associated with the long-term use of cannabis

A major concern about the recreational use of cannabis has been whether it may lead to functional or structural neurotoxicity or "brain damage" in ordinary language. Fehr & Kalant (1983a) defined neurotoxicity as "functional aberrations qualitatively distinct from the characteristic usual pattern of reversible acute and chronic effects, and that may be caused by identified or identifiable neuronal damage". On this definition an enduring impairment of cognitive functioning could be interpreted as a manifestation of neurotoxicity if neuronal damage were also demonstrated. Cognitive deficits may be the end result of secondary changes associated with drug use, as opposed to a direct toxic effect on neurons. A thorough review of the cognitive literature in relation to long-term cannabis use is presented in Chapter 5. This chapter will concentrate on the direct investigations of neurological function and toxicity arising from exposure to cannabinoids.

The review begins with an examination of the evidence for functional neurotoxicity from animal behavioural studies. Neurochemical, electrophysiological and brain substrate investigations of functionality follow, and the chapter concludes with the findings of more invasive examinations of brain structure and morphology in animals, and of less invasive techniques for imaging the human brain.

Animal behavioural studies

Animal research provides the ultimate degree of control over extraneous variables; it is possible to eliminate factors known to influence research findings in humans, such as nutritional status, age, sex, previous drug history and concurrent drug use. The results, however, are often difficult to extrapolate to humans because of between species differences in brain and behaviour and in drug dose, patterns of use, routes of administration and methods of assessment. It is beyond the scope of this monograph to review that vast animal literature, particularly as most animal studies have involved acute administration only. It should be noted, however, that recent studies of that nature are helping to elucidate the actions of cannabinoids in the brain, which will in turn enable a more thorough understanding of its long-term effects (e.g. Heyser *et al.*, 1993; Hampson *et al.*, 1996; Lichtman & Martin, 1996; Sim *et al.*, 1996; Terranova *et al.*, 1996).

Animal research into the effects of cannabis on brain function has typically administered known quantities of cannabinoids to animals for an extended period of time and then examined performance on various tasks assessing brain function, before using histological and morphometric methods to study the brains of the exposed animals. In general, the results of studies with primates produce results that most closely resemble the likely effects in humans; the monkey is physiologically similar to humans while rats, for example, metabolize drugs in a different way, and monkeys are able to perform complex behavioural tasks. Nevertheless, every animal species examined to date has been found to have cannabinoid receptors in the brain (see Chapter 2). In animal models, nontargeted staring into space following administration of cannabinoids is suggestive of psychoactivity comparable to that in humans. The most characteristic responses to cannabinoids in animals are mild behavioural aberrations following small doses, and signs of gross neurotoxicity manifested by tremors and convulsions following excessively large doses. Where small doses are given for a prolonged period of time, behavioural evidence of neurotoxicity has emerged (Rosenkrantz, 1983). Chronic exposure produces lethargy, sedation and depression in many species and/or aggressive irritability in monkeys.

A clear manifestation of neurotoxicity in rats, which has been called the "popcorn reaction" (Luthra *et al.*, 1976), is a pattern of sudden vertical jumping in rats exposed to cannabinoids for 5 weeks or longer. It is also seen in young animals exposed to cannabinoids in utero and then given a small dose challenge at 30 days of age. Several studies of prenatal exposure indicate that the offspring of cannabis treated animals show small delays in various stages of postnatal development, such as eye opening, various reflexes and open field exploration, although after several weeks or months their development is indistinguishable from normal (e.g. Fried & Charlebois, 1979). This means that either the developmental delay was not chronic, the remaining damage is too subtle to be detected by available measures or the "plasticity of nervous system organization in the newborn permitted adequate compensation for the loss of function of any damaged cells" (Fehr & Kalant, 1983a).

Behavioural tests in rodents have included conventional and radial arm maze learning, operant behaviour involving time discriminations, open field exploration and two-way shuttle box avoidance learning. Correct performance on these tests is dependent on spatial orientation or on response inhibition, both of which are believed to depend heavily on intact hippocampal functioning and the involvement of prefrontal cortex. Nakamura *et al.* (1991) used an eight-arm radial maze to measure the effects of acute and chronic THC administration on working memory in the rat. In the investigation of chronic effects, rats were tested 18 hours after each drug administration of 5 mg/kg THC 6 days per week for 90 days. There was gradual deterioration of performance, measured by the number of errors, in delayed memory conditions, but this impairment was reversible only after 30 days of discontinuation of the drug. Some studies have found decreased learning ability on such tasks several months after long-term treatment with cannabinoids (see Fehr & Kalant, 1983b). For example, Stiglick & Kalant (1982a, b) reported altered learning behaviour in rats 1–6 months after a 3 month oral dosing regimen of marijuana extract or THC. Both they and Nakamura *et al.* (1991) claimed that the deficits observed in their studies were reminiscent of behavioural changes seen after damage to the hippocampus. Long lasting impairment of learning ability and hippocampal dysfunction suggests that long lasting damage may result from exposure to cannabis. Some studies have been carried out too soon after the final drug administration to exclude the possibility that the observed effects may still be acute or subacute effects, or may be due to the continued action of accumulated cannabinoids.

Memory function in rats and monkeys has often been assessed by delayed matching to sample tasks. A recent study with rats (Heyser *et al.*, 1993) found that an acute THC induced disruption of performance on such a task was similar to that produced by damage to the hippocampus, and was associated with a specific decrease in hippocampal cell discharge only during the encoding phase of the task. The effects were completely reversible within 24 hours of dosing, but this does not rule out the possibility of a neurotoxic effect following repeated or prolonged administration. Continuing studies from this group have shown that THC induced impairments on a delayed nonmatch to sample task were the same as those resulting from complete removal of the hippocampus and, furthermore, that these effects were completely blocked by coadministration of the cannabinoid antagonist SR141716A, thus confirming that the disruption in memory processes occurs via cannabinoid receptor mediated effects on hippocampal neural activity (Hampson *et al.*, 1996).

Deadwyler *et al.* (1995) showed that initially severe disruption of performance on a delayed match to sample task following administration of 10 mg/kg THC, was completely eliminated after 30–35 days of continuous exposure to the drug, thus reflecting tolerance. Withdrawal from the drug temporarily impaired performance, but this resolved within 2 days and no further effects on performance were apparent up to 15 drug free days later. The authors discussed these results in terms of their consistency with recovery from a hippocampal deficit, and postulated a receptor coupled biochemical mechanism (this was supported by a study reported by Sim *et al.*, (1996), see below). These results should not be taken to imply that there would be no long-term deleterious effects developing gradually over a period of much longer exposure to the drug, and it must be remembered that these rats would have been very well practised at the task.

Research in progress by the same team is using a variety of techniques including selective lesions of hippocampus and cannabinoid treatment and blockade, ensemble (many neuron) recordings, and specific types of error and sequential dependency analyses of delayed nonmatch to sample performance, in working toward a unified theory of cannabinoid actions on hippocampal ensemble firing, encoding of task relevant information and receptor mediated effects (S.A. Deadwyler, personal communication; see also Deadwyler *et al.*, 1996a, b; Hampson & Deadwyler, 1996a, b; Hampson *et al.*, 1996; Deadwyler & Hampson, 1997). Essentially, the data suggest that cannabinoids make the animal susceptible to proactive interference from prior trials, an interference effect so enhanced that confusion as to what is sample on one trial and what was nonmatch on the last trial are not decipherable after several trials. Thus, in the short-term, exogenously administered cannabinoids affect delayed match and nonmatch to sample performance in the same manner as a hippocampal lesion: they operate to screen out relevant "to be remembered" information at an inappropriate time (during the sample phase) rather than at the appropriate time (during the intertrial interval) to reduce proactive interference (S.A. Deadwyler, personal communication).

Other studies have provided evidence that cannabinoids impair working memory through a cannabinoid receptor mechanism. Lichtman *et al.* (1995) reported that intracerebral administration of cannabinoids such as CP55,940 into the cannabinoid receptor rich hippocampus disrupted working memory in the radial arm maze task. Lichtman & Martin (1996) argued that more compelling support for receptor mediated THC induced memory impairment would be provided by the reversal of such impairment by a cannabinoid antagonist. Previously, Collins *et al.* (1995) had shown that the inhibitory effects of the potent cannabinoid HU-210 on long-term potentiation in the rat hippocampus, a neural model for a cellular substrate underlying learning or memory processes, were blocked by SR141716A. Lichtman & Martin (1996) were able to show that SR141716A in a dose dependent manner prevented THC induced impairment of spatial working memory assessed by radial arm maze performance. Furthermore, Terranova *et al.* (1996) have demonstrated in rats and mice actual improvement of short-term working memory and of memory consolidation, and the abolishment of memory disturbance induced by retroactive inhibition or that associated with aging, by the administration of the above antagonist in a dose dependent fashion in the absence of any pretreatment with cannabinoids. The authors commented that SR141716A did not enhance retrieval but facilitated the memory processes involved immediately after acquisition and during consolidation. The results of this research suggest that the endogenous cannabinoid system is involved in forgetting and in the memory deterioration associated with aging. It should be noted, however, that this facilitation of memory was partially antagonized by scopolamine, a muscarinic antagonist that impairs memory, which implies a connection between the blockade of cannabinoid receptors and the facilitation of cholinergic transmission (Terranova *et al.*, 1996). Gifford & Ashby (1996) have suggested that an endogenous substance might inhibit the release of acetylcholine through activation of the cannabinoid receptor (see also Gifford *et al.*, 1997). Lichtman & Martin (1996) found that SR141716A did not alleviate scopolamine induced impairment on the radial arm maze in rats and concluded that cannabinoids and cholinergic drugs do not impair spatial memory through a common serial pathway. Some recent studies have reported that while THC and several other psychoactive cannabinoids impaired memory function in rats, anandamide failed to do so (Crawley *et al.*, 1993; Lichtman *et al.*, 1995). The lack of demonstrable memory impairment following administration of anandamide, however, may be due either to the nature of the tasks employed in different studies, or to its rapid metabolism (Deutsch & Chin, 1993). When rats were pretreated with a protease inhibitor, anandamide dose dependently impaired working memory in a delayed nonmatch to sample task (Mallet & Beninger, 1995). The possibility also exists that endogenous ligands other than anandamide may be more specific to cognition (anandamide may represent one member of a family of endogenous compounds, see Chapter 2).

In a series of studies described by Slikker *et al.* (1992), rhesus monkeys were trained for 1 year to perform five operant tasks before 1 year of chronic administration of cannabis commenced. One group was exposed daily to the smoke of one standard joint, another on weekends only and control groups received sham smoke exposure (*n* = 15 or 16 per group). Performance on the tasks indicated the induction of what the authors referred to as an "amotivational syndrome" during chronic exposure to cannabis, manifested in a decrease in motivation to respond, regardless of whether the monkeys were exposed daily or only on weekends. This led the authors to suggest that motivational problems can occur at relatively low or recreational levels of use (in fact, the effect was maximal with inter-mittent exposure). Task performance was grossly impaired for more than a week following last exposure, although performance returned to baseline levels 2–3 months after cessation of use. Thus, the effects of chronic expo-sure were slowly reversible with no long-term behavioural effects. The authors concluded that persistent exposure to compounds that are very slowly cleared from the brain could account for their results. This hypothe-sis is consistent with the long half life of THC in the body.

One of the problems with studies such as these is that animals are often only exposed for a relatively short period of time, for example 1 year or less. Slikker and colleagues acknowledge that it remains to be determined whether longer or greater exposures would cause more severe or additional behavioural effects. It may be that chronic dysfunction is manifest only after many years of exposure, as suggested by human research (see Chapters 5 and 8). Although it is of concern that behavioural impairments have been shown to last for several months after exposure, it is reassuring that they have generally resolved over time.

A further difficulty with animal studies is a consequence of differences between animals and humans in route of cannabinoid administration. In humans the most common route of exposure to THC is via the inhalation of marijuana smoke, whereas most animals studies have relied on the oral administration or injection of THC because of the difficulty in efficiently delivering smoke to animals and the concern about the complications introduced by carbon monoxide toxicity. While it may well be impossible to evaluate the pharmacological and toxicological consequences of expo-sure to the hundreds of compounds in cannabis simultaneously, it is argu-ably inappropriate to assess the long-term consequences of human cannabis smoking by administering THC alone (Abood & Martin, 1992).

Hundreds of additional compounds are produced by pyrolysis when marijuana is smoked, which may contribute either to the acute effects or to long-term toxicity. Future studies need to address these issues for comparability to human usage. Appropriate controls, including those which mimic the carbon monoxide exposure experienced during the smoking of marijuana, may be necessary.

Neurochemistry

The discovery of the cannabinoid receptor and its endogenous ligand anandamide revolutionized previous conceptions of the mode of action of the cannabinoids. Much further research is required before the interactions between ingested cannabis, anandamide or other endogenous ligands, and the cannabinoid receptor are fully understood, nor should the anandamide pathways be seen as responsible for all of the central effects of the psychoactive cannabinoids. There is good evidence that cannabinoids affect the concentration, turnover or release of other endogenous substances (Pertwee, 1988, 1992). Much research has been devoted to examining the interactions between cannabinoids and several neurotransmitter receptor systems (e.g. norepinephrine (noradrenaline), dopamine, serotonin, acetylcholine, gamma-aminobutyric acid (GABA), histamine, opioid peptides and prostaglandins) (Pertwee, 1992). The results suggest that all these substances have some role in the neuropharmacology of cannabinoids, although little is known about the precise nature of this involvement. Cannabinoids may alter the activities of neurochemical systems in the central nervous system by altering the synaptic concentrations of these mediators through an effect on their synthesis, storage, release, or metabolism, and/or by modulating mediator–receptor interactions. There have been numerous reports of neurotransmitter perturbations in vitro and after short-term administration of cannabinoids (for reviews see Dewey, 1986; Martin, 1986; Pertwee, 1988, 1992).

Relatively few studies have examined whether long-term exposure to cannabinoids results in lasting changes in brain neurotransmitter and neuromodulator levels. An early study examined cerebral and cerebellar neurochemical changes accompanying behavioural manifestations of neurotoxicity (involuntary vertical jumping) in rats exposed to marijuana smoke for up to 87 days (Luthra et al., 1976). Sex differences emerged in the neurochemical consequences of chronic exposure. In females, acetylcholinesterase showed a cyclic increase and cerebellar enzyme activity declined. For both sexes, cerebellar RNA increased, but at different times for each sex, and at 87 days remained elevated only in females. Some of these neurochemical changes persisted during a 20-day recovery period, but the authors predicted the return to normality after a much longer recovery period. Cannabinoids administered prenatally not only impaired developmental processes in rats but produced significant decrements in RNA, DNA and protein concentrations and reductions in dopamine and norepinephrine concentrations in mice, which could be important in the role of protein and nucleic acids in learning and memory (see Fehr & Kalant, 1983b). Bloom (1984) reported that chronic exposure to cannabinoids has been shown to lead to increased activity of tyrosine in rat brain. Mailleux & Vanderhaeghen (1994) demonstrated that THC modulates gene expression of neuropeptides: a 3-week treatment with THC significantly increased the messenger RNA levels for substance P and enkephalin in the rat caudate-putamen. The authors reported this as opening the possibility that cannabis abuse might induce long-term effects on the physiology of the brain. These same authors had previously shown that dopamine, glucocorticoids and glutamate regulated cannabinoid receptor gene expression in the caudate-putamen (see Mailleux & Vanderhaeghen, 1994).

Recent evidence suggests, however, that there are few, if any, irreversible effects of THC on known brain chemistry. Ali *et al.* (1989) administered various doses of THC to rats for 90 days and then assessed several brain neurotransmitter systems at 24 hours or 2 months after the last drug dose. Examination of dopamine, serotonin, acetylcholine, GABA, benzodiazepine and opioid neurotransmitter systems revealed that no significant changes had occurred. A larger study with both rats and monkeys examined receptor binding of the above neurotransmitters and the tissue levels of monoamines and their metabolites (Ali *et al.*, 1991). No significant irreversible changes were demonstrated in the rats chronically treated with THC. Monkeys exposed to chronic treatment with marijuana smoke for 1 year and then sacrificed after a 7-month recovery period were found to have no changes in neurotransmitter concentration in frontal cortex, caudate nucleus, hypothalamus or brainstem regions. The authors concluded that there are no significant irreversible alterations in major neuromodulator pathways in the rat and monkey brain following long-term exposure to the active compounds in marijuana.

Slikker *et al.* (1992), reporting on the same series of studies, noted that there were virtually no differences between placebo, low dose or high dose groups of monkeys in blood chemistry values. The general health of the monkeys was unaffected but the exposure served as a chronic physiological stressor evidenced by increases in urinary cortisol levels which were not subject to tolerance (although plasma cortisol levels did not differ). Urinary cortisol elevation has not been demonstrated in other studies with monkeys. Slikker *et al.* reported a 50% reduction in circulating testosterone levels in the high dosed group with a nonsignificant rebound 1–4 weeks after cessation of treatment. It is worthy of note that these monkeys were 3 years of age at the commencement of the study and would have experienced hormonal changes over the course of entering adolescence during the study.

A recent pilot study compared monoamine levels in cerebrospinal fluid in a small sample of human cannabis users and age and sex matched normal controls (Musselman *et al.*, 1994). The authors' justification for the study was that THC administered to animals has been shown to produce increases in serotonin and decreases in dopamine activity. No differences were found between the user and nonuser groups in the cerebrospinal fluid concentration of homovanillic acid, 5-hydroxyindoleacetic acid, 3-methoxy-4-hydroxyphenylglycol, adrenocorticotropic hormone (ACTH) or corticotropin releasing factor. The authors proposed a number of explanations for these results: (1) cannabis use has no chronic effect on levels of brain monoamines, (2) those who use cannabis have abnormal levels of brain monoamines which are normalized over long periods of time by cannabis use, or (3) those who use cannabis have normal levels of brain monoamines that are transiently altered with cannabis use and then return to normal. There were insufficient data in this study to permit a choice between these hypotheses. The frequency and duration of cannabis use and the time since last use in the user group could not be determined. All users had denied using cannabis, having been drawn from a larger normative sample and identified as cannabis users by the detection of cannabinoid metabolites in urine screens. Further research is required to properly assess neurotransmitter levels in human cannabis users.

Electrophysiological effects

Cannabis is clearly capable of causing marked changes in brain electrophysiology as determined by electroencephalographic (EEG) recordings. Long-term abnormalities in EEG tracings from cortex and hippocampus have been shown in cats (Hockman *et al.*, 1971; Barratt & Adams, 1972, 1973; Domino, 1981), rats (see Fehr & Kalant, 1983b) and monkeys (Adams & Barratt, 1975; Harper *et al.*, 1977; Heath *et al.*, 1980) exposed to cannabinoids. Some sleep EEG abnormalities, such as a decrease in slow wave sleep, have also been observed. Stadnicki *et al.* (1974) demonstrated increased EEG synchrony and high voltage slow wave activity in the occipital cortex, amygdala, septum and hippocampus of implanted rhesus monkeys following several days administration of oral THC, but tolerance developed to these EEG effects. Withdrawal effects are sometimes apparent in the EEG (Fehr & Kalant, 1983b) with epileptiform and spike like activity most often seen.

Shannon & Fried (1972) related EEG changes in rat to the distribution of bound and unbound radioactive THC. Disposition of the tracer was primarily in the extrapyramidal motor system and some limbic structures and 0.8% of the total injected drug which was weakly bound in the brain accounted for the EEG changes. In monkeys, serious subcortical EEG anomalies were observed in monkeys exposed to marijuana smoke for 6 months (Heath *et al.*, 1980). The septal region, hippocampus and amygdala were most profoundly affected, showing bursts of high amplitude spindles and slow wave activity. Such early studies often lacked critical quantitative analysis. The definition of abnormal spike-like waveforms in EEG were not made to rigorous criteria and EEG frequency was not assessed quantitatively.

More recent studies have examined the effects of acute THC on extracellular action potentials recorded from the dentate gyrus of the rat hippocampus (Campbell *et al.*, 1986a, b). THC produced a suppression of cell firing patterns and a decrease in the amplitude of sensory evoked potentials, also impairing performance on a tone discrimination task. The evoked potential changes recovered rapidly (within 4 hours), but the spontaneous and tone evoked cellular activity remained significantly depressed, indicating an abnormal state of hippocampal/limbic system operation. The authors proposed that such changes could account for decreased learning and memory function and generally impaired cognitive performance following exposure to cannabis. The long lasting effects of prolonged cannabis administration on animal electrophysiology have not been investigated to any degree of specificity.

Most recently, the cannabinoid receptor antagonist SR141716A was shown to have arousal enhancing properties as assessed by analysis of the sleep–waking cycle and of EEG spectra in rats (Santucci *et al.*, 1996). There was a dose dependent increase in time spent in wakefulness at the expense of slow wave sleep and rapid eye movement sleep, but no change in motor behaviour. The spectral power of EEG signals typical of slow wave sleep were reduced. The authors claim their results suggest that an endogenous cannabinoid system is involved in the control of the sleep–waking cycle. Further evidence that anandamide may mediate the induction of sleep is reported by Mechoulam *et al.* (1997).

The waking or sleep EEG is increasingly recognized as a particularly sensitive tool for evaluating the effects of drugs in humans, especially drugs that affect the central nervous system as EEG signals are sensitive to variables affecting the brain's neurophysiological substrate. The recording of the EEG is one of the few reasonably direct, nonintrusive methods of monitoring central nervous system activity in humans. Alterations in EEG activity, however, are difficult to interpret in a functional sense. Struve & Straumanis (1990) provide a review of the human research dating from 1945 on the EEG and evoked potential studies of acute and chronic effects of cannabis use. While the data have often been contradictory, the most typical human alterations in EEG patterns include an increase in alpha activity and a slowing of alpha waves with decreased peak frequency of the alpha rhythm, and a decrease in beta activity (Rodin *et al.*, 1970; Heath, 1972; Fink, 1976a; Fink *et al.*, 1976; Volavka *et al.*, 1977). In general, this is consistent with a state of drowsiness. Desynchronization, variable changes in theta activity, abnormal sleep EEG profiles and abnormal evoked responses have also been reported (Fehr & Kalant, 1983b). Cannabis has been reported to reduce the duration of REM sleep (Feinberg *et al.*, 1976; Jones, 1980), although this may only occur early in administration studies, followed by a resolution and then an increase in REM sleep above baseline levels as smoking continues (Kales *et al.*, 1972).

Campbell (1971) compared EEG abnormalities observed in chronic cannabis users who had developed psychotic reactions to the EEG patterns of schizophrenics, neurological patients and nonproblematic cannabis users, and claimed that the incidence of EEG abnormalities was higher in the two groups of cannabis users than in either patient sample. These included excess sharp and theta activity, severe dysrhythmia and epileptiform spikes in frontal and temporal regions. In contrast, Dornbush *et al.* (1972) reported increased EEG alpha activity in the intoxicated state but no persistent changes following 21 day administration of cannabis to human volunteers. Koukkou & Lehman (1976, 1977) examined EEG frequency spectra during self reported THC induced hallucinations and found slower alpha and more theta. Subjects with a high tendency toward "cannabis induced experiences" exhibited resting spectra both before and after THC injection with higher modal alpha frequencies, reminiscent of subjects with high neuroticism scores, than subjects with a low tendency. Fink *et al.* (1976) suggested that the acute effects of cannabis on EEG are similar to those of anticholinergics, but differ from those of opiates and hallucinogens. Jones (1975) reviewed the data on EEG characteristics of over 200 marijuana users from a number of studies, mostly during acute intoxication, and reported very few EEG abnormalities being detected in those studies that were well controlled.

Clinical reports have associated cannabis with triggering seizures in epileptics (Feeney, 1979) and experimental studies have shown that THC triggers abnormal spike waveforms in the hippocampus whereas cannabidiol had the opposite effect. Yet there is suggestive evidence that cannabis may be useful in the treatment of convulsions. Feeney (1979) discusses these paradoxical effects.

A number of studies have investigated EEG in chronic cannabis users. No abnormalities were found in the resting EEG of chronic users from Greek, Jamaican or Costa Rican populations compared to controls (Rubin & Comitas, 1975; Karacan *et al.*, 1976; Stefanis, 1976). These early studies were flawed in many respects (see Chapter 5) and only subjects who were in good health and who were functioning adequately in the community were selected, thereby systematically eliminating subjects who may have been adversely affected by cannabis use and who may therefore have shown residual EEG changes. Furthermore, quantitative techniques for analysing EEG spectra were not applied.

The evidence from many other studies has been contradictory: users have been found to show either higher or lower percentages of alpha components than nonusers and to have higher or lower visual evoked response amplitudes (Deliyannakis *et al.*, 1970; Richmon *et al.*, 1974; Cohen, 1976). In a 94 day cannabis administration study (Cohen, 1976), lasting EEG abnormalities were more marked in subjects who had taken heavier doses but it was observed that even in abstinence, cannabis users had more EEG irregularities than nonusing controls. It was not determined for how long after cessation of use the EEG changes persisted. The equivocal results of many EEG studies may have been more consistent had quantitative methods been employed (early studies relied on visual inspection but by the mid-1970s power spectral analyses were sometimes being performed).

It has also been reported that chronic users develop tolerance to some of the acute EEG changes caused by cannabis (Feinberg *et al.*, 1976). Fried (1977) reviewed the literature pertinent to the development of tolerance to EEG effects in animals and humans, which again produced many inconsistent results. The question as to why chronic cannabis users can continue to display changes in EEG when tolerance is known to develop to such alterations remains unanswered.

In a recent series of well controlled studies, Struve *et al.* (1992, 1993, 1994, 1995) have used quantitative techniques to investigate persistent EEG changes in long-term cannabis users, characterized by a "hyperfrontality of alpha". Significant increases in absolute power, relative power and interhemispheric coherence of EEG alpha activity over the bilateral frontal-central cortex in daily marijuana users compared to nonusers were demonstrated and replicated several times. The quantitative EEGs of subjects with very long cumulative exposures (> 15 years) appear to be characterized by increases in frontal-central theta activity in addition to the hyperfrontality of alpha found in cannabis users in general (or those with much shorter durations of use). These very long-term users have shown significant elevations of theta absolute power over frontal-central cortex compared to short-term users and controls, and significant elevations in relative power of frontal-central theta in comparison to short-term users. Over most cortical regions, ultra long-term users had significantly higher levels of theta interhemispheric coherence than short-term users or controls. Thus, excessively long duration of cannabinoid exposure (15–30 years) appears to be associated with additional topographic quantitative EEG features not seen with subjects using cannabis for short to moderately long time periods.

These findings have led to the suspicion that there may be a gradient of quantitative EEG change associated with progressive increases in the total cumulative exposure (measured in years) of daily cannabis use. Infrequent, sporadic or occasional use did not seem to be associated with persistent quantitative EEG change. As daily use begins and continues, the topographic quantitative EEG becomes characterized by the hyperfrontality of alpha (Struve *et al.*, 1993, 1994). While it is not known at what point during cumulative exposure it occurs, at some stage substantial durations of daily cannabis use become associated with a downward shift in maximal EEG spectral power from the mid-alpha range to the upper theta/low alpha range. Excessively long duration cumulative exposure of 15–30 years may be associated with increases of absolute power, relative power and coherence of theta activity over frontal-central cortex (Struve *et al.*, 1992). One conjecture is that the EEG shift toward theta frequencies, if confirmed, may suggest organic change (Struve *et al.*, 1992). These data are supplemented by neuropsychological test performance features separating long-term users from moderate users and nonusers (Leavitt *et al.*, 1993), but the relation between neuropsychological test performance and EEG changes has not yet been investigated.

While the EEG provides little functionally interpretable information about the brain, event-related potential measures are more direct electro-physiological markers of cognitive processes. Relatively few studies have utilized event-related potential measures in research into the long-term effects of cannabis. Studies by Herning *et al.* (1979) demonstrated that THC administered orally to volunteers alters event-related potentials according to dose, duration of administration and the complexity of the task. This and other event-related potential studies are reviewed in Chapter 6. The original research reported in Part 2 of this monograph utilized event-related potential measures to demonstrate long lasting functional brain impairment and subtle cognitive deficits in chronic cannabis users and ex-users in the unintoxicated state.

Cerebral blood flow studies

Brain cerebral blood flow (CBF) is closely related to brain function. The study of CBF may help to identify brain regions responsible for the behavioural changes associated with drug intoxication. As psychoactive drugs may induce CBF changes through mechanisms other than alteration in brain function (e.g. by increasing carbon monoxide levels, changing blood gases or vasoactive properties, affecting blood viscosity, autonomic activation or inhibition of intraparenchymal innervation, acting on vasoactive neuropeptides), any conclusions drawn from drug induced CBF changes must be treated with caution.

Mathew & Wilson (1992) report several studies of the effects of cannabis on CBF. Acute cannabis intoxication in inexperienced users produced a global decrease, whereas in experienced users CBF increased in both hemispheres but primarily at frontal and left temporal regions. There was an inverse relation between anxiety and CBF. The authors attributed the decrease in CBF in naive subjects to their increased anxiety after cannabis administration, while the increased CBF in experienced users was attributed to the behavioural effects of cannabis. A further study showed that the largest increases in CBF occurred 30 minutes after smoking. The authors concluded that cannabis causes a dose related increase in global CBF, but also appears to have regional effects, with a greater increase in the frontal region and in particular in the right hemisphere. The following variables were positively correlated with frontal CBF increases and inversely correlated with parietal flow: the "high", plasma THC levels and pulse rate, loss of time sense, depersonalization, anxiety and somatization scores.

The authors claimed their results suggested that altered brain function was mainly, if not exclusively, responsible for the CBF changes. The time course of CBF changes resembled that of mood changes more closely than plasma THC levels. Global CBF was closely related to levels of arousal mediated by the reticular activating system. High arousal states generally show CBF increases while low arousal states show CBF decreases. Of all cortical regions, the frontal lobe has the most intimate connections with the thalamus which mediates arousal, and CBF increases after cannabis use were most pronounced in frontal lobe regions. The right hemisphere is generally associated with the mediation of emotions and the most marked changes after cannabis were seen there. Time sense and depersonalization which are associated with the temporal lobe were severely affected but there were no significant correlations between these scores and temporal flow. CBF techniques are probably not sensitive enough in terms of spatial resolution to detect such effects and may well be limited to superficial layers of cortex. The parietal lobes are associated with perception and cognition. Cannabis reduces perceptual acuity, but during intoxication subjects report increased awareness of tactile, visual and auditory stimuli. It is possible that their altered time sense and depersonalization is related to such altered awareness.

The possibility remains that the CBF changes reflect drug induced vascular changes and not an alteration of specific brain functions. Acute administration of cannabis also increased cerebral blood velocity, but on prolonged standing after smoking, a dramatic reduction in cerebral blood velocity with reports of dizziness but with normal blood pressure suggested that cannabis may impair cerebral autoregulation. Carbon monoxide increased after both cannabis and placebo but did not correlate with CBF, and cannabis induced "red eye" lasted for several hours while the increased CBF declined significantly within 2 hours of smoking, lending support to the functionality hypothesis.

There have been a few investigations of the long-term effects of cannabis on CBF. Tunving *et al.* (1986) demonstrated globally reduced resting levels of CBF in nine chronic heavy users of 10 years, 1–12 hours after last use, compared to nonuser controls, but no regional flow differences were observed. Four of these subjects were assessed again between 9 and 60 drug free days later and showed a hemispheric CBF increase of 12%, indicating reduced CBF in heavy users immediately after cessation of cannabis use with a return to normal levels with abstinence. This study was flawed in that some subjects were given benzodiazepines, which are known to lower CBF, prior to the first measurement. Mathew *et al.* (1986) assessed chronic users of at least 6 months (mean 83 months) after 2 weeks of abstinence. No differences in CBF levels were found between users and nonuser controls. The subjects of this study, however, were not regular heavy users as were those in Tunving et al's (1996) study, and they were not impaired in any identifiable way as a result of their use (Mathew & Wilson, 1992). In contrast, the experienced subjects of Mathew and Wilson's acute studies (1992) were chronic heavy users and they had also shown lower baseline CBF levels compared to the inexperienced subjects. The number of studies available on the effects of cannabis on CBF are relatively small and the findings of reduced CBF levels in chronic heavy users clearly require replication. Further application of techniques with better spatial resolution, such as positron emission tomography (PET) which also enables quantification of subcortical flow, may provide better information.

Positron emission tomography studies

Positron emission tomography (PET) is a nuclear imaging technique that allows the concentration of a positron labelled tracer to be imaged in the human brain (Raichle, 1983). PET can measure the regional distribution of positron labelled compounds in the living human brain, and to some extent their time course. Some PET studies have labelled oxygen and measured blood flow, while many others have utilized an analogue of glucose to measure regional brain glucose metabolism (as nervous tissue uses glucose as its main source of energy).

Measurement of glucose metabolism reflects brain function as activation of a given brain area is indicated by an increase in glucose consumption. PET may be used to assess the effects of acute drug administration by using regional brain glucose metabolism to determine the areas of the brain that are activated by a given drug. Assessment of brain glucose metabolism has been useful in identifying patterns of brain dysfunction in patients with psychiatric and neurological diseases. It is a direct and sensitive technique for identifying brain pathology because it can detect abnormalities in the functioning of brain regions in the absence of structural changes, such as may occur with chronic drug use. It is accordingly more sensitive than either computer assisted tomography (CAT) scans or magnetic resonance imaging (MRI) in detecting early pathological changes in the brain.

Only one set of studies to date has used the PET technique to investigate the effects of acute and chronic cannabis use. Volkow *et al.* (1991b) reported data from a preliminary investigation comparing the regional brain metabolic effects of acute cannabis administration in three control subjects (who had used cannabis no more than once or twice per year) and in three chronic users (who had used at least twice per week for at least 10 years). The regions of interest were the prefrontal cortex, the left and right dorsolateral, temporal, and somatosensory parietal cortices, the occipital cortex, basal ganglia, thalamus and cerebellum. A measure of global brain metabolism was obtained using the average for the five central brain slices, and relative measures for each region were obtained using the ratios of region/global brain metabolism. Due to the small number of subjects, descriptive rather than inferential statistical procedures were used for comparison. The relation between changes in metabolism due to cannabis and the subjective sense of intoxication was tested using regression analysis.

In the control subjects, administration of cannabis led to an increase in metabolic activity in the prefrontal cortex and cerebellum; the largest relative increase was in the cerebellum and the largest relative decrease was in the occipital cortex. The degree of increase in metabolism in the cerebellar cortex was highly correlated with the subjective sense of intoxication. The cannabis users reported less subjective effects than the controls and showed less changes in regional brain metabolism, reflecting tolerance to the actions of cannabis. The authors did not report comparisons of baseline levels of activity in the users and controls, perhaps due to the limitations of the small sample size. In a larger sample, such a comparison would enable an evaluation of the consequences of long-term cannabis use on resting levels of glucose metabolism. The increases in regional metabolism in Volkow *et al.*'s study are in accord with the increases in cerebral blood flow reported by Mathew & Wilson (1992). The regional pattern of response to cannabis in this study is consistent with the localization of cannabinoid receptors in brain.

Further studies with eight infrequent cannabis users (range: once every 2 weeks to once a year) (Volkow *et al.*, 1991a) or 11 subjects with a wide range of experience with cannabis (Volkow *et al.*, 1995) found a variable response to acute intravenous THC administration in terms of global cerebral glucose metabolism, with some subjects showing an increase, others a decrease or no change. Nevertheless, the regional metabolic changes replicated those of their preliminary study, but the only significant changes were an increase in metabolic activity in the cerebellum, which correlated significantly with both the subjective sense of intoxication and with plasma THC concentration, and activation of prefrontal cortex which was most prominent in those subjects with a history of frequent use of cannabis (Volkow *et al.*, 1995). Interestingly, however, there was a negative

correlation between plasma THC concentration and the degree of metabolic change in prefrontal cortex – the higher the plasma THC, the higher
the metabolic values in cerebellum, but the lower the values in prefrontal
cortex (Volkow *et al.*, 1991a, b). The authors discussed the implications of
their findings in terms of the reinforcing properties of drugs of abuse,
citing the role of the cerebellum in emotion and reinforcement and emphasizing its anatomical interconnections with the limbic system and prefrontal cortex.

A recently reported study by the same team (Volkow *et al.*, 1996) investigated brain glucose metabolism in chronic cannabis users at baseline and
during intoxication. At baseline, the eight chronic users (mean 5.5 years of
use of between 1 and 7 days per week) showed lower cerebellar metabolic
activity than the eight controls, which was suggested to reflect changes in
the cannabinoid receptors, possibly attributable to chronic cannabis use.
Thirty to 40 minutes after intravenous administration of 2 mg THC, all
subjects showed significantly increased metabolism in prefrontal cortex,
left and right frontal cortices, right temporal cortex and cerebellum.
Cerebellar metabolism was correlated with the degree of subjective intoxication, but not with plasma THC concentration. Chronic users showed
significantly greater increases in prefrontal cortex, orbitofrontal cortex
and basal ganglia, while controls showed a decrease in the latter two
regions. The increased prefrontal activation during intoxication is consistent with Mathew & Wilson's (1992) findings of prefrontal CBF increases
in regular but not infrequent cannabis users. Volkow *et al.* (1996) interpreted the altered metabolic function observed in orbitofrontal cortex and
basal ganglia in their chronic users to be similar to that found in cocaine
abusers, alcoholics and patients with obsessive-compulsive disorders, and
postulated the importance of a dysfunction in these regions in the regulation of initiation and termination of behaviours, loss of control and
compulsion. Unlike other drugs of abuse which have consistently been
shown to decrease regional brain metabolism following a single acute
administration (e.g. cocaine, heroin, amphetamines, alcohol and benzodiazepines), cannabis consistently produced increases.

A further application of PET would be to label the cannabinoids themselves: labelling of THC with a positron emitter has been achieved and
preliminary biodistribution studies have been carried out in mice and in
the baboon (Charalambous *et al.*, 1991; Marciniak *et al.*, 1991). More
recently, an iodinated analogue of SR141716A, the cannabinoid receptor
antagonist, has been characterized for PET or SPECT (single photon
emission computerized tomography) studies in mice, but does not bind in

baboons (Gatley *et al.*, 1996; Lan *et al.*, 1996). Research in progress from
this team is developing a new radiotracer with better blood–brain barrier
penetration that binds to the CB1 receptor in vivo and does permit SPECT
brain images in baboons (S.J. Gatley, personal communication). The use of
PET in future human studies is promising.

Brain histology and morphology

Animal studies

Early attempts to investigate the effects of chronic cannabinoid exposure
on brain morphology in animals failed to demonstrate any effect on brain
weight or histology under the light microscope. Electron microscopic
examination, however, has revealed alterations in septal, hippocampal and
amygdaloid morphology in monkeys after chronic treatment with THC or
cannabis. A series of studies from the same laboratory (Harper *et al.*, 1977;
Myers & Heath, 1979; & Heath *et al.*, 1980, discussed below) reported
widening of the synaptic cleft, clumping of synaptic vesicles in axon termi-
nals and an increase in intranuclear inclusions in the septum, hippocampus and amygdala. These findings incited a great deal of controversy and
the studies were criticized for possible technical flaws (Institute of
Medicine, 1982) with claims that such alterations are not easily
quantifiable.

Harper *et al.* (1977) examined the brains of three rhesus monkeys 7
months after 6 months of exposure to marijuana, THC or placebo, and
two nonexposed control monkeys. In the treated group, one monkey was
exposed to marijuana smoke three times each day, 5 days per week,
another was injected with THC once each day and the third was exposed
to placebo smoke conditions. The latter two had electrode implants for
EEG recording and had shown persistent EEG abnormalities following
their exposure to cannabis. Morphological differences were not observed
by light microscopy, but electron microscopy revealed a widening of the
synaptic cleft in the marijuana and THC treated animals with no
abnormalities detected in the placebo or control monkeys. Further,
"clumping" of synaptic vesicles was observed in pre- and postsynaptic
regions in the cannabinoid treated monkeys, and opaque granular material
was present within the synaptic cleft. The authors concluded that chronic
heavy use of cannabis alters the ultrastructure of the synapse and proposed that the observed EEG abnormalities may have been related to these
changes.

Myers & Heath (1979) examined the septal region of the same two cannabinoid treated monkeys and found the volume density of the organized rough endoplasmic reticulum to be significantly lower than that of the controls, and fragmentation and disorganization of the rough endoplasmic reticulum patterns, free ribosomal clusters in the cytoplasm and swelling of the cisternal membranes was observed. The authors noted that similar lesions have been observed following administration of various toxins or after axonal damage, reflecting disruptions in protein synthesis.

Heath *et al.* (1980) extended the above findings by examining a larger sample of rhesus monkeys ($N = 21$) to determine the effects of marijuana on brain function and ultrastructure. Some animals were exposed to smoke of active marijuana, some were injected with THC and some were exposed to inactive marijuana smoke. After 2–3 months of exposure, those monkeys given moderate or heavy exposure to marijuana smoke developed chronic EEG changes at deep brain sites, which were most marked in the septal, hippocampal and amygdaloid regions. These changes persisted throughout the 6–8 month exposure period as well as the postexposure observation period of between 1 and 8 months. Brain ultrastructural alterations were characterized by changes at the synapse, destruction of rough endoplasmic reticulum and development of nuclear inclusion bodies. The brains of the placebo and control monkeys showed no ultrastructural changes. The authors claimed that at the doses used, which were comparable to human usage, permanent alterations in brain function and ultrastructure were observed in these monkeys.

Brain atrophy is a major nonspecific organic alteration which must be preceded by more subtle cellular and molecular changes. Rumbaugh *et al.* (1980) observed six human cases of cerebral atrophy in young male substance abusers of primarily alcohol and amphetamines. They then conducted an experimental study of six rhesus monkeys treated chronically with various doses of cannabis extracts orally for 8 months and compared them to groups that were treated with barbiturates or amphetamines or untreated. No signs of cerebral atrophy were demonstrated in the cannabis exposed group and light microscopy revealed no histological abnormalities in four of the animals, but "equivocal" results for the other two. Brains were not examined under the electron microscope. The amphetamine treated group showed the greatest histological, cerebrovascular and atrophic changes.

More recently, McGahan *et al.* (1984) used high resolution computerized tomography scans in three groups of four rhesus monkeys. One was a control group, a second was given 2.4 mg/kg of oral THC per day for 2–10 months and a third group received a similar daily dose over a 5 year period. The dosage was considered the equivalent of smoking one joint per day. The groups receiving THC were studied 1 year after discontinuing the drug. There was a statistically significant enlargement of the frontal horns and the bicaudate distance in the brains of the 5-year treated monkeys compared to the control and short-term THC groups. This finding suggests that the head of the caudate nucleus and the frontal areas of the brain can atrophy after long-term administration of THC in doses relevant to human exposure.

A number of rat studies have found similar results to those in rhesus monkeys described above. Investigators have reported that after high dose cannabinoid administration there was a decrease in the mean volume of rat hippocampal neurons and their nuclei, and after low dose administration there was a shortening of hippocampal dendritic spines. Scallett *et al.* (1987) used quantitative neuropathological techniques to examine the brains of rats 7–8 months after 90 day oral administration of 10–60 mg/kg THC. The anatomical integrity of the CA3 area of rat hippocampus was examined using light and electron microscopy. High doses of THC resulted in striking ultrastructural alterations, with a significant reduction in hippocampal neuronal and cytoplasmic volume, detached axodendritic elements, disrupted membranes, increased extracellular space and a reduction in the number of synapses per unit volume (i.e. decreased synaptic density). These structural changes were present up to 7 months following treatment. Lower doses of THC produced a reduction in the dendritic length of hippocampal pyramidal neurons 2 months after the last dose, and a reduction in GABA receptor binding in the hippocampus although the ultrastructural appearance and synaptic density appeared normal. The authors suggested that such hippocampal changes may constitute a morphological basis for the persistent behavioural effects demonstrated following chronic exposure to THC in rats, effects which resemble those of hippocampal brain lesions. These findings are in accord with those of Heath *et al.* (1980) with rhesus monkeys and the doses administered correspond to daily use of approximately six joints in humans.

A study by Landfield *et al.* (1988) showed that chronic exposure to THC reduced the number of nucleoli per unit length of the CA1 pyramidal cell somal layer in the rat hippocampus. The brains of rats treated five times per week for 4 or 8 months with 4 or 8 mg/kg injected subcutaneously were examined by light and electron microscopy. Significant THC induced changes were found in hippocampal structure: pyramidal neuronal cell density decreased and there was an increase in glial reactivity reflected by cytoplasmic inclusions similar to that seen during normal aging or following experimentally induced brain lesions. No effects were observed on ultrastructural variables such as synaptic density. Adrenal–pituitary activity increased, resulting in elevations of ACTH and corticosterone during acute stress. The authors claimed that the observed hippocampal morphometric changes produced by THC exposure were similar to glucocorticoid dependent changes that develop in rat hippocampus during normal aging. They proposed that, given the chemical structural similarity between cannabinoids and steroids, chronic exposure to THC may alter hippocampal anatomical structure by interacting with adrenal steroid activity. More recently, Eldridge *et al.* (1992) reported that delta-8-THC bound with the glucocorticoid receptors in the rat hippocampus and was displaced by corticosterone or delta-9-THC. A glucocorticoid agonist action of delta-9-THC injections was demonstrated. Injection of corticosterone increased hippocampal cannabinoid receptor binding. These interactions suggest that cannabinoids may accelerate brain aging. Eldridge & Landfield (1990), Eldridge *et al.* (1991) and Landfield & Eldridge (1993) further discuss this research and its implications.

It should be noted that where THC has been administered to monkeys for 6 months, this represents only 2% of their life span and may not have been long enough to detect the gradual effects that could arise from interactions with steroid systems (and affect the aging process). In contrast, 8 months administration to rats represents approximately 30% of their life span. The differences in the ultrastructural findings of Landfield's and Scallett's studies may be due to the largely different doses administered; the 8 mg/kg of Landfield's study was not sufficient to produce any marked behavioural effects. Furthermore, the two studies examined slightly different hippocampal areas (CA1 or CA3).

Most recently, Slikker *et al.* (1992) reported the results of their neurohistochemical and electron microscopic evaluation of the rhesus monkeys whose dosing regimen, behavioural and histochemical data were reported above. They failed to replicate earlier findings: no effects of drug exposure were found on the total area of hippocampus, or any of its subfields, nor were there any differences in hippocampal volume, neuronal size, number, length or degree of branching of CA3 pyramidal cell dendrites. There were no effects on synaptic length or width, but there were trends toward increased synaptic density (the number of synapses per cubic mm), increased soma size, and decreased basilar dendrite number in the CA3 region with cannabis treatment. Slikker *et al.* were able to demonstrate an

effect of enriched environments upon neuroanatomy: daily performance
of operant tasks increased the total area of hippocampus and particularly
the CA3 stratum oriens, producing longer, more highly branched dendrites
and less synaptic density, while the reverse occurred in the animals
deprived of the daily operant tasks. The extent of drug interaction with
these changes was not clear and may explain some of the inconsistencies
between this study and those described above. Clearly, the question of
whether prolonged exposure to cannabis results in structural brain
damage has not been fully resolved.

Human studies

There is very little evidence from human studies of structural brain
damage. In their controversial paper, Campbell *et al.* (1971) were the first
to present evidence suggestive of structural/morphological brain damage
associated with cannabis use in humans. They used air encephalography to
measure cerebral ventricular size and claimed to have demonstrated evidence of cerebral atrophy in 10 young males who had used cannabis for 3
to 11 years, and who complained of neurological symptoms, including
headaches, memory dysfunction and other cognitive impairment.
Compared to controls, the cannabis users showed significantly enlarged
lateral and third ventricular areas. Although this study was widely publi-
cized in the media because of its serious implications, it was heavily criticized on methodological grounds. Most subjects had also used significant
quantities of LSD and amphetamines, and the measurement technique
was claimed to be inaccurate, particularly as it is difficult to assess ventricular size and volume to any degree of accuracy using the air encephalo-
graphic technique (e.g. Bull, 1971; Fink *et al.*, 1972; Susser, 1972).
Moreover, the findings could not be replicated. Stefanis (1976) reported
that echoencephalographic measurements of the third ventricle in 14
chronic hashish users and 21 nonusers did not support Campbell *et al.*'s
pneumoencephalographic findings of ventricular dilation.

The introduction of more accurate and noninvasive techniques, in the
form of computed tomographic (CT) scans, (also known as computer-
assisted tomographic (CAT) scans), permitted better studies of possible
cerebral atrophy in chronic cannabis users (Co *et al.*, 1977; Kuehnle *et al.*,
1977). Co *et al.* (1977), for example, compared 12 cannabis users recruited
from the general community, with 34 nondrug using controls, all within
the ages of 20–30 years. The cannabis users had used cannabis for at least
five years at the level of at least 5 joints per day, and most had also con-

sumed significant quantities of a variety of other drugs, particularly LSD. Kuehnle *et al.*'s (1977) subjects were 19 heavy users aged 21–27 years, also recruited from the general community who had used on average between 25 and 62 joints per month in the preceding year, although their duration of use was not reported. CT scans were obtained presumably at the end of a 31 day study, which included 21 days of ad libitum smoking of marijuana (generally five joints per day), and were compared to a separate normative sample. No evidence for cerebral atrophy in terms of ventricular size and subarachnoid space was found in either study. Although these studies could also be criticized for their research design (e.g. inappropriate control groups, and the fact that cannabis users had used other drugs), these flaws would only have biased the studies in the direction of detecting significant differences between groups, yet none was found. The results were interpreted as a refutation of Campbell *et al.*'s findings, and supporting the absence of cortical atrophy as demonstrated by Rumbaugh *et al.*'s (1980) CAT scans of monkeys. A further study (Hannerz & Hindmarsh, 1983) investigated 12 subjects who had smoked on average 1 g of cannabis daily for between 6 and 20 years by thorough clinical neurological examination and CT scans. As in the studies above, no cannabis related abnormalities were found on any assessment measure.

Recent research on cannabinoid receptor alterations

The development of tolerance following chronic administration of psychoactive compounds is often mediated by a downregulation of receptors. Thus, chronic exposure to THC could lead to receptor downregulation or receptor internalization (both resulting in a decreased number of cannabinoid receptors in the brain) or to conformational changes in the receptor which produce an altered receptor structure, each of which result in decreased receptor–ligand interaction (Adams & Martin, 1996). Receptor downregulation and reduced binding (particularly in the striatum and limbic forebrain) have been demonstrated in rats (Oviedo *et al.*, 1993; Rodriguez de Fonseca *et al.*, 1994); however, Westlake *et al.* (1991) reported that cannabinoid receptor properties were not irreversibly altered in rat brain 60 days following 90 day administration of THC, nor in monkey brain 7 months after 1 year of exposure to marijuana smoke. It was argued that these recovery periods were sufficient to allow the full recovery of any receptors that would have been lost during treatment. Abood *et al.* (1993) had also demonstrated the development of tolerance to THC without any alteration of cannabinoid receptor binding or mRNA levels in whole brain. More recently, Romero *et al.* (1995) reported increased binding in the cerebellum and hippocampus after acute or chronic exposure to either anandamide or THC. Increased binding following acute administration was attributed to changes in receptor affinity, but that following chronic administration was attributed to an increase in the density of receptors. Following chronic exposure to THC only, a downregulation of receptors in the striatum was observed. Mackie *et al.* (1997) demonstrated rapid internalization of cannabinoid receptors following agonist binding. The research suggested that longer term treatment with cannabinoids may cause the receptor to progress to lysosomes where it is degraded and the recovery of surface receptors requires new protein synthesis. The precise parameters of any alterations in cannabinoid receptor number and function that may result from chronic exposure to cannabinoids, and the extent of reversibility following longer exposures have not yet been determined to any degree of accuracy.

A recent study has demonstrated large decreases in G-protein activation throughout the brain following chronic treatment with THC, showing that effects on receptor function may occur without consistent changes in the number of receptor binding sites. Sim *et al.* (1996) investigated the alterations in signal transduction that mediate the production of tolerance. They pointed out that changes in receptor binding may not reflect changes in receptor function. They showed that a specific treatment regimen, which had previously been shown to produce complete adaptation to the debilitating effects of large doses of cannabinoids on a delayed matching to sample task (Deadwyler *et al.*, 1995), produced a functional "uncoupling" of the cannabinoid receptor from the G-protein that links it to cyclic AMP and other cellular mechanisms. Cannabinoid stimulated [S-35]GTP gamma S binding was substantially reduced in brain regions rich in cannabinoid receptors, and most dramatically in the hippocampus. This finding is consistent with the impairing effects of cannabinoids on short-term memory tasks (Heyser *et al.*, 1993). The uncoupling of the receptor from the G-protein by chronic drug treatment explains the cessation of the disruptive acute effects of THC on such tasks, which may be adaptive in certain circumstances, but the receptor-G-protein uncoupling may have profound effects on potassium A channels and all other effectors downstream from the receptor transducer coupling. The loss in agonist activity is analogous to desensitization and the findings consistent with the concept that desensitization and down-regulation are separate processes, with the former preceding the latter. The results of this study suggested that "profound desensitization of cannabinoid activated signal transduction mechanisms occurs after chronic delta(9)-THC treatment" (Sim *et al.*, 1996). The chronic treatment in this study was only 21 days. Studies such as this, in combination with research investigating the role of cannabinoid receptors in memory dysfunction (e.g. Heyser *et al.*, 1993; Hampson *et al.*, 1996; Lichtman & Martin, 1996; Terranova *et al.*, 1996) lead the way for revolutionizing our understanding of the mechanism of action of both endogenous and exogenous cannabinoids.

Two studies of human brain post-mortem have investigated changes in cannabinoid receptor binding or density with disease and normal aging. Westlake *et al.* (1994) showed that binding of the potent cannabinoid agonist CP-55,940 was substantially reduced in the caudate and hippocampus of Alzheimer's brains, with lesser reductions in the substantia nigra and globus pallidus. Reduced binding was associated also with increasing age and/or general disease processes resulting in cortical pathology and thus not specific to Alzheimers'. They claimed that receptor losses were not associated with overall decrements in levels of cannabinoid receptor gene expression. Biegon & Kerman (1995) found that increasing age is associated with a decrease in the density of cannabinoid receptors in prefrontal cortex, particularly in cingulate cortex and the superior frontal gyrus. The authors discussed their findings in terms of possible indirect modulation of dopaminergic activity by cannabinoids and suggested that the age-related decline in receptor density in prefrontal regions may contribute to decreased drug seeking behaviour with increasing age. As this age-related decrease in cannabinoid receptors was found in the normal human brain, it would be interesting for further research to examine receptor density in the prefrontal cortex of chronic cannabis users. These findings reinforce the possible role for the cannabinoid receptor in higher order cognitive functions and may have implications for elucidating the cognitive decline that occurs with age. Animal research has also examined changes in cannabinoid receptors with age. Mailleux & Vanderhaeghen (1992) reported age-related losses in cannabinoid receptor binding sites and mRNA in the rat striatum. Belue *et al.* (1995) demonstrated progressively increased binding capacity in rat striatum, cerebellum, cortex and hippocampus from birth through to adulthood, which they interpreted as reflecting either "an increased differentiation of neurons into cells possessing cannabinoid receptors, or an increase in the number of receptors on cell bodies or projections in regions undergoing developmental changes". Once the adult levels had been reached, binding activity in a whole brain preparation neither increased nor declined with normal aging; it would be interesting to see if the same results would have been obtained had specific sites such as prefrontal cortex been examined and if rats had been chronically administered cannabinoids. These studies require replication and pave the way for further exploration of aging phenomena as they may interact with chronic exposure to the drug.

Evidence for neurotoxicity in animals and subtle brain dysfunction in humans

Overall, surprisingly few studies of neurotoxicity have been published and the results have been equivocal. There is convincing evidence that chronic administration of large doses of THC leads to residual changes in rodent behaviours which are believed to depend on hippocampal function. There is evidence for long-term changes in hippocampal ultrastructure and morphology in rodents and monkeys. Animal neurobehavioural toxicity is characterized by long lasting impairment in learning and memory function, EEG and biochemical alterations, impaired motivation and impaired ability to exhibit appropriate adaptive behaviour. Although direct extrapolation to humans is not possible, the results of these experimental animal studies have demonstrated cannabinoid toxicity at doses comparable to those consumed by humans using cannabis several times a day. There is sufficient evidence also from human research to suggest that cannabinoids act on the hippocampal region producing behavioural changes similar to those caused by injury to that region (e.g. Drew *et al.*, 1980; see Chapter 5).

Human research has defined a pattern of acute central nervous system changes following cannabis administration. Altered brain function and metabolism in humans have been demonstrated following acute and chronic use by EEG, CBF and PET techniques; however, the cognitive, behavioural and functional responses to long-term cannabis consumption in humans continue to be the most consistent manifestation of its potential toxicity. It is possible that the extent of damage could be more pronounced at two critical stages of central nervous system development: in neonates when exposed to cannabis during intrauterine life (e.g. Fried, 1993, 1995, 1996; see Chapter 5) and in adolescence, during puberty when neuroendocrine, cognitive and affective functions and structures of the brain are in the process of integration. As discussed in Chapter 5, research is needed to investigate the possibility that more severe consequences may occur in adolescents exposed to cannabinoids than in those who commence cannabis use at a later age.

Human studies of brain morphology have yielded generally negative results, failing to find gross signs of "brain damage" after chronic exposure to cannabis. Nevertheless, the results of many human studies are indicative of more subtle brain dysfunction. It may be that existing methods of brain imaging are not sensitive enough to establish subcellular alterations produced in the central nervous system. Many psychoactive substances exert their action through molecular biochemical mechanisms which do not distort gross cell architecture. The most convincing evidence on brain damage would come from post-mortem studies. The post-mortem finding of age related decline in the density of cannabinoid receptors in prefrontal cortex of the normal human brain (Biegon & Kerman, 1995) holds promise for interesting future research to examine such changes as they interact with the chronic use of cannabis.

In 1983, Fehr and Kalant concluded that "The state of the evidence at the present time does not permit one either to conclude that cannabis produces structural brain damage or to rule it out". In 1984, Nahas wrote "The brain is the organ of the mind. Can one repetitively disturb the mental function without impairing brain mechanisms? The brain, like all other organs of the human body, has very large functional reserves which allow it to resist and adapt to stressful abnormal demands. It seems that chronic use of cannabis derivatives slowly erodes these reserves". In 1986, Wert and Raulin proposed that on the available evidence "there are no gross structural or neurological deficits in marijuana using subjects, although subtle neurological features may be present. However, the type of deficit most likely to occur would be a subtle, functional deficit which could be assessed more easily with either psychological or neuropsychological assessment techniques". By 1998, little further evidence has emerged to challenge or definitively refute these earlier conclusions.

This conclusion was anticipated as early as 1845 by the Parisian physician Moreau when he wrote of his observations of chronic hashish smokers:

unquestionably there are modifications (I do not dare use the word "lesion") in the organ which is in charge of mental functions. But these modifications are not those one would generally expect. They will always escape the investigations of the researchers seeking alleged or imagined structural changes. One must not look for particular, abnormal changes in either the gross anatomical or the fine histological structure of the brain; but one must look for any alterations of its sensibility, that is to say, for an irregular, enhanced, diminished or distorted activity of the specific mechanisms upon which depends the performance of mental functions.
(Moreau (de Tours), 1845).

What Moreau was suggesting was that we find other ways of assessing the subtle changes in cognition that occur with prolonged use of cannabis. Traditionally, this has entailed the application of neuropsychological tests and such studies are reviewed extensively in the next chapter. Nevertheless, the vastly advanced techniques of today ensure that research will continue to investigate the minute changes in brain ultrastructure and the functioning of the cannabinoid receptor which would no doubt underly the cognitive and behavioural dysfunction.

5

Chronic effects of cannabis on cognitive functioning

One of the well-known acute effects of cannabis is to impair cognitive processes. Therefore, it has long been suspected that cognitive dysfunction may persist well beyond the period of acute intoxication and that chronic cannabis use may cause lasting cognitive impairments. Although considerable research has been conducted into the acute cognitive effects of cannabis, there is a paucity of well-controlled studies of the long-term effects of chronic cannabis use on cognitive function. This chapter reviews the literature from each of several methodological approaches that have been used to investigate the chronic effects of cannabis on human cognitive functioning. Clinical observations will only be covered very briefly, with discussion restricted to either key papers or recent research. The priority in this chapter will be given to those human studies which made some attempts to scientifically control for extraneous variables. These have largely concentrated on neuropsychological assessments of brain function in chronic cannabis users.

The terms acute, subacute and chronic, when used to describe drug effects, have been defined in Chapter 1. Some effects may also be due to drug residues that remain in the body. Because of the slow clearance of THC and its metabolites from the body, repeated administration results in the accumulation of cannabinoids. There is no conclusive evidence for effects associated with accumulated cannabinoids, but the possibility that they continue to exert an effect remains nevertheless.

A caveat must be born in mind while critically assessing this literature; it is difficult to assess the long-term consequences of the use of any psychoactive drug. Many factors other than drug use must be controlled in order to confidently attribute any effects to the drug in question. In the case of assessing the long-term effects of drugs on cognitive function these difficulties include: differentiating cognitive impairment that preceded

drug use from that which may have been drug induced, accurately determining the duration and frequency of past drug use, and taking account of
the cognitive effects of multiple drug use. All these issues contribute to
uncertainty in the attribution of any observed impairment to the use of a
particular drug (Carlin, 1986).

Clinical observations

Concerns about the possibility that chronic cannabis use affected mental
processes were reinforced by early clinical reports of mental deterioration
in long-term cannabis users. Fehr & Kalant (1983b) provide a historical
review of early clinical observations. In general, the clinical literature suggests that cognitive dysfunction is most often observed in persons who
have used heavily (at least daily) for more than 1 year (Fehr & Kalant,
1983b).

The most widely cited evidence for clinically significant impairment due
to cannabis is the work of Kolansky & Moore (1971, 1972). These authors
initially reported 38 cases of psychiatric symptomatology ranging from
mild apathy, through personality disturbance, to psychosis which was
observed in adolescents and young adults (aged 13–24 years) who had
used marijuana at least twice per week. They later presented 13 case
reports of adult psychiatric patients (aged 20–41 years) who had used marijuana or hashish three to ten times per week or more for between 16
months and 6 years.

The clinical picture was one of "very poor social judgement, poor attention span, poor concentration, confusion, anxiety, depression, apathy,
passivity, indifference and often slowed and slurred speech" (Kolansky &
Moore, 1971). Various cognitive symptoms began with cannabis use and
disappeared within 3–24 months after cessation of drug use. These
included apathetic and sluggish mental and physical responses, emotional
lethargy, mental confusion, difficulties with recent memory, incapability of
completing thoughts during verbal communication, loss of interest in life
and goalessness.

The course and remission of symptoms appeared to be correlated with
past frequency and duration of cannabis smoking. Those with a history of
less intensive use showed complete remission of symptoms within 6
months; those with more intensive use took between 6 and 9 months to
recover while those with chronic intensive use were still symptomatic 9
months after discontinuation of drug use. Symptoms were also more
marked in users of hashish than in marijuana smokers.

Tennant & Groesbeck (1972) monitored the medical and psychiatric consultations of 720 hashish smoking US soldiers in West Germany. Just over half of the sample were occasional users who consumed between 0 and 12 g hashish per month. This group only complained of respiratory ailments. The heavy using group ($n = 110$) who consumed between 50 and 600 g hashish per month were described as "chronically intoxicated", generally apathetic and displaying impaired memory, judgement and concentration. Tennant and Groesbeck followed up nine heavily using patients after periods of abstinence, providing one of the few prospective studies to date. Six of the nine reported improvement in memory, alertness and concentration following discontinuation of use, while the other three complained of confusion and impaired memory for many months after ceasing use of the drug.

Both Kolansky and Moore, and Tennant and Groesbeck, emphasized the similarity between the symptoms they observed in long-term heavy cannabis users and those of organic brain damage. Kolansky and Moore (1972) hypothesized that the use of cannabis "adversely affects cerebral functioning on a biochemical basis. In the mildest cases there appears to be a temporary toxic reaction when small amounts of cannabis are consumed over a short period of time. However, in those individuals who demonstrate stereotyped symptomatology after prolonged and intensive cannabis use, the possibility of structural changes in the cerebral cortex must be raised". They called for investigation to assess structural and functional alterations in the brains of chronic cannabis users.

These clinical reports, together with a report of cerebral atrophy in young cannabis users which appeared around the same time (Campbell *et al.*, 1971), incited substantial controversy. Critics were quick to fault the experimental designs and to raise objections to the conclusions and extrapolations based on the evidence. Among these were the lack of objective measures of impairment and the biased sampling from psychiatric patient populations. The clinical observations, however, have been largely unchallenged and the consistency of symptoms across reports and cultures is particularly striking. For example, the clinical descriptions of chronic users in India have matched those from North America (Chopra, 1971, 1973; Chopra & Smith, 1974; Chopra & Jandu, 1976).

While clinical observations may raise concerns, they do not provide definitive evidence of causality because they are unable to rule out alternative explanations of an apparent association between drug use and symptoms. Altman & Evenson (1973), for example, examined 158 psychiatric patients and found 38 cases in which cannabis use had preceded such symptoms as confusion, depression, poor judgement, anxiety and apathy. In an exploration of possible relations between other factors and psychiatric problems, they found 10 other events (such as use of tobacco and beer, sexual intercourse, etc.) which preceded the onset of psychiatric symptoms more frequently than did cannabis use. The authors criticized Kolansky and Moore's failure to include in their sample individuals who had used cannabis and did not develop psychiatric symptoms. They warned of the scientifically unsound practice of using the case history technique to test hypotheses about causal relationships.

The clinical observations reported in the early 1970s were not new. Reports of adverse mental effects of cannabis use have appeared throughout history (see Abel, 1980; Fehr & Kalant, 1983a; Nahas, 1984). While the frequency of clinical reports of cognitive dysfunction has diminished in the past decade, this may reflect a decline in their novelty and noteworthiness rather than any reduction in the incidence of clinical disorders resulting from the chronic use of cannabis. Kalant (1996) shows a decline in the numbers of publications on cannabis in general as indexed by the *Cumulative Index Medicus* from 1971 to 1994 and argues that this is a reflection of political trends and lack of funding. There is plenty of evidence, anecdotal and research based (e.g. Stephens *et al.*, 1993), that chronic cannabis users continue to seek treatment (or would if they knew that it was available to them). They present complaining primarily of dependence on the drug, but often give as their prime reason for wanting to cease using, a concern that they are experiencing mental deterioration, a "dulling" of cognitive abilities, or difficulties with concentration and memory.

In recent years, clinicians have sought to characterize the specific deficits they observe with chronic cannabis users by integrating these into cognitive theory and evidence from empirical research (e.g. Lundqvist, 1995a, b, c). Treatment programmes for chronic cannabis users have been established which focus upon specific areas of cognitive dysfunction, such as verbal and logical-analytic abilities, abstraction, psychomotility and memory (Tunving *et al.*, 1988; Lundqvist, 1995a, c). Clinical observation suggests that the use of cannabis more often than every 6 weeks for approximately 2 years leads to changes in cognitive functioning, but clinical improvement in cognitive functioning can be seen within 14 days of abstinence and following 6 weeks of therapy users may function normally (Lundqvist, 1995a, c). The cannabis induced cognitive dysfunction was likened to the prefrontal syndrome, which is difficult to measure due to its complex effects on human behaviour (Stuss & Benson, 1986).

The clinical reports which appeared in the early 1970s served to alert the community at large to the possible risks involved in using cannabis at a time when the substance was becoming increasingly popular among the young. This in turn prompted field studies and better controlled empirical research.

Studies of users in countries with a long history of cannabis use within their culture

A logical starting point for the investigation of cognitive function in chronic cannabis users is to assess populations of users in countries where chronic daily use of cannabis has been an integral part of the culture for many decades, if not centuries. This kind of research was pioneered by Soueif (1971) in the largest scale study to date of 850 Egyptian hashish smokers and 839 controls. In response to public anxiety about the epidemic increase in marijuana use in the late 1960s, the National Institute on Drug Abuse (NIDA) commissioned three studies in countries with long histories of cannabis use, namely, Jamaica, Greece and Costa Rica. These studies have been the most widely quoted and considered to be comprehensive. This is not so much due to their sample sizes, which were quite small and therefore limit the conclusions that can be drawn, but mainly because each study was multidisciplinary, investigating not only cognitive function, but also medical-physiological status. Aside from the small sample size, each of these studies suffered from a number of other methodological difficulties which limited the conclusions that could be drawn. These studies will each be briefly discussed, along with the Egyptian study and several studies conducted in India.

Egypt

Soueif's Egyptian sample was from a male prison population which was poorly educated, largely illiterate and of lower socioeconomic status and hence unrepresentative of the general cannabis using populations in most other cultures. Significant differences were found between users and controls on 10 out of 16 measures of perceptual speed and accuracy, distance and time estimation, immediate memory (digit span backwards), reaction time and visual–motor abilities, including the Trail Making Test (Part A) and the Bender Gestalt test (Soueif, 1971, 1975, 1976a, b). These differences in performance were more marked in the youngest ($<$ 25 years) and best educated urban users than in the older, illiterate and rural subjects. Soueif concluded that prolonged cannabis use produces subtle deficits in the cortical level of arousal (Soueif, 1976a). He argued that high cortical levels of arousal are associated with high levels of proficiency, and "the lower the nondrug level of proficiency on tests of cognitive and psychomotor performance the smaller the size of function deficit associated with drug taking" (Soueif, 1976b).

Soueif's Egyptian study was subsequently criticized for methodological reasons (Fletcher & Satz, 1977). Soueif replied to these criticisms (Soueif, 1977) and maintained that long-term use of cannabis may lead to deficits in speed of psychomotor performance, distance and time estimation, immediate memory and visuomotor coordination, particularly in young, educated and urban users. The validity of these findings, however, remains under doubt because some of the tests used by Soueif do not have established neuropsychological validity (Carlin, 1986).

Jamaica

Bowman & Pihl (1973) conducted two field studies of chronic cannabis use in Jamaica, one with a small sample of 16 users and 10 controls from rural and semi rural areas, and the other with a small urban slum sample of 14 users and controls. Users had been very heavy daily consumers of cannabis for a minimum of 10 years (current use of about 23 high potency joints/day), while controls had no previous experience with cannabis. Tests were selected on the basis of having previously been shown to be sensitive to impairment following chronic heavy alcohol use (or other chemical insult). They were generally described as "measures of the efficiency of concept formation and memory" (Bowman & Pihl, 1973). The groups were matched for age, sex, social class, alcohol use, education and "intelligence", but most subjects were illiterate or semiliterate, with an average age of 30 years. No differences were found between the users and nonusers of either study, or when the rural and urban samples were combined.

A more extensive study of 60 male labourers in Jamaica (Rubin & Comitas, 1975) came to be regarded as the main Jamaican project (NIDA funded). It was hailed as a major breakthrough in cultural drug research because it used a combination of field based social-scientific evaluation and hospital based clinical evaluation (Rubin & Comitas, 1975). The neuropsychological and personality assessments were much more extensive than those conducted in Egypt or Greece. This study compared 30 users and 30 nonusers matched on age, socioeconomic status and residence. The user group which was aged between 23 and 53 years with a mean age of 34 years, had used cannabis for an average of 17.5 years (range 7–37 years) at around seven joints per day (range 1–24 joints), estimated to contain 60 mg of THC. They had not used any substances other than alcohol and tobacco. While it was stated that no control subject had used cannabis heavily in recent years, whether there had been heavy use in the past was not reported. At least nine of the controls were current "occasional" users of cannabis and all but 12 of the controls had some experience with cannabis.

A battery of 19 psychological tests were administered, generally after 3 days of abstinence, as part of a 6 day inpatient drug free hospitalization period during which many other clinical and physiological examinations were performed. The test battery included three tests of intellectual and verbal abilities (Wechsler Adult Intelligence Scale (WAIS), Ammons Full-Range Picture Vocabulary Test and the Reitan Modification of the Aphasia Screening Test) and 15 neuropsychological tests measuring abilities previously shown to be affected by acute cannabis intoxication. Simple and complex motor functions were tested by dynamometer, finger tapping, maze steadiness, graduated holes and pegboard. Sensory perception was assessed by tests of tactile and auditory stimulation, and tactile form and finger-tip writing recognition. Memory and attention were measured by the Tactual Performance Test (child's version), the Time-Sense-Memory Test and the Seashore Rhythm Test. The Indiana-Reitan Category Test (child's version) assessed concept formation. Portions of the WAIS, such as the Information, Vocabulary and Picture Arrangement subtests, were omitted as they were judged to be culturally inappropriate.

Comparisons of the users and nonusers on 47 subtest variables failed to reveal any consistently significant differences. There was no strong suggestion of differences that failed to be detected because of a small sample size since the user group scored better than the nonuser group on 29 variables, albeit nonsignificantly. The authors considered their results to be consistent with Bowman and Pihl's Jamaican study, and concluded that "in a wide variety of human abilities, there is no evidence that long-term use of cannabis is related to chronic impairment" (Rubin & Comitas, 1975).

The interpretation of these null results as evidence of an absence of effect of cannabis on cognitive functioning is complicated by a number of factors that may have attenuated differences between users and controls. First, the tests used were not standardized for use in Jamaica. Second, there are problems with the interpretation of test scores with the possibility of floor and ceiling effects obscuring any drug effects (particularly as children's versions of some tests were used), and test score means were not published. Third, the inclusion of cannabis users in the control group may have further contributed to the lack of significant group differences. No attempt was made to evaluate any long-term neuropsychological effects as a function of frequency or duration of use. Fourth, a number of other cultural differences may have confounded the results of this study. Jamaican society at the time had a tradition of cannabis use within which many viewed the drug as medicinal, benign or even as a work enhancer. Cannabis users were not viewed as amotivated "drop outs" from society, as they were in North America, for example. The cannabis users of this Jamaican sample were mainly farmers, fishermen and artisans from rural areas or casual urban labourers who claimed to increase their work output by using cannabis to relieve the monotony of dull, repetitive and laborious work (Comitas, 1976). If only the higher cognitive functions are affected by cannabis, the work performance of rural or manual labourers would not necessarily be affected. This does not exclude the possibility that the long-term use of cannabis may impair the performance of workers who have more complex tasks or those who come from higher socioeconomic groups for whom mental operations may predominate (Fink, 1976b). This sample was poorly educated, with a mean of 4.5 years of schooling (equivalent to third grade) so that if Soueif (1976a) is correct, there would only be small functional deficits associated with cannabis use.

Greece

The Greek NIDA study (Stefanis *et al.*, 1977) examined a sample of 47 chronic hashish users and 40 controls matched for age, sex, education, demographic region, socioeconomic status and alcohol consumption. The subjects were mostly refugees from Asia Minor, residing in a low income, working class area of Athens. The average duration of use was 23 years of an estimated daily use of 200 mg per day, and most users had smoked hashish on the day before testing, and some had smoked several hours before the test session. Controls were slightly better educated than users.

The WAIS and Raven's Progressive Matrices were administered to assess general intelligence and mental functioning (Kokkevi & Dornbush, 1977). Subtests of the WAIS were used to evaluate the possibility of impairment in specific cognitive and perceptual functions. While the WAIS was not standardized on a Greek population it had been used by the authors in a translated form for many years. The Raven's test was considered to be a more culture free assessment of intelligence and was used for reliability and validity purposes. The groups did not differ in global IQ score on either the WAIS or Raven's Progressive Matrices, but nonusers obtained a higher verbal IQ score than users. The users' performance was worse than controls on all but one of the subtests of the WAIS (Digit Span), even if not significantly so. Significant differences in performance between the two groups were obtained in three subtests of the WAIS: Comprehension, Similarities, and Digit Symbol Substitution. Impaired performance in the Comprehension and Similarities subtests indicates a possible defect in verbal comprehension and expression, verbal memory, abstraction and associative thinking. A low score on Digit Symbol Substitution (consistently shown to be affected by cannabis acutely) indicates a possible defect in visual–motor coordination and memorizing capacity. A trend toward inferior performance in the Picture Arrangement test may indicate a dysfunction in logical sequential thought.

The interpretation of these results was complicated by the lack of a requirement that subjects abstain from hashish prior to testing. Consequently, it was not clear whether the impairment found on these subtests was related to long-term use of hashish or whether it was due to the persistence of an acute drug effect at the time of testing. The poorer performance by users was assumed to "reflect their recent use of hashish, as the test was given within 2 hours of smoking hashish by some users" (Kokkevi & Dornbush, 1977), an interval that coincided with increased pulse rates, a reliable sign of acute intoxication. The differences between verbal and performance IQ were similar in both groups so the authors argued that there was no evidence of deterioration in mental abilities in the hashish users. They attributed the poorer performance by users to "acculturational and adaptational processes" rather than to "logical reasoning abilities", however, in line with the Egyptian and Jamaican studies, they conceded that "it is possible that the detection of subtle intellectual dysfunctions in groups with initially low levels of mental functioning are less easily observed" (Kokkevi & Dornbush, 1977).

A subsample of 20 of the Greek chronic users were administered a brief psychometric battery after smoking a given dose of cannabis (Dornbush & Kokkevi, 1976). These subjects had smoked for over 25 years and were assessed on simple tests of perceptual–motor ability. This study demonstrated the acute response of chronic users to be similar to that of short-term users in the USA: psychological test performances were adversely affected by cannabis in a way similar to that observed in naive subjects or short-term users under acute intoxication. The adverse effects on mental functioning were short lived, persisting for approximately 70 minutes after commencing smoking. Thus, no evidence was provided for tolerance or withdrawal effects. The only effect to be inferred was that practise effects, although not abolished by the consumption of marijuana, were less than those observed under placebo conditions. Furthermore, no differences were found in the EEG changes produced by an acute dose of cannabis in this Greek sample and a group of American volunteers; nor were there differences between the two samples in resting EEG patterns.

Costa Rica

The NIDA study of chronic heavy cannabis users in Costa Rica was modelled upon the Jamaican project but with greater sensitivity to cultural issues. It involved an intensive physiological, psychological, sociological and anthropological study of matched pairs of users and nonusers (Carter, 1980). Satz *et al.* (1976) reported the results of comparing 41 male long-term heavy cannabis users (on average 9.6 joints per day for 17 years) with matched controls on an extensive test battery designed to assess the impact of chronic cannabis use on neuropsychological, intellectual and personality variables. The educational level of the Costa Rican sample was slightly higher than that of either the Greek or the Jamaican populations, although more than half of the user group had not completed primary school and both users and nonusers had commenced employment at 12 years of age on average. The users were working class, mostly tradesmen with lower than average income, who reported that they often used cannabis to augment their work performance in a similar fashion to the Jamaican sample.

The tests included Finger Localization and Finger Oscillation (tapping) Tests, the Tactual Performance Test, the Rey-Davis test of nonverbal memory and learning and the Word Learning and Delayed Recall tests from the Williams Memory Battery, Logical Memory from the Wechsler Memory Scale, the Milner Facial Recognition Memory Test, the Benton Visual Retention Test, and a short form of the WAIS. These tests were translated into Spanish and standardized on a separate sample of the Costa Rican population. They were found to be free of cultural bias, and no floor or ceiling effects were demonstrated. All data were subjected to appropriate multivariate statistical analyses.

Despite their long duration and heavy use, the Costa Rican users did not differ significantly from controls on any test. Users scored consistently lower, if not significantly so, than nonusers on 11 of 16 variables in the neuropsychological test battery. These included the Word Learning, Delayed Recall and the Rey-Davis subtests of the Williams Memory

Battery, the Logical Memory test of the Wechsler Memory Scale and the Facial Recognition Memory Test. Although users' performance was poorer, particularly in the mean number of errors made, learning curves were similar for both groups. A multivariate analysis of the 14 variables comprising the WAIS also revealed no significant differences between groups. Users performed slightly better on 6 of the 11 subtests and had a slightly higher verbal and full scale IQ. An attempt to correlate test results with level of marijuana use yielded no consistent findings. The authors concluded that there was no evidence for irreversible brain damage, significant impairment of memory function or other cognitive impairment due to the chronic use of cannabis.

A 10 year follow up of the Costa Rican sample was conducted by Page *et al.* (1988). By the time of follow up, the users had an average 30 years experience with cannabis, but the sample size had dropped to 27 of the 41 original users and 30 of the 41 controls. The test protocol included some of the original tests as well as a number of additional tests measuring short-term memory and attention, which were selected for their sensitivity in detecting subtle changes in cognitive functioning. The new tests included the Rey-Osterrieth Complex-Figure Test, Buschke's Verbal Selective Reminding Test, the Self-Paced Continuous Performance and Underlining Tests, Mazes and Trail Making Test Part A.

No differences were detected on any of the original tests, but three tests from the new battery yielded significant differences between users and controls. In Buschke's Selective Reminding Test, the user group retrieved significantly fewer words from long-term storage than the nonuser group, although the groups did not differ on a measure of storage. Users performed more slowly than nonusers in the Underlining Test, with particularly poor performance in the most complex subtest. Differences between groups were not a function of practice or purely motor speed. The Continuous Performance Test also revealed users to be slower than controls on measures requiring sustained attention and effortful processing, although there were no differences in correct hits nor false alarm rates.

Page *et al.* interpreted their results as providing evidence that long-term consumption of cannabis is associated with difficulties in sustained attention and short-term memory. They hypothesized that such tests require more mental effort than the tests used in the original study and, as such, the results imply that long-term users of cannabis experience greater difficulties with effortful processing. They provided anthropological data to further support their hypotheses: users exhibited lower levels of mental effort at work than nonusers, although this was confounded by the choice of job. Users tended to work as labourers, street vendors or in the service industry, while nonusers tended to be craftsmen, store tenders or office managers. Page *et al.* claimed that if users "found it difficult to concentrate, especially on tasks that require attention to detail", they might be expected to choose jobs that are less demanding in mental performance than the jobs chosen by nonusers.

This study differs from its predecessors in that it did find differences between users and nonusers in tests of information processing, sustained attention and short-term memory. Nevertheless, Page *et al.* emphasized that the differences they found were "quite subtle" and "subclinical". Only a small number of subjects were classified as clinically impaired. The differences are so small and subtle, it is difficult to exclude several other alternative explanations before concluding that they reflect the longer duration of use by the sample, or the greater sensitivity and specificity of tests used. These alternative possibilities include that the differences were due to the inclusion of the few clinically impaired subjects within the sample and that some of the differences were due to acute intoxication or recent use as 24 hour abstinence was requested, but was not verified.

Most recently, a further follow-up of 17 of the original users and 30 of the original controls was reported by Fletcher and colleagues (1996). These subjects (mean age 45 years) were compared with a younger cohort (mean age 29 years) of 37 Costa Rican cannabis users (mean duration of use of 8 years) and 49 nonuser controls on tests of short-term and working memory and attention following a 72-hour period of abstinence verified by the analysis of two urine samples. Older long-term users performed worse than older nonusers on complex short-term memory tests involving learning lists of words and on complex tasks of selective and divided attention associated with working memory. No differences were found between younger users and nonusers.

India

Studies of long-term cannabis use in India commenced with Agarwal *et al.*'s (1975) examination of chronic bhang drinkers. Bhang is a tea like infusion of cannabis leaves and stems which is drunk, sometimes for medicinal purposes. The 40 subjects had used bhang daily for about 5 years, were less than 45 years of age, reasonably well educated with 65% having completed high school and none were illiterate. There was no control group so scores were compared to normative data on the tests used. By comparison with these norms, 18% of the bhang users had memory impairment on the Wechsler Memory Scale, 28% showed mild intellectual impairment on the Bhatia Battery of Intelligence (IQs less than 90) and

20% showed substantial cognitive disturbances on the Bender-Gestalt Visuo-Motor Test. The authors concluded that bhang may cause mild impairment in cognitive functions.

Wig & Varma (1977) administered a test battery to 23 long-term male users of cannabis (comprised of both daily charas (hashish) smokers and bhang drinkers of at least 5 years). Eleven of these were matched to a non-using control group with respect to sex, education, income, marital status and occupation. The entire sample was compared to the 11 controls on scores from Raven's Progressive Matrices, Malin's Intelligence Scale for Indian Children (adapted from the WAIS), PGI Memory Scale (adapted from the WMS), Bender-Gestalt, speed and 'H' marking tests from the General Aptitude Test Battery, a colour cancellation test and a time perception test. Users scored significantly lower on the tests of intelligence, memory, speed and accuracy, replicating Agarwal *et al.'s* findings, and pointing to problems in memory and concentration associated with long-term cannabis use.

The results of these studies are limited by either the absence of controls or the use of poorly matched controls, inadequate consideration of pre-morbid variables, unreliable measurement of the duration and severity of cannabis and other drug use, and the use of culturally inappropriate psychometric tests or tests that had not been adequately validated in the sample population. Nonetheless, many of the subjects in these studies were extremely heavy users, and the differences in cognitive performance could not always be explained by the uncontrolled confounding variables.

Mendhiratta *et al.* (1978) compared 50 heavy cannabis users (half bhang drinkers, half charas smokers of at least 25 days per month for a mean of 10 years) with matched controls. The entire sample was of low socioeconomic status. Tests were administered after 12 hours abstinence which was verified by overnight admission to a hospital ward. The tests included digit span, a recognition test, pencil tapping test, speed and accuracy tests, a time perception test, a reaction time test, a size estimation test (most of which were not standardized for the population studied) and the Bender-Gestalt Test.

The cannabis users reacted more slowly and performed more poorly in concentration and time estimation. The charas smokers were the poorest performers, showing impaired memory function, lowered psychomotor activity and poor size estimation. The fact that the smokers were most impaired may reflect a contribution by other compounds formed by pyroly-sis in the production of cognitive impairment; on the other hand, it may simply be a function of the higher potency of charas preparations. Nine to 10 years later, Mendhiratta *et al.* (1988) followed up 11 of the original bhang drinkers, 19 charas smokers and 15 controls. Repeat administration of the original tests showed significant deterioration on digit span, speed and accuracy tests, reaction time and on the Bender-Gestalt.

Ray *et al.* (1978) assessed the cognitive functioning of 30 chronic cannabis users (aged 25–46 years) who had used bhang, ganja (leaf and heads) or charas for a minimum of 11 times/month for at least 5 years, comparing their performance to that of 50 randomly selected nonuser controls of similar age, occupation, socioeconomic status and educational background. Few differences were found on tests of attention (e.g. digits backwards, serial addition/subtraction), visuomotor coordination (e.g. the Minnesota Perceptuo-Diagnostic Test) or memory (the PGI Memory Scale). Cannabis users' performance was impaired on only one of the subtests of the memory scale; however, the matching of subjects was not rigorous and the fact that all subjects were illiterate may have produced a floor effect masking differences between groups.

Varma *et al.* (1988) administered 13 psychological tests selected to assess intelligence, memory and other cognitive functions to 26 heavy marijuana smokers and 26 controls matched on age, education and occupation. The average daily intake of the cannabis users was estimated as 150 mg THC, with a frequency of at least 20 times per month and a mean duration of use of 6.8 years (minimum 5 years). Twelve hours abstinence was ensured by overnight hospitalization. The tests included pencil tapping, time perception, reaction time, size estimation, Trail Making (Form A), Bender-Gestalt, Nahor and Benson visuospatial reproduction, Standard Progressive Matrices, WAIS-R Verbal Scale, Bhatia's Short Scale (measure of IQ), PGI Memory Scale, and a disability assessment schedule. Varma *et al.* reported that the PGI Memory Scale was a locally developed and validated adaptation of the Wechsler Memory Scale which assessed memory function in 10 different domains.

Cannabis users were found to react more slowly on perceptuomotor tasks such as the pencil tapping and reaction time tests, but did not differ from controls on the tests of intelligence. When the scores of all the memory tests were combined, there was no difference between the total scores of cannabis users and controls, although cannabis users scored significantly more poorly on a subtest of recent memory. There were trends toward poorer performance on subtests of remote memory, immediate and delayed recall, retention and recognition. Users suffered disability in personal, social and vocational areas. The authors concluded that impairment of cognitive functions associated with long-term heavy use of cannabis was more apparent in perceptuomotor tasks than in tests of intelligence or memory. Nevertheless, the perceptuomotor tests employed in this study were of questionable validity, with particularly poor measures of reaction time and speed of responding, while the measures of memory function may have reached significance had a larger sample been tested. This suggests that any cognitive deficits due to cannabis may be specific to particular aspects of short-term memory.

Concerns mostly allayed but methodology flawed

The results of these culture specific studies of long-term heavy cannabis users served to allay concerns about the consequences of cannabis use since overt signs of "brain damage" as measured by psychological tests were not found. There was equivocal evidence for an association between cannabis use and more subtle long-term cognitive impairments.

Given that cognitive impairments are most likely to be found in subjects with a long history of heavy use, it is reassuring that most such studies have found few and small differences. It is unlikely that the negative results of these studies can be attributed to an insufficient duration or intensity of cannabis use within the samples studied. For example, the duration of cannabis use averaged 17.5 years and the daily THC level consumed ranged from an estimated 20–90 mg daily in Rubin and Comitas's Jamaican study, 23 years and 120–200 mg daily in the Greek sample and 16.9 years and 20–160 mg daily in the initial Costa Rican study.

The absence of differences is all the more unexpected since a number of factors may have biased these studies toward finding poorer performance among cannabis users. These include higher rates of polydrug use, poor nutrition, poor medical care and illiteracy among users, and the failure in many studies to ensure that subjects were not intoxicated at the time of testing, which would have increased the likelihood of detecting impairment. The use of a laboratory test to detect recent marijuana ingestion in studies with positive results would have been helpful in ruling out acute effects as the cause of the apparent impaired performance among users. Given the generally positive biases in these studies it has been argued that if cannabis use did produce cognitive impairment, a larger number of these studies should have shown positive results (Wert & Raulin, 1986b).

The force of this argument is weakened, however, by the fact that most of these studies suffered from numerous other methodological difficulties which may have operated against finding a difference. First, the instruments most often used for assessment have been developed and standardized mostly on North American populations. Second, many of these studies were based on small samples of questionable representativeness and subject to sampling bias, because only subjects who could be reached and were willing to participate were included in the studies while others possibly not equally resistant to drug-induced impairments might have been missed. Third, a number of studies failed to include a control group while others used inappropriate controls. Fourth, generalization of the results of these studies to users in other cultures is difficult, given the predominance of illiterate, rural, older and less intelligent or less educated subjects in these studies. Fifth, the studies were limited by their investigative instrumentation which may only be capable of detecting gross deficits at a group level. Sixth, few attempts were made to examine the relation between neuropsychological test performance and frequency and duration of cannabis use. Such an evaluation would rule out possible within group differences in chronic users.

In terms of the specific deficits reported, slower psychomotor performance, poorer perceptual motor coordination, and memory dysfunction were the most consistently reported deficits. Of the studies that specifically included tests of memory function, four detected persistent short-term memory and attentional deficits in chronic cannabis users (Page *et al.*, 1988; Soueif, 1976a; Varma *et al.*, 1988; Wig & Varma, 1977), while three detected no such deficits (Bowman & Pihl, 1973; Satz *et al.*, 1976; Mendhiratta *et al.*, 1978). Impairments were most frequently found on such tests as the Wechsler Memory Scale, the Bender-Gestalt test, Buschke's Selective Reminding Test and the Continuous Performance Test. The measures of short-term memory were often inadequate, failing to determine which processes may be impaired (e.g. acquisition, storage, encoding, retrieval) and often with an exclusion of higher mental loads and conditions of distraction. A proper evaluation of the complexity of effects of long-term cannabis use on higher cognitive functions requires greater specificity in the selection of assessment methods as well as the use of more sensitive tests.

Studies of young American or Canadian users with a relatively short history of cannabis use

The cognitive performance of American or Canadian cannabis users was also assessed in a number of studies in the 1970s. Most of the subjects in these studies were young and well-educated college students with relatively short-term exposure to cannabis in comparison to the long history of use among chronic users in the studies reviewed above. In 1970, Hochman & Brill (1973) surveyed a large sample of college students ($n = 1400$). The sample comprised nonusers (65.5%), occasional users (26%) and chronic users (8.5%) defined as those who had used three times/week for 3 years or had used daily for 2 years. They found no evidence of an "amotivational syndrome" in terms of lethargy or social and personal deterioration, but did demonstrate significant psychosocial differences between users and nonusers. Marijuana users were more rebellious, reckless, questioning and anti-authoritarian. Chronic users were less certain of long-term life plans than nonusers, although there was no relation between either frequency or duration of use and academic achievement. About 1% of marijuana users were estimated to suffer from impaired ability to function due to their use, but such loss of ability was subject to large individual differences and variability.

In a follow-up of the original sample over 2 consecutive years (1971: $n =$ 1133; 1972: $n = 901$), Brill & Christie (1974) assessed nonusers, occasional users (< 2 / week), frequent (2–4 / week), and regular users (≥ 5 / week) by a self report questionnaire. The majority of users perceived no effect of cannabis use on most areas of psychosocial adjustment. Just over 12% reported that their academic performance had declined and they were more likely to reduce their frequency of use or to quit. There were no significant differences found between users, nonusers or former users in grade point average. Cannabis users were more likely to drop out of college and had greater difficulty formulating life and career goals; fewer users planned to seek advanced academic degrees and more considered themselves to have poorer academic adjustment. Whether these attributes preceded cannabis use or were caused by it is impossible to determine. It may be argued that such differences do not necessarily reflect impairment or that they are not harmful. Indeed, the authors concluded that in a "functioning, intelligent undergraduate university population", few deleterious effects could be attributed to the use of the drug.

Entin & Goldzung (1973) conducted two studies of the residual impact of cannabis use on memory processes. In the first study, verbal memory was assessed by the use of paired associate nonsense syllable (CVC) learning lists. Twenty-six cannabis users (defined as daily for at least 6 months, but the range of use was not reported) were compared to 37 nonusers drawn from a student population. Cannabis users scored significantly more poorly on both free recall (the number of syllables recalled after a delay) and on acquisition, measured as improvement in recall over repeated trials.

In the second study, verbal and numerical memory were tested by the presentation of word lists, interspersed with Wendt three step arithmetic problems prior to recall. Cannabis users ($n = 37$) recalled significantly fewer words than nonusers ($n = 37$), but did not differ from controls on arithmetic test scores. The lack of an effect on the arithmetic tests was interpreted as a function of the short length of time during which numeric information must be stored for further manipulation, rather than being due to any numerical memory functions per se, i.e. the verbal memory tasks required longer term storage of information prior to retrieval.

These findings were interpreted as residual impairment of both the acquisition and recall phases of long-term memory processes. The authors attributed the impairments to either an enduring residual pharmacological effect on the nervous system or to an altered learning or attention pattern due to repeated exposure to cannabis. No details were provided with regard to the length of abstinence prior to testing, however. The authors stated that subjects were assumed "not to be under the influence of marihuana or any other drug during the testing situation. Any who were suspected were asked to return at another time for testing" (Entin & Goldzung, 1973).

Grant *et al.* (1973) studied the effects of cannabis use on test performance using eight measures from the Halstead-Reitan Battery among medical students. They found no differences between 29 cannabis users (of median 4 year duration and frequency three times/month) and 29 age and intelligence matched nonusers on seven of the eight measures. Users performed more poorly on the localization subtest of the Tactual Performance Test. These subjects were very select in that they were only light users, and as medical students were obviously functioning well. The failure to find any difference in sensorimotor integration or immediate sensory memory was later replicated by Rochford *et al.* (1977) in a comparison of 25 users (of at least 50 times over a mean 3.7 years) and 26 controls matched on sex, age and scholastic aptitude scores. By limiting their samples to populations of successful students, these studies are flawed in the reverse direction to the reports of Kolansky & Moore (1971, 1972).

Weckowicz & Janssen (1973) compared 11 male college students who smoked cannabis three to five times/week for at least 3 years with nonusers who were matched on age, education and socioeconomic and cultural backgrounds. They were assessed on a variety of tasks designed to measure field dependence, personality traits, social attitudes and values, as well as cognitive function. Users performed better than controls on eight of the 11 cognitive tests but performed more poorly on the Guilford Number Facility, which suggests that chronic use may affect sequential information processing. Otherwise, there was no evidence of organic brain damage or gross impairment of cognitive functioning. Weckowicz and

Janssen interpreted their findings in terms of social deviance, lack of conformity, rebelliousness and alienation.

In a cross validation of their previous findings, Weckowicz *et al.* (1977) compared 24 heavy smokers (at least daily for 3 years) belonging to the "hippie subculture" with nonuser controls matched for age (mean 22.5 years), education (mean 13.5 years) and social background. Cognitive functioning, personality traits and social values were assessed using the same test battery as used previously, with the addition of a selective listening task, the Wechsler Memory Scale, Miller Analogies Test, Utility Test, Word Association Test and Association Test. Cannabis users once again performed better on tests of "originality and cognitive ability", and scored significantly better on the selective listening task, leading the authors to interpret this as users having "better control of attention processes" and showing no signs of cognitive impairment. The measures analysed in the selective listening task were not reported. The cannabis users were also more likely to be current polydrug users and to have used LSD, psilocybin, cocaine, amphetamines and heroin.

Culver & King (1974) used the Halstead-Reitan Battery, the WAIS, the Trail Making Test, the Laterality Discrimination Test and three tests of spatial–perceptual abilities to examine the neuropsychological performance of three groups of undergraduates ($n = 14$) from classes in 2 successive years. These were marijuana users (of at least twice/month for 12 months), marijuana plus LSD users (LSD use of at least once/month for 12 months) and nondrug users. Significant differences appeared, disappeared and reappeared among the groups and classes in different years. The only consistent difference was on the Trail Making Test, in which the cannabis group performed significantly better than the cannabis plus LSD group, who also used more cannabis, but cannabis users did not differ from nonusers.

Gianutsos & Litwack (1976) compared the verbal memory performance of 25 cannabis smokers who had used for 2–6 years and at least twice/week for the last 3 months, with 25 nonsmokers who had never smoked cannabis. Subjects were drawn from an undergraduate university student population and were matched on age, sex, year at university, major and grade average. Cannabis users were "asked not to smoke before the experiment" and gave verbal report that they had not "smoked recently" prior to the time of testing, although the length of abstinence was not reported.

The task was a modification of the Peterson-Peterson paradigm which allows examination of short versus long-term storage of verbal information. In the original version of the task, arithmetic manipulations intervened between word presentation and recall. The modified task substituted further word reading for the arithmetic, arguing that such an interference task would prevent rehearsal of words and displace the to be recalled words from short to long-term storage. In interference tasks of this kind, the number of words recalled is a function of the number of post-list interference task words. Subjects were required to recall the first three words from a list of five, nine or 13 words read aloud, and the forced reading of two, six or 10 words constituted the post-list reading task. Cannabis users recalled significantly fewer words overall than nonusers, and the difference in performance increased as a function of the number of post-list words. Users also generated significantly more intrusion errors than nonusers. The authors concluded that the chronic use of cannabis interfered with the transfer of information from short to long-term storage.

Carlin & Trupin (1977) assessed 10 normal subjects who smoked marijuana daily for at least 2 years (range 2.5–8, mean 5; mean age 24 years; mean years education 14.6) and who denied other drug use. They administered the Halstead Neuropsychological Test Battery after 24 hours abstinence. No significant impairment was found by comparison with nonsmoking subjects matched for age, education and full scale IQ. Cannabis users performed faster on the Trailmaking Test Part B, a test sensitive to frontal damage. The authors concluded that "relatively long-term chronic marijuana use does not impair an individual's ability to solve complex cognitive tasks requiring recurrent observations of subtle stimulus characteristics, to manipulate complex visual motor problems, to answer questions dependent on prior learning, and to be accurate in identifying sensory stimulations, both unilateral and bilateral" (Carlin & Trupin, 1977). They acknowledged, however, that their sample was small and that perhaps less bright individuals may be at greater risk of developing impairments.

In 1981, Schaeffer, Andrysiak and Ungerleider reported no impairment of cognitive function in one of the first studies of a prolonged heavy cannabis using population in the USA. They assessed 10 long-term heavy users of ganja, aged between 25 and 36 years, all of whom were Caucasian and had been born, raised and educated in the USA (mean years of education 13.5). All had smoked between 30 and 60 g of cannabis (> 8% THC) per day for a mean of 7.4 years for religious reasons and were active members of a religious sect. They had not consumed alcohol or other psychoactive substances. While this sample contained cannabis users who had not used any other substances, it is not known what other confounding variables may have been introduced as a result of the peculiarities of belonging to a religious sect. Such a sample may not be representative of the general cannabis using population.

This study was also one of the first to use a laboratory test to assess levels of bodily cannabinoids. Schaeffer *et al.* reported that at the time of testing, all subjects had at least 50 ng/ml cannabinoids in their urines but they also stated that subjects smoked continuously, even during the testing session. It is expected that heavy users such as these would have developed tolerance to many of the effects of cannabis. The tests which were selected to assess intellectual function included the WAIS, the Benton Visual Retention Test, the Rey Auditory-Verbal Learning Test, Symbol-Digits Modalities Test, Hooper Visual Organization Test, Raven's Progressive Matrices and Trail Making (Parts A and B). As there was no control group, the data were compared with the standardized-normative information available for each test. An attempt was also made to obtain a measure of premorbid intellectual functioning. The authors obtained IQ measures from school assessments for two of the subjects, which were virtually identical to those measured in the study. Overall, WAIS IQ scores were in the superior to very superior range, and the scores of all other tests were within normal limits for age.

Despite the heavy and prolonged use of cannabis, there was no evidence of impairment in the cognitive functions assessed, namely language function, non-language function, auditory and visual remote, recent and immediate memory, or complex multimodal learning. The authors suggested that tolerance may develop to one or more of the constituents of cannabis, explaining the lack of impairment. Furthermore, it is possible that the superior to very superior intellect of these subjects may have allowed them to compensate for the effects of cannabis, and perhaps they would have performed not only within normal limits, but at a superior level had they not smoked cannabis.

The results of these empirical studies served to further allay fears that cannabis smoking caused gross impairment of cognition and cerebral function. The lack of consistent findings failed to support Kolansky & Moore's (1971, 1972) clinical reports of an organic like impairment. However, some critics (e.g. Cohen, 1982) have argued that the lack of evidence for impairment in these studies may be a function of their small sample sizes and potentially biased sampling techniques. By focusing on college students, it is suggested, these studies have sampled from a population unlikely to contain many impaired persons. The samples of younger, brighter and "successful" users may reflect the survivors whereas Kolansky and Moore reported on the casualties.

Such hypotheses, however, conflict with the explanations provided for the lack of evidence of impairment in the culture specific studies reviewed above. Soueif's proposition, for example, was that the lower the nondrug level of proficiency, the smaller the size of functional deficit associated with drug usage. This would imply maximal differences at the high end of cognitive ability. Perhaps the argument could be rephrased in terms of maximizing the possibility of detecting impairment by sampling from a broader range of ability, minimizing the possibility of sampling bias and floor and ceiling effects. In any case, Soueif's claim that the greatest drug induced impairment would occur in users with the highest levels of arousal, i.e. those for whom mental operations predominate (Fink, 1976b), was not supported by these studies of college students.

A more pertinent explanation for the lack of impairment is that the duration of cannabis use in these samples was quite brief, generally less than 5 years. It has been argued that at the time, cannabis smoking in North America had not existed long enough for impairments to emerge. Furthermore, when psychometric testing was used as a metric of cognitive function as opposed to self report questionnaires, sample sizes were often too small to permit the detection of any but very large differences between groups.

Not all studies found negative results. A small number of studies did find significant impairments in their cannabis using populations. What distinguished those studies that found differences between users and nonusers from those that did not? The answer may lie in the specificity of assessment methods. Rather than administering a standard psychometric test battery or tests of general intelligence, the studies that found differences selected tests to assess a specific cognitive function (memory), and attempted to determine the specific stages of processing where dysfunction occurred. Entin & Goldzung (1973), for example, found that users were impaired on both verbal recall and acquisition of long-term storage memory tasks, but not on arithmetic manipulations which require short-term storage of information. Gianutsos & Litwack (1976) used an interference condition in their verbal recall memory paradigm, thereby increasing the complexity of the task. Impairments became more apparent in the users as the interference increased, which suggests that cannabis use may affect the transfer of information from short- to long-term storage.

Given the lack of self awareness of such specific deficits, self-report questionnaires would probably not be able to detect such an impairment.

In the other studies, the only assessment of memory function was the inherent components of memory, alertness and concentration throughout all tests of the Halstead-Reitan Battery. Reitan himself acknowledged that this test battery "is probably not as specifically represented in terms of the memory factor as it might be" and that "it might be of value to include supplementary tests of memory" for proper evaluation (Reitan, 1986).

Controlled laboratory studies

A different approach to the investigation of the cognitive consequences of chronic cannabis use was taken in laboratory studies of the effects of daily administration of cannabis over periods of weeks to months. These studies have attempted to control for variation in quantity, frequency and duration of use, as well as other confounding factors such as nutrition and other drug use, by having select samples of subjects reside in a hospital ward while receiving known quantities of cannabis. All of these studies employed pre- and post drug observation periods, and could be thought of as a short form of longitudinal research. Because of the expense of such studies, sample sizes have generally been small and the duration of cannabis administration has ranged from 21 to 64 consecutive days.

Dornbush *et al.* (1972) administered 1 g of marijuana containing 14 mg THC to five regular smokers (all healthy young students) for 21 consecutive days. The subjects were tested immediately before and 60 minutes after drug administration. Data were collected on subjective ratings of mood, clinical observations, short-term memory and digit symbol substitution tests, and physiological signal recordings. Four subjects demonstrated partial tolerance to the euphoric effects of cannabis after the first week. Performance on the short-term memory test decreased on the first day of drug administration but gradually improved until by the last day of the study performance had returned to baseline levels. On the postexperimental day baseline performance was surpassed. Performance on the digit symbol substitution test was unaffected by drug administration and also improved with time, suggesting a practice effect. The authors interpreted their results as showing "the apparent safety of smoking 14 mg/day THC for 3 weeks".

Mendelson *et al.* (1974) reported a 31-day cannabis administration study in which 20 healthy, young male subjects (10 casual and 10 heavy users, mean age 23 years) were confined in a research ward and allowed 21 days of ad libitum marijuana smoking. A multidisciplinary battery of tests (psychiatric, psychological, physiological, biochemical and sociological) were administered during a 5-day drug-free baseline phase, the 21-day smoking period, and a 5-day drug-free recovery phase. Acute and repeat dose effects of marijuana on cognitive function were studied with a battery of psychological tests known to be sensitive to organic brain dysfunction (WAIS, Halstead Category Test, Tactual Performance Test, Seashore Rhythm Test, Finger Tapping Test, Trail Making Test). Overall, there was no overt impairment of performance prior to or following cannabis smoking nor was there any difference between the performance of the heavy and the casual users. Short-term memory function, as assessed by digit span forwards and backwards, was impaired while intoxicated and there was a relation between performance and time elapsed since smoking. An interesting finding was that subjects performed better when they were aware that the effects of cannabis smoking on memory were being assessed, than when they were not. This was interpreted as evidence that the: "acute deleterious effect of marihuana on ability to perform on a memory task may not be a reflection of direct impairment of neuronal systems sub-serving memory, but rather a reflection of what a person chooses to attend to while under the influence of the drug" (Mendelson *et al.*, 1974).

Reed (1974) reported that two of the subjects in each group from the above study showed "unequivocal evidence of impairment" in some aspect of cognitive or motor functioning. Two of the heavy users performed quite poorly on the Trail Making Test, and they and two casual users showed no consistent patterns of improvement on other tests. Their scores were lower than would have been predicted on the basis of their IQ scores and educational background. The probability of detecting such impairment in the normal population of healthy young adults would be low but it was not possible to find any relation to prior history of cannabis use. The authors claimed that tolerance did not develop to the impairing effect of cannabis over the 21 day period, but there were no indications that cannabis interfered with the ability of subjects to improve their performance with practice.

Rossi & O'Brien (1974) assessed memory and time estimation in the same sample of subjects. They aimed to explore the possible mechanisms of the observation that marijuana produces a subjective impression that time is passing slowly. One hypothesis is that of a direct pharmacological action on neuronal systems serving as a "biological clock". Another possibility is that altered time perception is incidental to the effects of cannabis on perception, memory and organization of thought, with a loosening of associations and the rapid flow of ideas speeding up the subjective sense of time. A further possibility is that short-term memory impairment may interfere with a sense of temporal continuity which is an essential element in time perception. The results of the study suggested that the effect on time perception was mediated directly through the action of THC on the central nervous system. They found a short-term acute effect on time perception (speeding up of the internal clock), and a longer lasting compensatory effect (slowing of the internal clock) which paralleled the stimulatory and depressant effects of the drug. Tolerance to the acute effect on time perception developed during the 21 day period.

Similar failures to detect cognitive effects have been reported by three other groups of investigators. Frank *et al.* (1976) assessed short-term memory and goal directed serial alternation and computation in healthy young males over 28 days of cannabis administration. Harshman *et al.* (1976) and Cohen (1976) conducted a 94 day cannabis study in which 30 healthy moderate to heavy male cannabis users, aged 21–35 years, were administered on average 5.2 joints per day (mean 103 mg THC, range 35–198 mg) for 64 days and were assessed on brain hemisphere dominance before, during and after cannabis administration. Psychometric testing was not employed, but subjects were given two work assignments with financial incentive; a "psychomotor" task involving the addition of two columns of figures on a calculator, and a "cognitive task" of learning a foreign language. No long-term impairments were detected with these somewhat inadequate assessment materials.

The experimental studies of daily cannabis usage for periods of up to 3 months in young adult male volunteers have consistently failed to demonstrate a relation between marijuana use and neuropsychological dysfunction. This is not surprising given the short periods of exposure to the drug in these studies. Furthermore, as subjects served as their own controls, and had all used cannabis for at least 1 year prior to the study, it would be surprising if an additional few months of cannabis use produced any significant decrements in performance. It may take many years for subtle impairments to be detected.

Studies of carry over effects

Most investigations of the acute effects of cannabis monitored performance on psychomotor tasks for a few hours following the onset of smoking on the assumption that performance decrements would last only for the duration of subjective intoxication. Impaired performance, particularly on tasks requiring divided attention among other cognitive abilities, has been reported to last from 2 to 8 hours following moderate doses (e.g.

Barnett *et al.*, 1985; Perez-Reyes *et al.*, 1988; Heishman *et al.*, 1989; Marks & MacAvoy, 1989). Chait *et al.* (1985) reported minimal evidence for a "hangover" effect the morning after smoking (9 hours later) on hand–eye coordination tasks, free recall and time perception. Few studies have investigated effects beyond 8 hours or attempted to determine the actual duration of the impairments observed.

By the mid 1980s, new evidence was mounting for lingering effects of cannabis beyond the period of acute intoxication. In particular, a report suggesting that cannabis may have residual detrimental effects on the performance of psychomotor tasks for up to 24 hours after smoking (Yesavage *et al.*, 1985) aroused some concern. This study monitored the performance of 10 pilots on a flight simulator task after smoking a single moderate dose of cannabis. Despite the pilots' lack of subjective awareness of any residual intoxicating effects or decrements in performance, they showed definite trends toward impairment on all variables measured 24 hours later. One of the criticisms of this study was that it failed to include a placebo control condition or group. In a follow up study, the task was modified somewhat and impairment was only manifest for up to 4 hours after smoking, leading the authors to suggest that performance decrements may only be apparent on more complex, as opposed to simple, psychomotor tasks (Leirer *et al.*, 1989). More recently, these authors replicated their original findings using a more difficult but realistic simulator task in a double-blind experiment (Leirer *et al.*, 1991). Those pilots who had smoked marijuana still experienced significant difficulty in aligning the computerized landing simulator and in landing the plane at the centre of the runway 24 hours later, with no subjective awareness of any carry over effects on their performance, mood or alertness. The authors interpreted their findings in terms of Baddeley & Hitch's (1974) framework of working memory as a "limited capacity work space for the temporary storage and processing of information coming from sensory input or from long-term memory" and suggested the carry over effects from cannabis may occur whenever "our limited capacity working memory is presented with more information than it is able to process" (Leirer *et al.*, 1991). The concept of working memory encompasses various other cognitive functions which require conscious integration and manipulation of information, such as divided and focused attention, short-term retention of information and reasoning (Baddeley, 1986).

Heishman *et al.* (1990) also reported preliminary findings to suggest that smoked marijuana can impair performance on cognitive tasks for up to 24 hours. Although based on a very small sample ($n = 3$), decreased accuracy and increased response time on serial addition/subtraction and digit recall tasks remained impaired the day after smoking, but the decrements were not as severe as they were whilst subjects were acutely intoxicated. They have since reported an extension of that study with nine subjects with a moderate history of cannabis use in a double blind experimental procedure with minimal exposure (eight puffs only) to two active doses (1.8% or 3.6% THC) (Heishman *et al.*, 1993). Psychomotor and cognitive performance measures included a circular lights (hand–eye coordination) task, serial addition/subtraction, logical reasoning, digit recall, and a manikin (spatial skills) task, and these were administered at nine set intervals before and up to 25 hours after smoking. Results indicated minimal acute performance impairment: response rate decreased, while response times increased on the serial addition/subtraction task, with a trend toward decreased accuracy, and similar effects on the logical reasoning and digit recall tasks. Not surprisingly, there was no evidence of residual impairment on any task the day after marijuana smoking. Few conclusions can be drawn from Heishman's studies, given the small sample size and the minimal exposure to low dose minimally impairing cannabis preparations, and the authors made no attempt to reconcile the likely effects of practice in their experimental design.

At best, these reports have provided some evidence for lingering impairments on complex cognitive tasks following the acute ingestion of cannabis.

Recent research

The equivocal results of the early investigations into the long-term effects of cannabis on cognitive function, together with the problem of relatively short exposure to the drug in many countries, led to something of a hiatus in research on the long-term cognitive effects of cannabis in the 1980s. Although the accumulated evidence indicated that cannabis did not severely affect intellectual functioning, uncertainty remained about more subtle impairments. Their study required advances in methodology and assessment techniques. Reports of mental deterioration and impaired cognitive functioning in cannabis users continued to be reported in the clinical literature (e.g. National Institute on Drug Abuse, 1982) and anecdotally.

In the meantime, considerable advances were made in the field of cognitive psychology and neuropsychology. There were substantial theoretical developments in the fields of cognition, memory function and information processing, and more sensitive measures of cognitive processes were developed. Moreover, by the late 1980s, cannabis use had become so wide-spread, and was being used at a progressively younger age, to revive interest in the issue.

Research from the late 1980s through the 1990s improved on the design and methodology of previous studies in a number of ways. It ensured the use of adequate control groups, attempted to verify abstinence from cannabis prior to testing, and attempted to precisely quantify the levels of cannabis use. In addition, there has to some extent been a narrowing of focus on the cognitive functions assessed, with greater attention to investigating specific cognitive processes and relating impairments in them to the quantity, frequency and duration of cannabis use.

Greater specificity in the focus of research was prompted by accumulating evidence from previous research, and advances in pharmacology and biochemistry which suggest that cannabis primarily exerts its effect upon those areas of the brain responsible for attentional and memory functioning. Miller & Branconnier (1983), for example, reviewed the literature and concluded that the detrimental effect of cannabis on human memory is the single most consistently reported psychological deficit produced by cannabinoids acutely, and the most consistently detected impairment in studies of long-term cannabis use. They proposed that the observed deficits in attention, memory consolidation and sequential-integration behaviours were mediated by the cholinergic limbic system, particularly in the septal-hippocampal pathway.

This proposal was supported by an earlier study which reported the similarity between cannabis induced impairments of memory and those due to hippocampal damage (Drew *et al.*, 1980). Performance of hippocampally lesioned patients on a battery of psychometric tests thought to assess various aspects of auditory and visual recent memory and mental set shifting were compared to retrospective data from cannabis intoxicated subjects. Tests for comparison included the Babcock Story Recall, digit span, paired-associate learning, and the Benton Visual Retention Test (for patients) or the similar Army Designs task (for marijuana intoxicated subjects). When compared to controls, the two groups exhibited similar impairments of memory function, although the cannabis intoxicated subjects produced significantly more intrusion errors.

Intrusion errors are one of the most robust phenomena of cannabis induced memory deficits in tasks of both recall and recognition (Miller & Branconnier, 1983). Such errors involve the introduction of extraneous items, word associations or new material during free recall of words, or the identification of false or previously unseen items in recognition. Miller and Branconnier conjectured that the mechanism causing intrusion errors was the failure to exclude irrelevant associations or extraneous stimuli during concentration of attention, a process in which the hippocampus may play a major role (Douglas, 1967; Kimble, 1968; Eichenbaum & Cohen, 1988). The finding of high densities of the cannabinoid receptor in the cerebral cortex and hippocampus (Herkenham *et al.*, 1990) supports the hypothesis that cannabinoids are involved in attentional and memory processes. Past studies of long-term effects of cannabis have not used sufficiently specific nor sensitive measures of such processes.

It is also important to note that most past studies have been conducted on adults, while the effects of long-term cannabis use on the young have not been adequately addressed. With an increase in the prevalence of cannabis use among adolescents and young adults, there has been a growing concern about its possible impact on the psychological development of young people. This is important because of the possibly deleterious effects of such a psychoactive substance upon psychosocial adaptation and maturation during their formative years, and the effects on cognition, learning and scholastic achievement.

In the first study of its kind with adolescents, Schwartz *et al.* (1989) reported the results of a small but carefully controlled pilot study of persistent short-term memory impairment in 10 cannabis dependent adolescents (aged 14–16 years). Schwartz's clinical observations of adolescents in a drug abuse treatment programme suggested that memory deficits were a major problem, which according to the adolescents persisted for at least 3–4 weeks after cessation of cannabis use. His sample was middle class, North American, matched for age, IQ and absence of any previous learning disabilities with 17 controls, eight of whom were drug abusers who had not been long-term users of cannabis, and another nine had never abused any drug. The cannabis users consumed approximately 18 g per week, smoking at a frequency of at least 4 days per week (mean 5.9) for at least 4 consecutive months (mean 7.6 months but the range was not reported). Subjects with a history of excessive alcohol or phencyclidine use were excluded from the study. Cannabinoids were detected in the urines of eight of the 10 users over 2–9 days.

Users were initially tested between 2 and 5 days after entry to the treatment programme, this length of time allowing for dissipation of any obvious short-term effects of cannabis intoxication on cognition and memory. Subjects were assessed by a neuropsychological battery which included the Wechsler Intelligence Scale for Children, and six tests "to measure auditory/verbal and visual/spatial immediate and short-term (delayed) memory and praxis (construction ability)" (Schwartz *et al.*, 1989). These were the Peterson-Peterson short-term Memory Paradigm, Buschke's Selective Remembering Test, the Benton Visual Retention Test, Wechsler Memory Scale Prose Passages, Rey-Osterrieth or Taylor's Complex Figure Drawing, and a Paired Associate Learning Test. After 6 weeks of supervised abstinence with biweekly urine screens for drugs of abuse, a parallel test battery was administered.

On the initial testing, there were statistically significant differences between groups on two tests: cannabis users were selectively impaired on the Benton Visual Retention Test and the Wechsler Memory Scale Prose Passages. The differences were smaller but were still detectable 6 weeks later. Analysis of test measures showed cannabis users to commit significantly more errors than controls initially on the Benton Visual Retention Test for both immediate and delayed conditions, but differences in the 6 week post-test were not significant. Users scored lower than controls on both immediate and delayed recall in the Wechsler Memory Prose Passages Test in both test sessions. The authors concluded that "cannabis dependent adolescents have selective short-term memory deficits that continue for at least 6 weeks after the last use of marijuana". Further testing beyond 6 weeks, while not possible in this study, would have provided useful information on the recovery of function. The fact that there was a trend toward improvement in the scores of cannabis users suggests that the deficits observed were related to their past cannabis use and that functioning may return to normal following a longer period of abstinence.

The authors discussed the clinical implications of their results in terms of the need to develop treatment strategies which address the possible long lasting cognitive deficits which affect both performance of complex tasks and the ability to learn. They referred to investigations which suggest that adolescents with learning disabilities are at high risk of cannabis abuse. Their own results heighten concerns about the effects of long-term cannabis use on learning impaired adolescents. For such individuals, regular use of cannabis, even to a lesser degree than that used by Schwartz's sample, may significantly contribute to worsening school performance. Furthermore, they suggest that individuals with learning disabilities and those who have a borderline or low IQ might be even more susceptible to cannabis induced deficits of short-term or recent memory.

Schwartz's study was the first well-controlled study to demonstrate cognitive dysfunction in cannabis using adolescents with a brief mean duration of use. The implications of these results are that young people may be more vulnerable to any impairments resulting from cannabis use.

Unfortunately, like many of its predecessors, Schwartz's team made little effort to interpret the significance of the selectivity of their results. There was nothing to suggest which specific elements of memory formation or retrieval were disrupted. The two tasks represented two different types of information processing. The Benton requires the retention of visual information in iconic or unprocessed form over very brief periods, whereas the Wechsler task requires the extraction of abstractions from stories, encoding these abstractions, retrieving information and complex responding. The authors acknowledged that their "data provide little guidance on which to formulate hypotheses concerning the neurologic substrates of the observed results" and suggested that the "isolation of the location and types of disruptions that account for the current results should therefore be one goal of future research in this area".

A more recent examination of memory and intellectual function in adolescents (Millsaps *et al.*, 1994) supported the findings of Schwartz *et al.* (1989). The Wechsler Memory Scale-Revised and the WAIS-R were administered to 15 adolescent users (mean age 16.9 years) who had used on average 8.9 g of cannabis per week for over 2 years (mean 29.1 months). They had completed a mean of 9.5 years of education, although some had fallen behind in their schooling due to delinquent behaviour. Subjects were excluded on the basis of abuse of or dependence on any other substances, ever having used phencyclidine (PCP), or any history of neurologic illness, seizures or head injury. All subjects met the criteria for cannabis dependence according to DSM-III-R (American Psychiatric Association, 1987). They were abstinent for a mean of 27 days prior to testing. Most, but not all subjects underwent urine drug screens, but for those who did not, information from collaterals was obtained to verify abstinence.

Each subject's premorbid IQ was calculated using a demographically based prediction equation. Subjects were then used as their own controls, comparing the premorbid estimated IQ to the obtained Full Scale IQ. Difference scores for each individual subject were also calculated by subtracting each the WMS-R General Memory Index and the Delayed Memory Index from the Full Scale IQ, and the former two measures from the Attention/Concentration Index. The authors reported that memory impairment due to central nervous system dysfunction has been investigated in this manner in the recent neuropsychological literature. Full Scale IQ was found not to be lower than the premorbid IQ estimate, consistent with all other findings to date that suggest that general intellectual function is not impaired by chronic cannabis use. In contrast, both the General and Delayed Memory Indices were significantly reduced when compared to Full Scale IQ, although remained in the low average range. Attention/Concentration was found to be relatively intact. These results suggest that long-term marijuana use in adolescents leads to subtle impairment of memory functions, still detectable following abstinence of about one month. Once again, this study made no attempt to identify the precise memory processes that might be impaired.

Leon-Carrion (1990) used the subscales of the WAIS to compare an older group of 23 male chronic cannabis users (aged 18–27 years, 2.5 joints/per day for 4.5 years) to a matched control group. The cannabis users had significantly lower scores than controls on six of the 11 sub-scales: Comprehension, Similarities, Vocabulary, Block Design, Picture Arrangement and Object Assembly. Overall, the cannabis users' scores were lower than would be expected for their age. Their Full Scale IQ, and both Verbal and Performance IQ, were lower than controls. These results suggest that the cannabis users may well have differed in ability from controls prior to their having commenced using cannabis, even though the author argues against this on the basis of socioeconomic, cultural and educational status. A vocabulary score alone is perhaps the single best indicator of original intellectual endowment, being the the most resilient to insult. Nevertheless, the author's interpretation of the results is in accord with many other observations: users were most impaired in their ability to learn from experience, their capacity for compromise, elaboration of adequate judgements and situational adaptation, and organizational, verbal and communication skills. Many of these abilities are thought to be under the control of the frontal lobes.

It appears that the same group of subjects were assessed on an 8 hour long version of the Trail Making Test to investigate cognitive styles and relations between both cerebral hemispheres (Leon-Carrion & Vela-Bueno, 1991). Cannabis users exhibited great fluctuation between cognitive styles and weaker dominance-subdominance hemispheric alternation which was clearly maintained over time in control subjects. The authors interpreted these findings to suggest that chronic consumption of cannabis "can affect cognitive styles and the brain, altering the Basic Rest Activity Cycle between the hemispheres". The significance of these findings is open to interpretation, although the tests may be tapping some aspect of frontal lobe function.

One crucial requirement for evaluating the performance of chronic marijuana users is comparison with an appropriately matched group of non-using subjects. Although most studies have made substantial progress in this regard, one concern remains that some of the impairments found may have been present in the cannabis users prior to their cannabis use. Short of an expensive longitudinal study that follows children over many years, the most desirable procedure is to match groups of users and nonusers on some measure of intellectual functioning, preferably obtained before the onset of drug use, or otherwise to obtain a valid measure that can be used to estimate the premorbid level of intellectual functioning, as was used in the study of Millsaps *et al.* (1994) with adolescents.

Block and colleagues (1990; 1993) have conducted a study in which they used scores on the Iowa Tests of Basic Skills collected in the fourth grade of grammar school. These are standardized ability tests that have been administered to almost all grammar school children in Iowa for several decades. They used these scores to establish that their user and nonuser samples were comparable in intellectual functioning before they began using marijuana. The study's aim was to determine whether chronic marijuana use produced specific cognitive impairments and, if so, whether these impairments depend on the frequency of use. Block and colleagues assessed 144 cannabis users (aged 18–42 years), 64 of whom were light users (1–4/week for 5.5 years) and 80 heavy users ($\geq$ 5/week for 6.0 years) (range 2–10+ years use), and compared them with 72 controls. Twenty-four hours of abstinence was required prior to testing.

Subjects participated in two sessions. In the first session they completed the 12th grade version of the Iowa Tests of Educational Development, which emphasize basic, general intellectual abilities and academic skills and effective utilization of previously acquired information in verbal and mathematical areas (subtests include Vocabulary, Correctness and Appropriateness of Expression, Ability to do Quantitative Thinking and Ability to Interpret Literary Materials plus a Short Test of Educational Ability). In the second session subjects were administered computerized tests that emphasise learning and remembering new information, associative processes and semantic memory retrieval (e.g. free and constrained associations, paired-associate learning, text learning, Buschke's Selective Reminding Task), concept formation and psychomotor performance (e.g. discriminant reaction time and critical flicker fusion). The tasks selected had been previously shown to be sensitive to the acute or chronic effects of cannabis. They were also relevant to the skills required in school and work performance.

The results showed that while users and nonusers were matched on 4th grade Iowa scores, heavy users showed impairment in two areas when tested on the 12th grade Iowa Test: verbal expression (Correctness and Appropriateness of Expression) and mathematical skills (Ability to Do

Quantitative Thinking). The results of the computerized tests, reported several years later (Block & Ghoneim, 1993), showed that heavy, chronic marijuana use of at least seven times/week did not produce overall impairments in Buschke's Test but selectively impaired the retrieval of words that were easy to visualise. The impairments in heavy users remained significant after controlling for the effects of lifetime and recent use of other drugs and alcohol. One test of abstraction (Concept Formation) showed superior performance in a particular test condition (fuzzy concepts) in users of moderate frequency (5–6/week). The authors were also able to show reasonable, albeit imperfect, agreement between acute and chronic effects of marijuana on cognition by comparison with the results of another study examining the acute effects of cannabis on the same battery of tests (Block *et al.*, 1992). The impairments associated with heavy, chronic use were much less pervasive than the immediate effects of marijuana smoking. Two tests showing a large degree of impairment acutely (Ability to Interpret Literary Materials, and Text Learning) showed no long-term adverse effect. This research has been among the first to directly compare the acute and chronic effects of cannabis upon the same test battery, and the authors point out that while acute and chronic effects of drugs are sometimes similar, they can also be markedly different.

Another recent study used self reported highschool Scholastic Aptitude Test scores as a measure of premorbid intellectual ability (Pope & Yurgelun-Todd, 1996). This well-controlled research detected specific impairments of attention, memory and frontal lobe function in heavy marijuana using college students by means of selected neuropsychological tests. Pope & Yurgelun-Todd (1996) tested two samples of undergraduate college students: 64 light and 65 heavy cannabis users of median age 21 years (range 18–28), and composed of equivalent numbers of males and females. Light users were those who reported using cannabis only occasionally (a maximum of 9 days in the past 30 days), while heavy users reported using regularly (a minimum of 22 days in the past 30 days). The duration of cannabis use was not reported nor were its effects investigated. Subjects were hospitalized overnight to ensure abstinence from cannabis of at least 19 hours prior to testing. The tests administered were the vocabulary subtest of the WAIS-R to obtain a measure of verbal IQ, digit span, the Stroop test, the Wisconsin Card Sorting Test (WCST), the Benton Verbal Fluency Test, the Wechsler Memory Scale, the California Verbal Learning Test (CVLT) and the Rey-Osterreith Complex Figure Test.

Heavy users and light users were equivalent on the verbal portion of the Scholastic Aptitude Test, but heavy users had lower scores on the quantitative portion and on the total score, as well as a lower verbal IQ. These variables were used as covariates in the analyses. No differences between the two groups were found on digit span. Male heavy users were slower than light users in the interference condition of the Stroop test. Heavy users of both sexes made more perseverative responses on the WCST than light users. On the verbal fluency test, heavy users of low verbal IQ produced significantly fewer words than light users of low verbal IQ, and five of the heavy users scored below the threshold of low normal scores. The memory quotient on the WMS did not differ between groups and nor did any of the subtests except that male heavy users performed significantly more poorly on the delayed recall of figures. Male heavy users also recalled significantly fewer elements of the Rey Figure on immediate recall. Heavy and light users differed significantly on recall of the first administration of the CVLT word list, and on each subsequent administration over five trials and in an interference condition involving short delay. There was a trend also toward poorer performance following a long delay. The sex differences found on certain subtests of this study are interesting in that they suggest that there may be differential effects of cannabis use on males and females. Sex differences have rarely been investigated in the research to date on the cognitive effects of cannabis.

The investigators performed a number of careful post hoc analyses in an attempt to establish that the poorer performance of the heavy users was an effect of cannabis and not attributable to, say, premorbid deficits or use of other substances. While these confounds were ruled out, the authors were unable to attribute their findings to either a temporary effect due either to drug residues lingering in the brain or to an abrupt withdrawal from heavy use or to a lasting alteration of central nervous system function as a result of lifetime exposure to cannabis. The authors have previously argued, quite correctly, that this attributional problem applies to all studies of cognitive function in long-term cannabis users (Pope *et al.*, 1995). Further analyses failed to support the hypothesis that poorer performance was related to total lifetime consumption of cannabis. However, no correlational analysis was reported nor were any effects associated with the actual duration of use tested. In fact, the mean duration of cannabis use of their samples was not reported and it is unlikely that their subjects had used for an extensive period of time as they were all college students with a mean age of 20–21 years. In fact the authors did state that "many" subjects had used for 2 years or more, and that none had used for more than a decade. It is possible that their heavy users had in fact used for a greater number of years than their light users. This is proposed in the light of accumulating evidence for effects associated with cumulative exposure to cannabis, or the duration of use. We have recently reported both verbal learning and memory function as measured by the RAVLT to be more impaired in long-term users than short-term users, with no effects associated with quantity/frequency of use, but our sample was a much more entrenched group of cannabis users seeking treatment for cannabis dependence (n = 100, mean duration of use = 14 years, 84% using daily) (Solowij et al., 1997). Perseverative responses on the WCST correlated significantly with the number of years of cannabis use.

Pope & Yurgelun-Todd's (1996) study was important in identifying with much greater precision and specificity those aspects of cognitive functioning that may be impaired by even relatively short-term but heavy use of cannabis. Their results suggested that heavy cannabis use "was associated with reduced function of the attentional/executive system, as exhibited by decreased mental flexibility and increased perseveration on the WCST, and reduced learning on the CVLT". They claimed that cannabis use may compromise some memory functions, but the principal effect is on the attentional/executive system, while recall per se remains relatively intact. They further claimed that the most pronounced effects may be on the abilities to shift and/or sustain attention, functions associated with the prefrontal cortex. A similar conclusion was drawn by the recently reported Costa-Rican follow-up (Fletcher et al., 1996).

Converging evidence for frontal involvement comes from a very different approach to assessing the long-term consequences of exposure to cannabis. The Ottawa Prenatal Prospective Study (OPPS) is an exceptionally well controlled longitudinal study of children who had been prenatally exposed to cannabis in utero. Summaries of the findings to date and a discussion of their interpretation and implications are presented by Fried (1993, 1995, 1996). For the purposes of this review, only assessments of the cognitive and central nervous system development of the children, and only those effects which remained statistically significant after controlling for many potentially confounding variables, such as birth weight, other drug use, socioeconomic status and nutrition, will be discussed.

The levels of exposure to cannabis in the sample were approximately as follows: 60% of the mothers used cannabis irregularly, 10% reported smoking two to five joints per week and 30% smoked a greater amount during each trimester of pregnancy. Prenatal exposure to cannabis was associated with high pitched cries, disturbed sleep cycles, increased tremors and exaggerated startles in response to minimal stimulation in newborn to 30 day old babies. The babies showed poorer habituation to visual stimuli, consistent with the sensitivity of the visual system to the teratogenic effects of cannabis demonstrated in rhesus monkeys and rats (e.g. Fried & Charlebois, 1979). Fried's interpretation of these findings was that exposure to cannabis may affect the rate of development of the central nervous system, with a particularly slow rate of maturation of the visual system. This hypothesis was supported by visual evoked potential studies of the children at 4 years of age. Children who had been exposed to cannabis in utero showed greater variability and longer latency of the evoked potential components, indicating immaturity in the system.

From 1 to 3 years of age, no adverse effects of prenatal exposure were found on the Bayley Scales, which provide mental and psychomotor developmental indices and assess infant behaviour. At 2 years it appeared that the children were impaired on tests of language comprehension as assessed by the Reynell Developmental Language Scale, but this effect did not persist after controlling for other factors such as ratings of the home environment. At 3 years of age, the McCarthy Scales of Children's Abilities also failed to detect any negative associations with prenatal exposure to cannabis. At 4 years of age, however, the children of cannabis using mothers were significantly inferior to controls on tests of verbal ability and memory as assessed by the McCarthy Scale and the Peabody Test of receptive vocabulary. The explanation for the gap in detecting impairments in the preceding age range, was that the degree and types of deficits observed may only be identifiable when cognitive development has proceeded to a certain level of maturity and when complex behaviour can be examined at a more specific rather than global level (Fried, 1996). It has been suggested that it is around this age that the frontal lobes begin to function.

At 5 and 6 years of age, the children were not impaired on global tests of cognition and language and the investigators speculate on the possible influence of schooling as an explanation for the "catching up" of the exposed children. By age 6 years, however, a deficit in sustained attention was detected in a computerized task that differentiated between impulsivity and vigilance. Fried (1993) proposed that "instruments that provide a general description of cognitive abilities may be incapable of identifying nuances in neurobehaviour that may discriminate between the marijuana exposed and nonmarijuana exposed children". He suggested the need for tests which examine specific cognitive characteristics and strategies, such as the test of sustained attention. From 6 to 9 years of age the children continued to be assessed on a battery of neurobehavioural tests. Preliminary analyses have suggested that cannabis exposed children scored more poorly than nonexposed children on parental behavioural ratings, visual perceptual and memory tasks, language comprehension and distractibility, although the extent to which these differences remain clinically significant following statistical control of (possibly inappropriate) confounding variables is uncertain (Fried, 1996). Fried warns that his sample came from a middle class, low risk population and that his results might therefore be interpreted as a somewhat conservative estimate of the potential risk, but also notes that any effects associated with prenatal exposure to cannabis are likely to be subtle and yet to affect the complex executive functioning that develops throughout childhood (Fried, 1995, 1996). Fried (1993) suggested that cannabis "may affect a number of neonatal behaviours and facets of cognitive behaviour under conditions in which complex demands are placed on nervous system functions". Most recently, Fried (1995; 1996) concludes that the areas of vulnerability that have emerged from this course of study are consistent with the cognitive construct termed "executive function" – the ability to maintain an appropriate problem solving set for attainment of a future goal, that involves the integration of a variety of cognitive processes and which is thought to be subserved by the prefrontal lobes.

Further evidence for an enduring deficit comes from a NIDA funded project (principal investigator F. Struve) to investigate persistent central nervous system sequelae of chronic cannabis exposure. This research has utilized both neuropsychological tests and quantitative EEG techniques. The latter determined significant increases in absolute power, relative power and interhemispheric coherence of EEG alpha and theta activity, primarily in frontal-central cortex, in daily cannabis users of up to 30 years duration compared to short-term users and nonusers (e.g. Struve *et al.*, 1994, see Chapter 4). The results suggest that there may be a gradient of quantitative EEG change associated with progressive increases in the total cumulative exposure (duration in years) of daily cannabis use which may indicate organic change. To date, correlations between the EEG changes and neuropsychological test performance have not been reported.

Preliminary analyses of the neuropsychological test data have been presented at conferences (e.g. Leavitt *et al.*, 1992, 1993). These investigations have been exceptionally well controlled. Subjects were extensively screened for current or past psychiatric or medical disease or central nervous system injury, and underwent extensive drug history assessments with 8 weeks of twice weekly drug screens. Groups were matched for age and sex. Daily cannabis users who had at least 3–6 years of use were compared to a group who had used for 6–14 years, a special interest group who had used on a daily basis for 15 years or more, and a nonuser control group. Sample sizes varied from study to study, but averaged approximately 15 per group.

An extensive battery of psychological tests included measures of simple and complex reaction time (using Sternberg's procedure), attention and memory span (e.g. digits forward and backward, continuous performance task, Trail Making, serial addition/subtraction, divided attention (Paced Auditory Serial Addition Test (PASAT), Stroop interference task), language and comprehension tasks, construction (complex Rey figure), verbal and visual learning/memory (Wechsler Memory Scale and California Verbal Learning Test (CVLT)) and "higher" mental abilities/concept formation/logical reasoning (WAIS-R, Category Test and Conceptual Level Analogies Test (CLAT)). The effects of age and education were addressed through a multiple regression procedure which removed expected values computed using only age and education from all outcome variables. Only nonusers were used to estimate regression weights and these were "jackknifed".

Preliminary analyses have shown test scores in general to show a gradation, with the best performance characterising nonuser controls, followed by the daily cannabis users and the worst mean scores shown by the ultra long-term special interest group (Leavitt *et al.*, 1992, 1993; J. Leavitt, personal communication). Neuropsychological measures which would not be expected to be affected by cannabis use (e.g. Information and Vocabulary subtests of the WAIS-R) were not significantly different between groups. Selected WAIS-R subtests did show significant differences between groups with, in each case, the daily cannabis users performing more poorly than controls and the greatest level of impairment being found in the ultra long-term group. Select subscales of the Revised Wechsler Memory Scale showed similar trends. Long duration users performed more poorly than short-term users and controls, and there were few differences between the latter two groups on complex reaction time, verbal learning/recall (CVLT), complex reasoning/conceptual abilities (Category, CLAT) and short-term memory (verbal, visual, delayed Wechsler Memory Scale subtests). There was a trend toward poorer performance on the complex mental tracking task (PASAT). The investigators claimed that duration of use was related to impaired performance, but did not report any correlations. Tests sensitive to mild cortical dysfunction were those most affected in the long-term user groups. The results attest to the importance of taking cumulative duration of exposure to cannabis into account when studying the cognitive functioning of chronic cannabis users.

One of the robust sequelae of acute intoxication is altered time sense and the underproduction of time estimations has been demonstrated and replicated in many studies. A further study from this group has investigated time production in chronic users after 24 hours abstinence (Webb *et al.*, 1993). Twenty eight daily users ($\geq$ 7 joints/week for $\geq$ 3 years) displayed greater time underproduction than 32 controls, which suggests that time distortion may persist beyond the acute phase of intoxication. Additional analyses suggested that time distortions were greater for long-term than short-term users.

Overall, this series of studies made an important advance in terms of its rigorous methodology, extensive range of neuropsychological assessment tests, and the analyses and interpretations of the results. The results suggested that long duration users seem to process some kinds of information more slowly as compared to nonusers, and that the effects of long-term cannabis use are most likely to surface under conditions of moderately heavy cognitive load. The authors acknowledge that small sample sizes dictate caution and that there were no data available to assess the premorbid cognitive capacity of these subjects. Nevertheless, the results allowed the following conclusions to be drawn (J. Leavitt, personal communication):

(1) while basic attentional processes appear to be intact, long-term cannabis users are less efficient when performing complex cognitive tasks or attempting to resist distraction;

(2) long-term users' ability to efficiently process information declines more rapidly under a moderate cognitive load when compared with controls or short duration users;

(3) while remote memory appears unaffected, long-term users are inefficient at learning and recalling information over the short-term, especially when the task is unfamiliar or complex; they show increased susceptibility to retroactive interference, whereby new information interferes with the retrieval of old information (which is consistent with difficulty in resisting distraction);

(4) long-term users are inefficient at performing complex tasks that require cognitive flexibility, recognition of unproductive planning strategies, and learning from experience, functions that have been clinically associated with the frontal area;

(5) because language and verbal intellectual abilities appear unaffected, long-term cannabis users may cope reasonably well with routine tasks of everyday life, but they may have difficulties with verbal tasks that are novel and/or which cannot be solved by automatic application of previous knowledge.

Further specific assessments are required to fully explore the scope and nature of deficits in long-term user populations.

A call for greater specificity and sensitivity

The weight of evidence suggests that the long-term use of cannabis does not result in any severe or grossly debilitating impairment of cognitive function. There is sufficient evidence from the studies reviewed above that the long-term use of cannabis leads to a more subtle and selective impairment of cognitive functioning. Impairments appear to be specific to higher cognitive functions, which include the organization and integration of complex information involving various mechanisms of attention and memory subprocesses. The evidence suggests that prolonged heavy use may lead to progressively greater impairment. It is not known to what extent such impairment may recover with prolonged abstinence.

Our understanding of the long-term cognitive effects of cannabis is far from complete. Researchers in the field have continued to recommend that these effects be examined with greater sensitivity and specificity. It was the aim of the research reported in this monograph to do precisely that: in an attempt to isolate with greater specificity the nature of cognitive dysfunction in long-term cannabis users, a series of studies utilized very sensitive techniques to examine specific stages of information processing, focusing on attentional mechanisms (Solowij *et al.*, 1991, 1995a, b, c; Solowij, 1995). Few of the more recent studies described above had been published when the series of original research studies conducted by this author commenced in 1989. Nevertheless, in line with the conclusions reached from the more recent studies of others, a thorough examination of the literature had also lead the author to suspect that deficient attentional mechanisms may well underlie many of the functions where impairments had been detected in the past. The particular susceptibility to distraction, the loosening of associations and the intrusion errors seen in memory tasks all pointed to a problem with distractibility, perhaps an inability to maintain a focus of attention. It was clear that any deficit would only manifest under a moderate cognitive load in a complex task. Selective attention was selected as a specific aspect of cognitive functioning for assessment, as the technique of recording brain event-related potentials had advanced to the extent of enabling a sensitive measure of the processes of selective attention. This technique, while being applied widely in the field of cognitive psychology, was an as yet underutilized tool in the cannabis research arena. The combination of a complex task with a sound normative base and careful experimental design would provide the opportunity to explore with validity, reliability and greater specificity the long-term cognitive effects of cannabis.

Before proceeding to describe the series of original research studies, one final review chapter is devoted to introducing the theoretical conception of the processes involved in selective attention and discussing the practicalities, interpretation of and validity of the technique of recording brain event-related potentials.

6

Selective attention and event-related potentials (ERPs)

Selective attention

Selective attention is one of a number of processes which collectively comprise the state of attending to the environment. William James described the essence of this process more than a century ago:

Everyone knows what attention is. It is the taking possession by the mind, in clear and vivid form, of one out of what seem several simultaneously impossible objects or trains of thought. Focalization, concentration of consciousness are of its essence. It implies withdrawal from some things in order to deal effectively with others.
(*James, 1890*).

Thus, selective attention could simply be defined as those processes which allow some stimuli to be processed more rapidly and effectively than others, or "the predisposition of an organism to process selectively relevant, as compared to irrelevant, environmental information" (Harter & Aine, 1984). An entirely adequate model of selective attention has not yet been formulated. Selective attention may be viewed as a facilitatory mechanism that enhances the processing of relevant stimuli, or it may be viewed as a filtering mechanism protecting a limited capacity central processor from overload by irrelevant sources of information.

Early behavioural research and theorizing in the area was initiated by Broadbent (e.g. 1958). The aim of continuing research has been to elucidate the processes involved in the selection of relevant from irrelevant information, to determine where, how and when differential processing occurs, and to establish the fate of the irrelevant information or to what extent it is processed. The main models of selective attention have been based on "early" versus "late" selection theories. Early selection theories propose that the selection of the to be attended stimulus occurs at a very early stage of processing and is based on the physical feature differences between the to be attended and the to be ignored stimuli. Late selection theories propose that all incoming information is fully analysed before selection of the to be attended stimulus occurs, and selection is based on the representation of an appropriate stimulus in a short-term memory store. Each theory has variously been supported or discredited by experimental evidence.

Much of the discrepancy from behavioural data may have arisen from the fact that there were two types of dichotic listening tasks generally used in selective attention experiments which were assumed to invoke the same processes. In the first, subjects are required to shadow information presented in the relevant channel (e.g. an attended ear) while ignoring competing prose or words in the irrelevant channel (e.g. the other, unattended ear). The degree of interference and intrusions from the irrelevant channel provide a measure of the processing of the irrelevant stimuli and their distractibility value. In the second type of paradigm subjects are required to attend to a particular channel and respond to a predetermined stimulus or class of stimuli. Measures of reaction time were thought to indicate the amount of processing required for correct selection of targets in the presence of competing distractors. Kahneman & Treisman (1984) pointed out that these paradigms may not necessarily tap the same underlying processes.

Broadbent's (1958) "early selection" theory proposed that selection is achieved by a filter which screens irrelevant input based on differences between physical features of the to be attended and the to be ignored stimuli at a very early stage, before conscious perceptual analysis has even taken place. One problem with this model was that while it allowed for switching between channels, it did not allow for simultaneous processing of more than one channel, such as in divided attention tasks, yet various dichotic listening studies established that deeper processing of stimuli from the to be ignored channel did occur (e.g. Treisman, 1964a, b; evidence also came the Stroop effect). Broadbent argued that irrelevant stimuli were completely eliminated from the information processing system, while Treisman proposed that unselected messages were merely attenuated.

According to "late selection" models (e.g. Deutsch & Deutsch, 1963) all incoming information is processed in parallel and fully analysed before selection of the to be attended stimulus occurs. Selection is based on a comparison of incoming information with a representation of the physical characteristics of a stimulus in a short-term memory store. The late selection models, however, were unable to explain why a semantic change, for example, would be more difficult to detect than a physical change. Johnston & Dark (1982) cited many examples of experimental evidence that did not fit either early or late selection theories. A number of intermediate models were developed to account for the seemingly discrepant findings of behavioural research.

Broadbent (1971), for example, modified his original all or none theory in proposing two different processes: "stimulus set" or filtering in which relevant stimuli are distinguished from irrelevant stimuli at an early stage on the basis of a simple physical feature (e.g. colour); and "response set" when the difference between relevant and irrelevant stimuli is less discriminable (e.g. semantic) and relevant stimuli are distinguished by a common set of responses. With further revision, these terms were dispensed with and replaced by a model of early filtering, which was passive, and occurred in the pre-attentive stage, a later, active attentional phase of verification, termed "pigeonholing", and a third phase of "categorizing" complex stimulus configurations (Broadbent, 1977, 1982). All of these modifications nevertheless assumed discrete, limited capacity stages of information processing of limited speed. Early selection of a single channel achieved by a filter was a requirement in order to not overload the system. Neither early nor late selection theories were able to adequately explain the intrusion of irrelevant information at certain times and not others.

Kahneman (1973) proposed an allocation model of selective attention in which attentional processing resources from a limited capacity pool are flexibly distributed amongst competing tasks. The amount allocated depends on the nature of the task and may facilitate the processing of some stimuli at the expense of others; "spare" capacity resources may be allocated to the processing of irrelevant stimuli. Little spare resources are available for irrelevant stimuli in complex and demanding tasks. This model allowed for concurrent performance of a number of tasks with flexible allocation of resources according to task demands, which may change (or the perception of which may change) momentarily. Only if the combined processing demands of the tasks exceeded the limited capacity available was performance on one or the other or both tasks impaired.

The variation in cognitive processing requirements implied that some processes must occur automatically and can hence occur in parallel while others entail controlled, conscious and effortful processing drawing upon the limited resources (e.g. Schneider & Shiffrin, 1977; Shiffrin & Schneider, 1977). These distinctions could not adequately explain how attentional resources are selectively allocated or the fate of irrelevant information.

The extent of automaticity of information processing was contentious also between the early and late selection models: late models assumed far more automaticity. The issue of automaticity is central to the debate concerning the processes of selective attention, for the more that can be explained by automatic processing the less that needs to be attributed to attentional mechanisms (Näätänen, 1988).

A different school of thought described selective attention in terms of encoding, schema theory and priming effects (e.g. Neisser, 1976; Hochberg, 1978). In this facilitatory conceptualization, certain information is primed for processing whereas irrelevant stimuli are neither filtered, inhibited nor attenuated, but are simply not analysed further because they fail to match the schema. Tipper & Cranston (1985) proposed that active inhibition of distractors, as opposed to passive decay, may be one mechanism of successful selective attention; initially targets and distractors are processed in parallel up to categorical levels of representation from which point targets receive further processing but distractors are actively inhibited. Cowan (1988) proposed a habituation model of selective attention whereby a physical representation of the irrelevant stimuli is formed in memory and following repeated presentations allows habituation to such stimuli. When a physical change occurs in the irrelevant channel, a mismatch with the representation causes orientation to that stimulus or channel. This mismatch is supported by psychophysiological evidence of "mismatch negativity" (MMN) (Näätänen, 1985; Näätänen & Picton, 1986) (see below). This model assumes that perceptual analysis takes place automatically and that controlled activation by a central executive processor directing attention to relevant stimuli prevents their habituation. *How* the central executive does so is not explained.

Aside from these traditional cognitive theories, selective attention has also been explained in terms of connectionist models (e.g. Grossberg & Stone, 1986; McClelland, 1988). These theories focus on parallel, distributed processing that occurs very quickly but they cannot yet explain those processes that take longer and have a serial component. Broadbent (1985) has argued that connectionist models are inappropriate in cognitive psychology because they are on a different computational explanatory level, intermediate between cognitive and neural models.

The argument over whether the processing of multiple attributes of stimuli proceeds in parallel or in a serial manner has been around for decades and also remains unresolved, with much experimental evidence to support or discredit either theory. The data suggest that processing begins in parallel, with some attributes processed independently and some simultaneously, some features extracted earlier than others (Posner, 1978). Some have argued that processing in a novel task is initially serial and that parallel processing only develops with practice (e.g. Shiffrin & Schneider, 1977). Treisman & Galade (1980) developed a feature integration theory in which it was proposed that the processing of complex multidimensional stimuli occurred in two stages: In the first, simple analysis of stimulus features (e.g. colour, orientation) occurred rapidly, in parallel and automatically; the second stage involved the conjunction of these features into objects, which occurred slowly in a serial fashion and required focal attention. Woods *et al.* (1994) recently reported brain event-related potential (ERP) evidence that feature conjunction in the auditory modality occurs very early, before the analysis of individual features is complete. Most of these theoretical developments, however, arose from research into visual selective attention.

In contrast, auditory attention research was dominated by dichotic listening type tasks which continued to be interpreted in terms of filtering models. While this research provided some information regarding the nature of selective attention, the debates about early versus late selection, the extent of automaticity and the extent of processing of irrelevant stimuli were not resolved. This was due to the fact that theories could only be developed and tested by reliance on behavioural data obtained during performance of such tasks as dichotic listening, signal detection and priming tasks. As overt responses are withheld for irrelevant stimuli, behavioural data cannot reveal the extent of automaticity or to what extent unattended information is processed. The advent of sensitive new techniques of recording the electroencephalograph (EEG) while subjects were engaged in dichotic listening tasks, for example, provided a way of re-evaluating the nature of selective attention processes. Such techniques based on event-related potential (ERP) interpretations, discussed below, have amassed a wealth of data over the past 15 years which has generally been interpreted as resolving the debate in favour of early selection theories (Hansen & Hillyard, 1983; Mangun & Hillyard, 1995).

Early selection models generally implied serial dependency between the early and later stages of analysis; however, Hansen & Hillyard (1983) pointed out that equivalent economy of processing is possible under parallel or holistic models of feature analysis, "provided that analyses terminate as soon as sufficient evidence accrues that a stimulus is irrelevant". This interpretation implied contingent or hierarchical information processing where "the level of one stimulus dimension influences the depth or extent of processing of other dimensions" (Hansen & Hillyard, 1983).

Hierarchical models of information processing predict that those stimulus features that are easily discriminable are initially selected for allocation of attention, followed by more complex, less discriminable features. This process continues until all stimuli that do not share every attribute of the relevant attended stimulus are gradually filtered out and not accorded any further processing. Thus, only those stimuli selected on the basis of having one relevant attribute would receive further processing for the presence of other relevant attributes. This model was well supported by ERP data. Late selection models, on the other hand, predicted an exhaustive search of all stimulus attributes, which was found not to occur from analysis of ERP traces to relevant attended and irrelevant unattended stimuli.

The selective attention task of Hansen & Hillyard (1983) has become a most widely researched paradigm, producing results consistent with a hierarchical information processing model across various experimental manipulations. It is a complex multidimensional auditory selective attention task in which tone pip stimuli vary on the dimensions of location, pitch and duration. In their 1983 paper, Hansen and Hillyard manipulated the physical dimensions of location and pitch such that one discrimination was more difficult than the other. For example, in the easy location/difficult pitch condition, tone pips were delivered randomly to the left or right ear, an easy discrimination, but within each ear, tone pips varied only slightly in pitch, either high or low, such that they were difficult to discriminate. In the difficult location/easy pitch condition, tone pips were delivered such that they were subjectively perceived to be occurring at some point towards the back of the head, making a decision as to whether they were occurring on the left or right quite difficult, but they were vastly different in pitch. In each case, the ERP pattern indicated that the rejection of the easy irrelevant dimension occurred early (e.g. rejecting half the stimuli on the basis of location), and that selection/rejection within the difficult dimension was contingent upon prior processing of the easy dimension and subsequently further processing of the selected stimuli (e.g. after half of the stimuli were selected on the basis of coming from the relevant location, they were further processed before half were rejected again on the basis of being of the wrong pitch).

Anatomical, neurophysiological and functional schema based models

Anatomical concepts of cerebral organization lend support to both parallel and hierarchical mechanisms in stimulus processing, but no single anatomical model has been able to fully explain the anatomy of selective attention, in terms of how the nervous system selects relevant stimuli and suppresses irrelevant stimuli. One theory claims that selection occurs at the periphery, say at the level of the cochlea in auditory selective attention (e.g. Hernández-Peón *et al.*, 1956; Hernández-Peón, 1966). According to this theory, involuntary attention occurs as a result of the transmission of sensory information controlled by the reticular formation; voluntary attention occurs through modification by the descending fibres of cortical origin, the cortico-reticular-sensory pathway, which is also thought to inhibit irrelevant information. This theory, however, was developed from animal research and further substantiation and replication with human data has proved elusive (e.g. Hirschhorn & Michie, 1990; Michie *et al.*, 1996). Evidence for selection at the thalamic level has also come from animal research. This theory proposes that the thalamic reticular nucleus regulates the transmission of sensory information by acting as an inhibitory gating mechanism in inhibiting thalamocortical circuits carrying irrelevant information (Skinner & Yingling, 1977).

The most favoured anatomical model of selective attention is the cortical model, based on a vast array of psychophysiological data from ERP studies, magnetoencephalography (MEG) and regional cerebral blood flow (rCBF) studies. Näätänen & Picton (1987) summarized the evidence for the auditory cortex as a possible selection site and Woods (1989) discussed the connections throughout the brain emphasising their activation through a progressively narrowing attentional spotlight, highlighting the hierarchical organization of information processing in the auditory system. While lower centres may be responsible for simple sensory feature detection, complex processing allowing the complete perception, integration and interpretation of complex stimuli occurs in the cortical regions of the brain. Woods (1989) also suggested that there may be separate selective attention mechanisms in different sensory modalities, and Woods *et al.* (1994) provided evidence that ERP components elicited by attention to different features of stimuli (e.g. frequency, location) had different scalp distributions consistent with generation in different cortical fields, although feature conjunction was found to occur before the analysis of individual features was complete. Recent animal research has demonstrated precise segregation of spatiotemporal firing along both contextual and behavioural dimensions in hippocampal neuronal ensembles, showing that conjunctions of task relevant features are represented effectively by ensembles of hippocampal neurons (Deadwyler & Hampson, 1995; Deadwyler *et al.*, 1996a).

The essence of the cortical model is that all auditory inputs undergo rapid, involuntary processing of their physical characteristics by a "permanent feature-detection system" (Näätänen, 1985, 1988, 1990). All physical features of stimuli, such as location, pitch, intensity and duration, are encoded in a passive neuronal trace. These passive neural representations may be responsible for involuntary attention switching which enables unattended stimuli to attain conscious processing momentarily, thus offering an explanation for the intrusion of irrelevant stimuli (as well as mismatch negativity, discussed below). Voluntary, effortful focusing of attention leads to the formation of a more permanent "attentional trace", a voluntarily maintained representation of the relevant stimulus characteristics. All other inputs are actively compared against this representation, and the duration of this matching process reflects the degree of similarity between the input and the attentional trace. Only those stimuli with a perfect match are selected for further processing, for updating and maintaining the attentional trace. These concepts are discussed further below, as indexed by various ERP components.

The prefrontal cortex is also an area known to be involved in attentional functions. Damage to the prefrontal area of the frontal lobe appears to cause attention related problems with ready formation of irrelevant associations and disturbances in the selectivity of action (Luria, 1966). Patients with frontal lobe lesions are often unable to suppress irrelevant information and have tendencies to perseverate, being unable to shift attention, but also having difficulties in focusing and sustaining attention (e.g. Damasio, 1979; Fuster, 1980). CBF increases in the region of the frontal lobe during auditory attention (e.g. Näätänen, 1987), consistent with evidence that the frontal lobes maintain and control the attentional trace. At least two ERP studies have reported dysfunction in selective attention and increased distractibility in patients with lesions of the dorsolateral prefrontal cortex (Knight *et al.*, 1981; Woods & Knight, 1986). Further ERP evidence of frontal activation is discussed below. The involvement of the anterior cingulate cortex in attentional processes was discussed in Chapter 2. It is unlikely, however, that selective attention can be localized to any one area, but most likely occurs as a result of numerous connections or networks in the brain (Mesulam, 1990).

Influenced by their observations of frontal lobe patients, Norman & Shallice (1980, 1986, but see 1980) formulated a model concerned primarily with the attentional control of action. This model proposed that most actions are controlled by schemata – collections of actions that given appropriate triggering are activated automatically. Conflicting schemata are avoided by a semi automatic conflict resolution system that rules according to priorities set by the supervisory attentional system (SAS), a limited capacity system of conscious attentional control. The SAS is called upon in tasks requiring planning and decision making, where novel or poorly learned sequences of acts are involved, in technically difficult or dangerous situations, or where a strong habitual response or temptation requires inhibiting. The SAS model explains that where two demanding tasks are performed simultaneously much of the coordination can be carried out through the low level conflict resolution procedures without overloading the SAS. When the SAS becomes overloaded by an excess number of incoming sources, errors occur (e.g. slips of action or of the tongue can occur because while the SAS is occupied with another task, various other automatic schema may be triggered). At slow rates the supervisor is able to perform effectively but its capacity to cope is overloaded at fast rates of incoming information or of responding. Baddeley (1986) equated the SAS with his concept of the central executive in working memory.

Recently, Houghton & Tipper (1994) advanced a neural network model of selective attention, formulated at cognitive, functional and neurophysiological levels which also emphasizes response activation, but in addition, the active inhibition of distracting information. Following from the theories and observations of Norman and Shallice, and the work of others such as Luria and Treisman, Houghton and Tipper acknowledged that attention must be considered in the global context of an organism's self organization of its goal directed behaviour. They suggested that schema based expectations facilitate the perception and comprehension of the environment without the need to focus attention serially on each object, and thus that a highly efficient parallel perceptual analysis takes place in familiar situations. Nevertheless, they proposed that internal representations of distractor objects are also required to achieve successful goal directed behaviour around a target object. Thus, "the role of attention . . . lies . . . in the linking of the appropriate action with the appropriate object in contexts which may afford an arbitrary number of such linkages, the great majority of which, at any time, will be disruptive to the organism's goal-seeking behaviour", and "selective attention acts to modulate . . . competition in favor of target objects" (Houghton & Tipper, 1994).

In contrast to the spotlight models of attention based on excitatory processes, Houghton and Tipper's model proposes a supplementary inhibitory component which acts to suppress competing information derived from the analysis of distractors. They argued that much neuropsychological evidence points to the role of areas of the prefrontal lobes in the direction and maintenance of attention, and to a strong inhibitory component in this function. They cited Fuster (1980), who had reviewed an extensive body of evidence on the subject and concluded that "the essential role of the orbitomedial prefrontal cortex in the suppression and control of interference . . . may be considered inhibitory and part of . . . the selective attention that the animal must direct and maintain for the proper conduct of behavioural sequence". They cited also the ERP research of Arnsten *et al.* (1983) who showed that naloxone improves selectivity by increasing the suppression of distractors rather than by changing the analysis of the attended targets. This naloxone induced facilitation of suppression of distracting stimuli was believed to occur in frontal cortex which is rich in naloxone binding sites.

Houghton and Tipper's model suggests that selective attention facilitates the maintenance of goal directed behaviour by "gating the flow of perceptual information into response systems (conceived to encompass both action and thought), emphasizing goal relevant information, and backgrounding irrelevant or contextual information". This involves the prefrontal lobes "gating the flow of activation from posterior (perceptual) systems through to frontal motor planning and execution systems" (Houghton & Tipper, 1994). Information from internally driven targets and externally driven perceptual object representations meets in a match/mismatch field that generates feedback signals leading to the foregrounding of objects which match the target specification. Objects which do not match the target specification are suppressed by inhibitory feedback mechanisms. The strength of specific inhibitory mechanisms is proposed to continually adapt to the strength of the to be ignored stimuli as a self regulating feedback loop. Their model may account for a variety of experimental phenomena that were unexplained by previous theories.

Event-related potential indices of selective attention

Event-related potentials or ERPs are scalp recorded electrical changes occurring in the brain in response to an event or stimulus. The procedure of recording ERPs is a sensitive technique which permits the simultaneous assessment of electrophysiology, cognition and behaviour and the detection of subtle dysfunction in specific stages of information processing. ERP techniques have become increasingly useful for the study of selective attention because of their ability to measure covert cognitive processes in the absence of any requirement that the subject attend or respond to stimuli, and because of their excellent temporal resolution (of the order of milliseconds) (Mangun & Hillyard, 1995; Rugg & Coles, 1995). In these factors alone ERP techniques can provide information otherwise unavailable from other behavioural or physiological methods (e.g. positron emission tomography (PET), functional magnetic resonance imaging (fMRI)). The functional significance of ERP effects and limitations on their interpretation are discussed by Rugg & Coles (1995); a complete understanding hinges upon a full integration of ERP research with research elucidating the neural bases of cognition. The problem of elucidating the functional significance of a physiological correlate of information processing is not unique to ERP data. Interpretation has been assisted by a vast amount of experimental and pharmacological manipulations, by source localization studies of ERP generators and by studies of clinical populations and patients who have suffered lesions (Rugg & Coles, 1995). Thus, progress on the fronts of identifying the cognitive correlates of ERPs and their neural origins is accelerating rapidly and ERP techniques have made significant contributions in a number of areas of cognitive enquiry (Rugg & Coles, 1995).

The procedure for generating ERPs is described in detail by Rugg & Coles (1995). Basically, this involves recording the electroencephalograph (EEG) while subjects are engaged in a cognitive task. Portions of the EEG, which are time locked to specific stimuli are extracted and averaged as depicted in Fig. 6.1. These represent the brain's response to an event or stimulus and are hence referred to as event-related potentials. As such, they are distinguished from the spontaneous potentials that make up the ongoing EEG in the absence of stimulation, thought to reflect the global state of the subject (e.g. the generalized psychological states of arousal or drowsiness). ERPs, on the other hand are evoked by, and hence time locked to, specific discrete environmental events open to a vast array of experimental manipulation. By averaging the response to repeated presentations of stimuli of a certain type, the background noise of the ongoing EEG is diminished while the constant ERP response to that stimulus type becomes increasingly distinct.

The typical ERP consists of a series of peaks and troughs, positive and negative deflections (see Figure 6.1), which reflect the synchronous activity of large neuronal populations, such as a localized area of cerebral cortex or thalamus, or specific auditory nuclei in the brainstem. What are referred to as ERP "components" can only be inferred from the results of experimental manipulation and measurement of the resultant ERP deflections (Näätänen & Picton, 1987). Thus, an ERP component constitutes a cerebral event reflecting a distinct cognitive process. While much research is

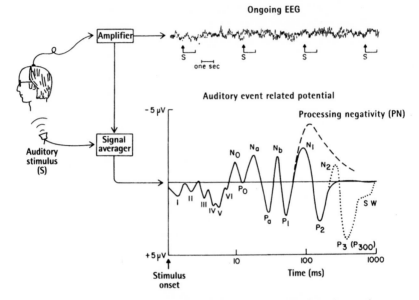

Figure 6.1 An idealized auditory ERP waveform depicting the process of recording the EEG and averaging around a stimulus, and the major early brainstem, middle latency and late "endogenous" components. (Adapted from Hillyard, S.A. & Kutas, M., 1983. Reprinted by permission of Annual Reviews Inc.)

being conducted into the neural generators of the various ERP components, the actual neural source of the component need not be the defining criterion for the differentiation of components, but rather the cognitive process itself (Donchin *et al.*, 1978; see also Rugg & Coles, 1995).

The focus of current ERP and cognitive research has been to identify ERP components as markers of specific stages of information processing. The amplitude and latency of ERP components are thought to reflect the nature, timing and duration of various cognitive processes. These are indexed by the "endogenous" components of the ERP waveform, as opposed to the early obligatory "exogenous" components. Rather than a strict dichotomy, this may be conceived of as "an exogenous-endogenous *dimension* that is coextensive with time. Thus, those ERP components that occur within the first 100 ms of stimulus presentation tend to be more exogenous, while those occurring later tend to be more endogenous" (Rugg & Coles, 1995), and thus tend to occur in order of increasing sensitivity to cognitive factors.

Exogenous components were conceived of as being evoked by factors extrinsic to the nervous system, sensitive to variations in physical stimulus characteristics regardless of their processing demands or task relevance. They have, however, been shown to be modifiable by cognitive manipulations (Rugg & Coles, 1995). They begin shortly after stimulus onset and last for up to the first 250 ms post-stimulus, varying in amplitude and latency according to the physical characteristics of stimuli, and varying across the scalp according to stimulus modality. They are comprised of early, middle and late components.

Early brainstem potentials occur within the first 10 ms post-stimulus and reflect the neural activity of auditory nuclei in the cochlea and brainstem. The middle latency thalamic potentials are evident between 10 and 50 ms post-stimulus and reflect the procession of auditory information through to the auditory cortex. Following the animal research of Hernández-Peón and colleagues (1956; 1966), much human research has been directed toward attempting to discover early signs of selective attention in early brainstem potentials, and where evidence has been demonstrated, this has proved impossible to replicate (e.g. Lukas, 1980, 1981 vs Hirschhorn & Michie, 1991). Evidence has emerged for an attention effect occurring in the mid-latency range of between 20 and 50 ms post-stimulus (Woldorff & Hillyard, 1991), thus providing compelling evidence for early selection models of attention, but this "P20-50 effect" was found to be generated in the auditory cortex (Woldorff *et al.*, 1993) .

While early and middle latency components are of very low amplitude, they are closely followed by large amplitude waves named according to their polarity and sequence: the P1-N1-P2 complex refers respectively to the first large positive wave occurring around 50 ms post-stimulus (also known as P50), the first large negative wave occurring around 100 ms post-stimulus (also known as N100), and the second large positive wave occurring around 200 ms post-stimulus. While these components will be elicited by stimuli in a passive task, in an active cognitive task these exogenous waves are overlapped by the appearance of endogenous components, signalling the beginnings of conscious effortful attentional processing.

P1 (or P50) has been implicated in the gating or inflow control of sensory information. A number of psychiatric patient populations, including schizophrenics, have shown increases in the amplitude of P1 in conditioning test paradigms, reflecting diminished gating (e.g. Waldo *et al.*, 1992). The mechanism responsible for sensory gating has been suggested to interact with the catecholaminergic system (Adler *et al.*, 1982).

The N1 component is viewed as a true onset response generated by cerebral systems responding specifically to stimulus onset (Näätänen &

Picton, 1987). N1 is thought to be made up of several components, each with different generators within the brain but all sensitive in amplitude and latency to the registration of various stimulus parameters. Its scalp distribution is modality specific and in the auditory modality N1 is larger in the hemisphere contralateral to the ear of stimulation. The P2 wave follows N1, and while it may have different neural generators, it appears to be similar to N1 in its sensitivity to various stimulus characteristics.

Numerous endogenous ERP components may be elicited in a variety of cognitive tasks, representing a wealth of cognitive operations. Only those components of relevance to auditory selective attention will be discussed here. Just as the so called exogenous components have been shown to be affected by cognitive factors, so too have the later endogenous components been shown to be influenced by the physical attributes of task parameters (Rugg & Coles, 1995).

N2

The N2 is the second major negative component peaking after stimulus onset. It is an endogenous component best seen when an occasional stimulus is either omitted from a train of stimuli delivered at a constant rate, or replaced by a physically deviant stimulus (Squires *et al.*, 1975; Näätänen, 1982). It is closely coupled with the P300 and particularly with P3a (see below) (Squires *et al.*, 1975; Picton & Stuss, 1980), reflecting the operation of a cerebral "mismatch detector" engaged by stimulus deviance (Snyder & Hillyard, 1976). Its morphology and topography were found to differ as a function of experimental manipulation, which suggests that the N2 is not a single entity but rather a number of different components that are active in the N2 range (Näätänen & Gaillard, 1983). Näätänen and Picton (1986) were able to identify eight N2 subcomponents; however, the two most well recognized are the mismatch negativity (MMN) and the N2b.

The MMN is a negative component which can overlap the N1 and P2 components and is observed when stimulus deviance is defined by changes in pitch, intensity, duration, spatial location and phonemic change (Näätänen, 1990). The larger the difference between the deviants and standards, the larger the MMN and the earlier it is elicited. MMN is best observed under nonattend conditions when subjects are asked to ignore auditory stimuli and perform a distractor task. As such it is considered to index an automatic process independent of attention, being generated by a cerebral process sensitive to stimulus change which compares the sensory input from a deviant stimulus to a stored neuronal representation of the physical features of previous standard stimuli (Näätänen, 1985; Alho *et al.*, 1989). It is argued that it serves the biologically vital function of causing attention to switch towards changes in unattended auditory input (Näätänen, 1990). The MMN has a fronto-central distribution and is larger at temporal than midline sites. There is continuing debate about whether the MMN is or is not enhanced by overt attention (Woldorff *et al.*, 1991; Alho *et al.*, 1992).

The other component in the N2 range is the N2b which is elicited under conditions of attention to deviants, being superimposed on the MMN. It has a longer latency than the MMN (approximately 220 ms), a centro-parietal distribution, is modality nonspecific and is closely coupled with P3a (Squires *et al.*, 1975; Picton & Stuss, 1980; Näätänen & Gaillard, 1983) reflecting the beginnings of cognitive stimulus evaluation, target selection and decision making processes. Some have suggested that the N2 may actually be a better index of decision processes than the later P300 wave (discussed below) (Ritter *et al.*, 1979).

Processing negativity (PN)

This is the ERP component most specifically related to selective attention. ERP studies of selective attention have primarily utilized the "cocktail party" paradigm, a version of the dichotic listening task described above, in which multiple channels of multidimensional auditory stimuli are presented to the subject at rapid rates. While the subject's task is to attend to one channel only, ERPs elicited by stimuli from every channel are recorded and differences between attended channel ERPs and unattended channel ERPs constitute the attention effect. This effect of attention is seen as a broad negativity in the ERP waveform, termed "processing negativity" (Näätänen, 1982; Hansen & Hillyard, 1983).

The early onset of PN (e.g. 60–80 ms post-stimulus) was the most convincing source of evidence for early selection in the auditory system. Originally this negativity was interpreted as an enhancement of N1 amplitude in attended as opposed to unattended stimuli (Hillyard *et al.*, 1973), but later studies isolated a separate endogenous negative component, PN, superimposed upon the N1 wave (Näätänen & Michie, 1979; Näätänen, 1982). The extent to which N1 itself is actually modulated by attention is still debated and under active investigation (Näätänen, 1992; Mangun & Hillyard, 1995). PN is elicited by all stimuli sharing the more salient properties of the relevant stimulus, generated when selective attention is directed toward the relevant sensory attributes of the passive neuronal trace. PN is argued to be the best index of the more permanent attentional trace (Näätänen, 1990).

PN may be clearly seen in the ERP waveform as a negativity in the trace to attended stimuli compared to unattended stimuli (see Figure 6.1), or it may be observed in difference waveforms (Nd) created by subtracting the unattended trace from the attended. This method has demonstrated two overlapping components: early PN (or Nd) which is maximal over fronto-central areas and reflects the selection of relevant from irrelevant sources of information by a matching process between the stimulus and the attentional trace, and a more prolonged negativity in the attended ERP, termed late PN (or Nd), which has a much more frontal distribution (Hansen & Hillyard, 1980; Näätänen, 1982; Woods, 1989). This late frontal component of processing negativity most likely reflects the maintenance and rehearsal of the attentional trace (Näätänen, 1982). PN may also be present in unattended ERPs if the discrimination is difficult, ie. a small physical separation between attended and unattended stimuli, although evidence is accumulating for a third component contributing to Nd: a positivity in the unattended ERP starting at about 170 ms (Alho *et al.*, 1987; Michie *et al.*, 1990a, 1993). This positivity may reflect active inhibitory processing of the irrelevant stimuli; an active suppression of processing when the irrelevant stimulus has been found to be incompatible with the attentional trace (Alho *et al.*, 1987; Michie *et al.*, 1993).

P300

If a conscious decision about the significance of a stimulus has to be made, or a response to a particular stimulus in the attended channel is required, the ERP waveform to that stimulus will show a large positive component, generally referred to as the P300 complex. P300 is one of the most researched, most easily elicited and largest of the endogenous ERP components (see Figure 6.1), but many years of research have failed to determine precisely its functional role (Picton, 1992; Rugg & Coles, 1995). P300 is elicited by task relevant, infrequently occurring target stimuli in the attended channel (Donchin, 1981; Pritchard, 1981). It occurs maximally at parietal scalp sites with a peak latency of 300–900 ms depending on task difficulty among other parameters (Rugg & Coles, 1995). There is evidence that P300 amplitude reflects the allocation of attentional resources for stimulus evaluation processes, inclusive of context or memory updating, while its latency is a sensitive index of stimulus evaluation time (Isreal *et al.*, 1980; Pritchard, 1981; Donchin & Coles, 1988). This component, now recognized as the P3b, is distinguished from the smaller, more fronto-central P3a which is elicited by unattended, task irrelevant and intermittent novel stimuli, reflecting the degree of contrast with frequently occurring stimuli and hence associated with the N2b component (Squires *et al.*, 1975, 1977; Näätänen & Gaillard, 1983). Recent evidence suggests that there may be multiple neural generators of the P300 component distributed throughout the brain (Johnson, 1993).

Contingent negative variation (CNV)

In paired stimulus paradigms where one stimulus acts as a warning signal that the other will soon follow, a slow negativity develops in the ERP during the interval between the two stimuli, reaching a maximal amplitude just prior to the presentation of the second stimulus. This anticipatory component is termed contingent negative variation or CNV (Walter *et al.*, 1964). It has variously been interpreted as a sign of expectancy, intention to act, attention and arousal (e.g. Tecce, 1972). Increased attention generally results in increased CNV amplitude, but general tonic arousal leads to CNV decrement. Tecce & Cole (1974) showed that reports of alertness following amphetamine administration correlated with larger CNV, while paradoxical drowsiness was associated with CNV reduction. A separate component nevertheless closely related to CNV is the post-imperative negative variation (PINV). This is a continuation of the CNV beyond the point of normal resolution, which has been observed in schizophrenics (Timsit-Berthier *et al.*, 1984), but also in normal subjects only when the second stimulus in the pairing is uncontrollable by the subject (e.g. when the subject is not able to terminate it by a motor response).

It is these cognitive or endogenous ERP components discussed above, primarily processing negativity and P300, that are of particular interest for the purposes of the research to be described in Part 2 of this book. The Hansen & Hillyard (1983) multidimensional auditory selective attention paradigm was selected for the study of selective attention processes in long-term cannabis users. There exists a wealth of normative data on the ERP patterns elicited by this paradigm, and it has been used to investigate information processing among other groups suspected of deficient attentional mechanisms, for example schizophrenics (Michie *et al.*, 1990b; Ward *et al.*, 1991). The paradigm has proved useful in the study of hierarchical models of information processing by manipulating the difficulty of discrimination of each dimension (Mangun & Hillyard, 1995), and has been extended to examine the processing of auditory features and their conjunctions (Woods *et al.*, 1994).

For the series of studies to be described herein, the version of the paradigm used was that where stimulus duration was the most difficult discrimination, followed by pitch and then location. In this paradigm, the subject's task is to selectively attend to a particular combination of these dimensions (e.g. right ear, high pitch) and to detection infrequent long duration target tones. The most efficient strategy in performing this task, is one where the subject rapidly rejects half the stimuli from further analysis on the basis of location, continues to process those stimuli entering the relevant attended ear and rejects half of those on the basis of pitch, before finally deciding whether the stimulus is of long or short duration. This strategy enables the formation of the attentional trace to the frequent short duration tones of relevant pitch in the attended ear, evidenced by PN in the ERP waveform to these tones. Hierarchical models predict that tones occurring in the unattended ear should be rejected rapidly, evidenced by a positive shift in the ERP following the N1 peak, whereas tones of irrelevant pitch in the attended ear would be processed for a little longer but rejected soon after with a later positive shift in the ERP waveform. Use of this paradigm would determine whether chronic cannabis users engage in a less efficient mode of information processing than do controls.

It was hypothesized that long-term cannabis users may adopt a less efficient mode of information processing than controls and show evidence of intrusion of irrelevant information in their ERP waveforms. Particularly strong evidence of this would be a lack of separation between relevant and irrelevant pitch ERPs to tones in the attended ear, with inappropriately large PN to the pitch irrelevant tones. Evidence of PN to tones in the unattended ear, with a large separation between relevant and irrelevant pitch ERPs, would suggest engagement in exhaustive analysis of independent stimulus dimensions.

As P300 reflects various processes associated with evaluating a stimulus, including the allocation of attentional resources, it was hypothesized that P300 may be delayed or reduced in amplitude in cannabis users compared to controls. P300 amplitude has consistently been found to be reduced in schizophrenics (Pfefferbaum *et al.*, 1984, 1989; Pritchard, 1986; Michie *et al.*, 1990b; Ward *et al.*, 1991; Ford *et al.*, 1994; Souza *et al.*, 1995) among other psychiatric groups (Pfefferbaum *et al.*, 1984; O'Connor *et al.*, 1994) and alcoholics and children of alcoholics (Porjesz & Begleiter, 1987; Williams, 1987; O'Connor *et al.*, 1994; Vanderstelt *et al.*, 1994). P300 amplitude has also been found to correlate with ratings of clinical symptoms of schizophrenia (Pfefferbaum *et al.*, 1989; Shenton *et al.*, 1989; Ward *et al.*, 1991) and with performance on perceptual-motor tests in alcoholics and controls (Parsons *et al.*, 1990).

Aside from these investigations of P300 amplitude, other ERP indices of altered cognitive functioning have been examined in a variety of clinical groups. Examples include P300 latency in schizophrenia and bipolar affective disorder (Souza *et al.*, 1995), N2 or MMN in schizophrenia (Salisbury *et al.*, 1994; Catts *et al.*, 1995), various ERP components in distinguishing schizophrenia subtypes (John *et al.*, 1994), P2 as a predictor of response to antidepressants in major depressive disorder (Paige *et al.*, 1994), PN and P300 in obsessive-compulsive disorder (Towey *et al.*, 1994), N1 and P2 auditory evoked potentials and antisocial tendencies in alcoholism (Hegerl *et al.*, 1995), ERP indices of memory functioning in social drinkers (Fox *et al.*, 1995). The use of ERPs as a tool in the study of the cognitive effects of cannabis has been virtually nonexistent.

Cannabis and event-related potentials

Most of the studies investigating the electrophysiological effects of cannabis were carried out in the 1970s, examining the EEG and producing equivocal results. These EEG studies have been reviewed in Chapter 4. Very few studies have investigated the effects of cannabis upon ERPs; most have been acute studies and none has investigated the processes of selective attention. The small literature on cannabis and ERPs is briefly reviewed here.

A number of the early EEG studies included a cursory examination of evoked responses without adequate description of how these were evoked or what components were measured. Generally, evoked responses are a reflection of exogenous components only, being passively elicited by the presentation of auditory or visual stimuli in the absence of any cognitive task demands. The effect of cannabis on evoked potentials has also been variable.

Rodin *et al.* (1970) found no consistent changes in auditory (AEP), visual (VEP) or somatosensory evoked potentials (SEP) during an induced "social high". Low *et al.* (1973) found no effect of low or high dose THC on VEP peak amplitude or latency. Stefanis *et al.* (1977) found no latency changes but reported an increased N150 peak amplitude after administering various doses of hashish to their Greek sample of chronic hashish smokers. Tinklenberg (1972) found an increase in amplitude of the N200 and P280 components of the VEP, and some prolongation of latency, following low dose THC, and Tassinari *et al.* (1974) reported similar increases in amplitude of the late VEP components. Lewis *et al.* (1973) reported significant latency prolongation of almost all VEP peaks with high dose THC, with a similar trend for low dose THC and a trend toward SEP peak latency prolongation. Additionally they reported a decrease in VEP N75-P100 peak amplitude at both high and low doses and a significant SEP N130-P200 amplitude reduction. These effects were evident in occasional and frequent cannabis users alike. Lewis *et al.* (1973) interpreted the prominence of evoked potential latency prolongation being due to an increase in "the threshold of cortical and subcortical neurons or neural networks involved in producing the evoked response" and claimed that there was no evidence of an excitatory action of THC on the central nervous system.

Two studies used a passive attention task with frequent and infrequent tone bursts which subjects were instructed to ignore. Roth *et al.* (1973) reported decreased P2 amplitude to frequent and infrequent stimuli following cannabis, but no effect on N1 amplitude and no latency differences. There was suggestive evidence for a reduction in P300 amplitude to the infrequent stimulus. Roth and colleagues interpreted their findings as indicating that subjects under the influence of cannabis may have an increased ability to "tune out" the outside world, substantiated by users' claims of dreamlike states with reduced attention to the environment, but the authors cautioned that this should not be interpreted as an enhanced ability to selectively ignore irrelevant stimuli. However, Kopell *et al.* (1978) used a similar paradigm but found neither amplitude nor latency changes.

Earlier, Kopell *et al.* (1972) had reported an enhancement of CNV with the oral administration of low dose THC, but not high dose. They interpreted this as an enhanced ability of mildly intoxicated subjects to selectively attend and suggested that this may be due to better exclusion of miscellaneous irrelevant stimuli while anticipating a relevant stimulus. Low *et al.* (1973) replicated these findings of increased CNV amplitude with low dose smoked THC using a similar simple reaction time task to that used by Kopell and colleagues, but they also employed a difficult discrimination task and found the high dose actually decreased CNV amplitude in this task. Both low and high doses increased PINV. Similarly, Braden, Stillman and Wyatt (1974) demonstrated no overall effect of moderate dose smoked THC on CNV amplitude in the simple reaction time task, but found that subjects who reported experiencing a below average "high" showed CNV amplitude increase, while those reporting above average "high" showed CNV amplitude decrease. They proposed that the relation between CNV amplitude and THC dose is probably in the form of an inverted U, suggesting possible enhancement of attentive mechanisms at low doses but impaired attentional functioning with high doses. They also proposed that since cannabis is often demonstrated to slow reaction time, the increase in CNV amplitude may be "due to a compensatory effort to concentrate". At higher doses "with more complete impairment of task orientation, this compensatory effort might not be possible". Alternately, they proposed that low dose cannabis might serve to make a dull task more interesting, which is not incompatible with greater difficulty in concentration.

Herning *et al.* (1979) studied 27 male regular users, aged 21–31 years, over a 3–4 week period as inpatients receiving various daily doses of THC. Auditory ERPs and CNV were recorded during a series of behavioural tasks of varying complexity pre-drug treatment, early and late during the inpatient treatment, and post-treatment. The auditory N1 component was significantly depressed in the high dose group during the first few days of treatment but resolved over time, remaining depressed only during the most demanding behavioural tasks. The CNV was depressed during all tasks for high and low dose groups early in treatment, but once again mostly resolved, remaining only in the high dose group during the most difficult task. These results suggest the development of tolerance to these effects. The authors suggested, however, that these changes may persist with high doses, and were more likely to manifest during complex stimulus processing tasks. The changes were hypothesized to be related to different aspects of a common attentional alteration during stimulus processing.

In one of the few studies to directly compare the effects of cannabis and alcohol on ERPs, Roth *et al.* (1977) incorporated a complex memory search task based on the Sternberg paradigm which presented 1–4 digits, and then a warning tone followed by a single digit probe. They found no drug effects on the amplitude or latency of auditory N1 or P2 to the warning tone, but P300 amplitude to the probe was reduced by both cannabis and alcohol. CNV amplitude between the warning tone and test digit showed no drug effects, but the latency of resolution of the CNV was longer under cannabis than alcohol or placebo and reaction time was significantly increased by cannabis alone.

The overall effects of acute administration on human evoked potentials are difficult to summarise due to the lack of consistency in routes of administration, doses given, tasks employed and indeed their variable results. Nevertheless, it can be surmised that cannabis may affect either the latency or amplitude or both of the evoked potential in an adverse manner. There has been insufficient research into the effects of cannabis on ERPs in well designed studies employing sensitive tasks that tap quite specific cognitive functions.

Recently, a series of evoked potential and ERP studies of chronic cannabis users have been reported from the same team, mostly in abstract form. Struve & Straumanis (1990) briefly mentioned the results of their pilot study of chronic cannabis users, abstinent for 5–7 days prior to testing, which found decreased VEP P100 amplitude, increased SEP N18-P30 amplitude and smaller and later P300 in an auditory oddball discrimination task. A pilot study of cannabis using psychiatric patients found longer latency and smaller amplitude auditory P300 than in cannabis naive psychiatric patients or controls (Straumanis *et al.*, 1991). The same study reported no difference in brainstem auditory evoked responses (BAER) between cannabis using and nonusing psychiatric patients, and a further study confirmed that any differences in BAER alterations were related more to psychiatric status and not marijuana or polydrug use (Patrick & Struve, 1994). Straumanis *et al.* (1993) found few differences in AEP, VEP or SEP components between long-term cannabis users (> 15 years), moderate users (3–6 years) and controls, but suggested a reduction of P300 amplitude with cannabis use. A full paper from this team described the results of simple auditory and visual oddball discrimination tasks (Patrick *et al.*, 1995) which negated their previous findings with psychiatric patients. Using particularly stringent inclusion/exclusion criteria for both the cannabis users and controls, no differences were found between groups for P300 latency, but apparently smaller P300 amplitudes in users were found not to be significant when groups were equated for age. The authors acknowledged that the simple nature of their task may have lead to the lack of differences between groups and that a more complex task may be required to detect any deficits associated with the long-term use of cannabis. This group has previously reported replicable topographic quantitative EEG correlates of daily cannabis use (see Chapter 4; Struve *et al.*, 1993, 1994).

Clearly, there is a need for further research into the long-term effects, and indeed the acute effects, of cannabis on human ERPs, particularly now that their interpretation is enhanced by more modern cognitive theories. For the purposes of the investigation described in Part 2 of this book, it was considered of greater urgency to investigate long-term cognitive effects than to contribute to the labyrinth of acute studies.

Part 2

Research

7

An event-related potential study of attentional processes in long-term cannabis users

Studies prior to the 1990s provided little information as to the nature of any specific deficits associated with the long-term use of cannabis, although attentional mechanisms were often implicated. As argued in Chapter 5, one reason for the equivocal nature of results from past studies may be that the tests used were insufficiently sensitive to detect subtle dysfunction of specific cognitive processes. There has been relatively little use of quantitative measures derived from experimental cognitive psychology in any studies of chronic drug-related deficits.

The advent of brain event-related potential (ERP) recording technology allowed for the simultaneous assessment of electrophysiology, cognition and behaviour and the detection of subtle dysfunction in specific stages of information processing. The interpretation of ERP components is based on modern theories of cognition and information processing. The series of studies described here employed these techniques to address the question of the existence and nature of attentional deficits in long-term cannabis users.

The paradigm selected to assess the efficiency of attentional mechanisms was a complex multidimensional auditory selective attention task based on that developed by Hansen & Hillyard (1983). This task was selected for two reasons. First, because of the inherent complexity of the task. An in depth examination of the literature suggested that impairments would most likely be detected only in cognitively demanding tasks involving interference. Second, because there exists a wealth of normative data on the ERP patterns elicited by this paradigm, as well as data from a number of other clinical groups suspected of deficient attentional mechanisms, for example schizophrenics (Michie *et al.*, 1990b; Ward *et al.*, 1991). The precise nature of the task is described in detail below.

Before proceeding with this complex task, it was considered useful to conduct a preliminary study measuring ERPs in cannabis users and controls in a standard "oddball" paradigm. The oddball paradigm is a discrimination task in which a rare target must be detected from a background of frequently occurring stimuli (e.g. tone pips). Correct identification of a target tone reliably elicits the P300 component of the auditory ERP. While it was predicted that use of a cognitively demanding task was required to evince any deficits associated with cannabis use, the simple oddball task was an appropriate starting point for measurement of the most basic electrophysiological indices of attention, which at the time of commencement of this research had not previously been investigated in this population. (Recently Patrick *et al.* (1995) have reported null findings using an easy version of this task; see Chapter 6.) This study will not be reported in full here but brief results are outlined below.

Two conditions were utilized, manipulating the difficulty of the auditory discrimination (1000 and 2000 Hz vs 1000 and 1100 Hz tones) and the results supported the hypothesis that any differences between cannabis users and controls are more likely to be detected in difficult and demanding tasks. Further, the results were suggestive of functional and electrophysiological differences between users and controls in frontal regions of the brain. In cannabis users, P300 peak amplitude was markedly reduced at frontal and central sites in the difficult condition compared to the easy condition ($p < 0.003$). Users showed an uncharacteristically large frontal P300 component in the easy condition. N2 peaked significantly later in the difficult condition in users compared to controls ($p < 0.005$), which suggests a possible delay in stimulus evaluation time with more difficult stimulus discriminations, although P300 was not significantly delayed in users ($p > 0.2$). Interestingly, N2 latency has been reported to increase as a function of age (Iragui *et al.*, 1993) and the same authors reported in their auditory oddball paradigm that aging is also associated with greater anterior positivity, in terms of larger frontal P300 components. Zeef & Kok (1993) and Friedman *et al.* (1993) have also demonstrated that the scalp distribution of P300 changes with age to a more frontal orientation. The latter authors point out that the shift to a more anterior distribution of P300 is one of the most robust age related findings in the ERP literature, and is consistent with a change in frontal lobe activity with increasing age. It is possible that the effects observed here on N2 latency and the large frontal P300 component in cannabis users may reflect accelerated aging in terms of cognitive decline. This hypothesis is in accord with the studies of Landfield *et al.* (1988, 1993) which examined the interactions between cannabinoids and the glucocorticoid system in the brain and suggested that cannabinoids may accelerate brain aging (see Chapter 4). The findings of altered N2 and P3 components were suggestive of some dysfunction in stimulus evaluation strategies and allocation of attentional resources, evident primarily in the region of the frontal cortex. It has recently been suggested that there may be multiple neural generators of the P300 component distributed throughout the brain (Johnson, 1993), and it is possible that cannabinoids may selectively disrupt neural sources in the frontal lobes.

The small sample size of this preliminary study ($n = 8$ for each of cannabis users and controls) dictates caution in the interpretation of results and formulation of speculative hypotheses. The lack of consistency between our study and that reported by Patrick *et al.* (1995) may variously be due to our smaller sample, our use of a substantially more difficult discrimination, our examination of ERPs to correctly detected targets (we used a button press while Patrick *et al.* required subjects merely to count targets) and our examination of frontal sites. Our results provided some clues as to possible deficits although the simple nature of this task may not permit the detection of any cognitive dysfunction. The auditory oddball task does not draw heavily upon attentional resources (ie. is not attentionally demanding); even in the difficult discrimination condition it required little more than simply responding to a deviant stimulus. The complex selective attention task was expected to engage attentional resources more fully, tapping specifically the ability to selectively attend to task relevant stimuli while suppressing task irrelevant information.

Experiment 1: effects of long-term cannabis use on ERPs recorded during an auditory selective attention paradigm

As stated above, in this experiment ERPs were recorded during a complex multidimensional auditory selective attention task based on a paradigm developed by Hansen & Hillyard (1983). This task involved the presentation of a random series of tone pips which varied on the dimensions of location, pitch and duration. Subjects were required to attend to tones of a particular location and pitch and to respond to infrequent target tones of slightly longer duration than the short duration background standards. The paradigm is useful for studying hierarchical modes of information processing by manipulating the difficulty of discrimination of each dimension. In this case, the duration discrimination was the most difficult, followed by pitch and then location. This enables the subject, whose task is to selectively attend to a particular combination of these dimensions, rapidly to reject half of the stimuli from further analysis on the basis of location.

Use of this paradigm would determine whether chronic cannabis users engage in a less efficient mode of information processing than do controls, and whether their ability to selectively attend and ignore irrelevant information is compromised. Processing negativity (PN) and P300 were the two components of particular relevance in this study.

Method

Subjects

For this and all experiments reported here, cannabis users and controls were recruited from university campuses and from the general community by advertising and all were paid for their participation. Ethnicity was not specifically determined but the great majority were white Caucasian and of Australian nationality. Subjects were initially screened in a telephone interview. The criterion for inclusion in the user group was a minimum of 3 years of regular use of cannabis. This was defined as using cannabis at least twice a week on average over the past 3 years. Subjects were asked specific questions relating to their general health (see Appendix A) and any respondents with a history of fits, febrile, neurological or psychiatric illnesses, multiple concussion or periods of unconsciousness were excluded from testing.

Subjects on any prescribed medication other than antibiotics were excluded from the sample. Subjects were screened for alcohol consumption with the following criteria for inclusion in the sample: less than 28 standard drinks per week on average for males and less than 14 for females, based on the National Health and Medical Research Council (1986) guidelines for levels of "safe" drinking. A standard drink in Australia contains 10 g of absolute ethanol. Further criteria for inclusion were no more than 1 month of continuous drinking above these levels in the past 3 years and no more than 6 months ever of drinking above these levels. Subjects were screened for other drug use and rejected on the basis of a history of regular use of any drug other than cannabis ("regular" defined as greater than or equal to once a month) or any subject having used any drug other than cannabis in the month prior to testing.

Ten cannabis users met the strict criteria for inclusion in this study, but one was unable to do the difficult selective attention task. Hence, the final sample in this experiment consisted of six male and three female cannabis users, aged 19–40 years (mean 29.4 years, s.d. = 8.5). These were matched on age (to within 2 years), sex and years of education with nine nonuser controls, aged 21–41 years (mean 29.5 years, s.d. = 7.8). The average number of standard drinks per week consumed by the user group was 11.4 (s.d. = 9.4) and 5.7 (s.d. = 5.7) by the control group. Alcohol consumption in the two groups was not significantly different (F(1,16) = 2.49, $p > 0.1$). (Any possible contributory effects of alcohol were examined in Experiment 2 reported in Chapter 8.)

The National Adult Reading Test (NART) (Nelson, 1982) was used as a measure of premorbid IQ. Cannabis users and controls did not differ in this regard (NART correct scores: users 39.9 (s.d. = 5.6) = Full Scale IQ 119.6; controls 39.6 (s.d. = 3.9) = Full Scale IQ 119.4; $p > 0.7$). All subjects had completed 13 years of school education and at least 1 year at tertiary level.

The mean years of cannabis use in the user group was 11.2 years (s.d. = 6.98, range 3–20 years) and the average level of use was 4.77 days per week (s.d. = 1.85, range twice/week to daily use). The mean weekly consumption was 766 mg THC (s.d. = 859, range 30–2400 mg/week), calculated as 15 mg THC per average cannabis cigarette. The longest period of abstinence from cannabis in the past 3 years ranged from 3 to 4 days to 3 months, mean 42 days (s.d. = 27.8). Of the controls, two had never tried cannabis, three had tried it once or twice and the remainder had used cannabis occasionally at parties between 3 and 7 years ago with the most experienced control having used 12 times in his entire life.

Subjects were instructed to abstain from cannabis and alcohol for at least 12 hours prior to testing. The day before the test session subjects were telephoned and reminded of these instructions and requested to provide a urine sample prior to going to bed. All subjects complied with this request.

Stimuli

Stimuli consisted of sequences of tone pips delivered randomly to the left or right ear via stereophonic headphones (TDH 49) at an intensity of 80 dB SPL. The tones varied in location (left ear/right ear), pitch (high/low) and duration (long/short). Half the tone pips presented to each ear were 1047 Hz and the remainder were of a higher pitch at 1319 Hz (representing C6 and E6 on the musical scale). Tones at each ear/pitch combination occurred with equal probability ($p = 0.25$). Within each ear/pitch combination, 19% of the stimuli were 51 ms in duration (the standards) and 6% were 102 ms (the targets), both having a 10 ms rise and fall time. The stimuli were presented as a random sequence lasting 160 seconds per run with a stimulus onset asynchrony (SOA) of 200 to 500 ms. All aspects of stimulus delivery and randomization were under computer control

(Data General Nova 4-C), the only constraint placed on the randomization procedure being that two target stimuli of the same type could not occur consecutively.

Event-related potential recording

Seven channels of electrophysiological data, six EEG (electroencephalogram) and one EOG (electrooculogram), were recorded using an electrode cap (Electro-cap International) and tin electrodes, respectively. The data were recorded using a Beckman Accutrace EEG machine with a time constant of 5 seconds and high frequency cut off of 30 Hz (3 dB down). Scalp electrodes were located over six lateral sites, F3, F4, C3, C4, P3 and P4. The EOG channel monitored vertical and horizontal eye movement via electrodes taped above and on the outer canthus of the left eye. All scalp electrodes were referred to linked earlobes. A light emitting diode 1 m away from the subject at eye level was used as a fixation point. The ground electrode was located on the forehead. EEG and EOG channels were continuously digitised at 5.76 ms/point (175 Hz) for the duration of a run and stored on disk with stimulus and response markers for later analysis. Stimulus presentation and data acquisition were controlled by a Data General NOVA 4-C computer.

Procedure

On arrival at the laboratory, subjects deposited their urine sample from the previous evening in a freezer. They were requested to provide a second urine sample sometime during the test session. Urine samples were subsequently analysed to confirm that the subject was not in an acutely intoxicated state during testing. The criterion on which this assertion was based was that the THC levels detected in the second sample were lower than those detected in the first. This ensured that no cannabis had been consumed during the time between provision of the two samples (presumably at least 12 hours).

Subjects participated in a single 3 hour test session. They were interviewed about their general health and detailed drug history according to a structured questionnaire (see Appendix) and they completed a number of other questionnaires designed to assess various aspects of anxiety and other psychopathologies. The results of these assessments are discussed in Chapter 11.

Subjects were tested for normal hearing by standard audiometric assessment. They sat in an armchair in a darkened, sound reduced room adjacent to the laboratory. The response button was mounted on the arm of the chair and they were instructed to use their index finger to depress the button. Subjects were given training on the selective attention task until they achieved the criterion level of performance of 50% hits and no more than 25% of responses being false alarms. This was generally achieved after two practice runs of 160 seconds each for both users and controls. The electrodes were then attached and the recording session commenced.

Subjects were instructed to attend to a particular location and pitch, and to respond as rapidly as possible to the long duration tones by pressing the response button mounted on the arm of the chair. There were four attention conditions: respond to left low long, left high long, right low long or right high long. Each subject completed two runs of each attention condition, one with a right hand response and one with a left hand response. The order of attention conditions and responding hand was randomised among subjects and counterbalanced across groups.

Data analysis

Button press responses were classified as correct detections or "hits" if they occurred within a 200–1200 ms response window after an attended target stimulus. Reaction time was measured as the latency in ms of the button press from the onset of the attended target. An attended target not followed by a response within the response window was regarded as an error of omission or "miss". Button presses at other times were regarded as errors of commission or "false alarms". The number of hits as a ratio of the number of attended targets provided an estimate of the hit rate, while the false alarm rate was calculated as a ratio of the total number of nontargets.

The digitised EEG data with stimulus and response markers were processed and analysed on a VAX11/780 using a program which extracted overlapping epochs of 1050 ms including a 150 ms prestimulus baseline. All epochs containing EOG artefact greater than 64 μV were rejected prior to averaging. Separate averages were created for hits and misses, and for the seven different nontarget stimuli, excluding those which were followed by a false alarm response. Averages to the same stimulus type were summed over runs with left and right hand responses. All amplitude measures were made relative to a 150 ms prestimulus baseline. Latency measures were relative to stimulus onset. The data were analysed using BMD-P2V analysis of variance. The Greenhouse-Geisser method of adjusting the degrees of freedom was used to determine the significance of main effects and interactions where appropriate (Vasey & Thayer, 1987) for all analyses reported in this book. Statistical analyses are described in more detail in the results section below.

Hansen & Hillyard (1983) adopted a procedure for stimulus classification to denote whether the stimulus matched (+) or did not match (−) the target of each run, on each of the stimulus characteristics of location (L), pitch (P) and duration (D). Thus, the attended target requiring a response was denoted by L+P+D+, whereas a stimulus presented to the same location but of a different pitch and of short duration, was denoted by L+P−D−. For purposes of simplicity, and also to emphasize the differences between cannabis users and controls that will become apparent later, the labels adopted here for each stimulus type will use Hansen and Hillyard's abbreviation for attended and unattended location as L+ and L−, respectively, but otherwise will denote the stimulus as being of relevant or irrelevant pitch. Thus, a stimulus notation of "L+ irrelevant pitch" denotes a stimulus presented to the ear to which the subject was to attend, but of a pitch the subject was to ignore. According to Hansen and Hillyard's classification system, such a stimulus would be denoted by L+P−D+ if it were of long duration, or by L+P−D− if it was a short-duration tone. Here, short duration tones will be referred to as standards and long duration tones as targets. Averages to the same stimulus type across different attention conditions were created, but collapsed across high and low pitched stimuli and runs with left and right hand responses, and sorted according to whether they were recorded from the hemisphere ipsilateral or contralateral to the stimulated ear.

Results

Performance data

Task performance measures of reaction time, percentage correct detections (hits) and percentage errors of commission (false alarms) from cannabis users and controls are presented in Table 7.1. The mean reaction time of the user group was longer than that of the control group but this difference failed to reach statistical significance ($p > 0.3$). Cannabis users had a significantly lower correct hit rate than controls ($F(1,16) = 4.67, p < 0.05$). Users made significantly more false alarms than controls ($F(1,16) = 6.10, p < 0.03$). Thus, most of the performance measures indicated that the performance of cannabis users in this selective attention task was poorer than that of the controls.

Table 7.1 *Mean task performance measures of reaction time (RT), hit rate and false alarm rate of cannabis users and controls (with SD in parentheses)*

	RT (ms)	Hit rate (%)	False alarm rate (%)
Users	573.06	71.94	1.64
	(67.63)	(16.04)	(1.58)
Controls	536.96	86.72	0.32
	(79.25)	(12.79)	(0.29)

Event-related potential data

The processes of selective attention were assessed by comparing the amplitudes of the various ERP components elicited by the four standard and four target stimuli distinguished on the basis of their location and pitch characteristics. These measures were subjected to a repeated measures analysis of variance (BMD-P2V), with factors of group, stimulus, electrode site and hemisphere. Here, and for the remainder of the studies reported in this book, analyses of the early components (P1, N1, P2) will only be reported if significant group effects or interactions were found. Similarly, the results reported from analyses of all other ERP components will focus on group differences and not effects due to experimental manipulation.

Figure 7.1 depicts grand average ERPs to long duration target stimuli recorded from frontal, central and parietal scalp sites of cannabis users and controls. The L+ relevant pitch trace represents the brain's response to the attended target tones which the subjects had to identify and respond to with a button press. The large positive component evident in this trace is the P300, and the most noticeable difference between groups on first inspection of the plots is the amplitude of this component. It appears greatly reduced in cannabis users compared to controls at all electrode sites.

The P300 component was measured as the mean amplitude between 300 and 900 ms. Analysis of variance confirmed that this component was smaller across all electrode sites in the user group compared to the control group ($F(1,16) = 4.37$, $p < 0.053$). When measured as the most positive peak occurring in the same range, there was a trend toward smaller peak

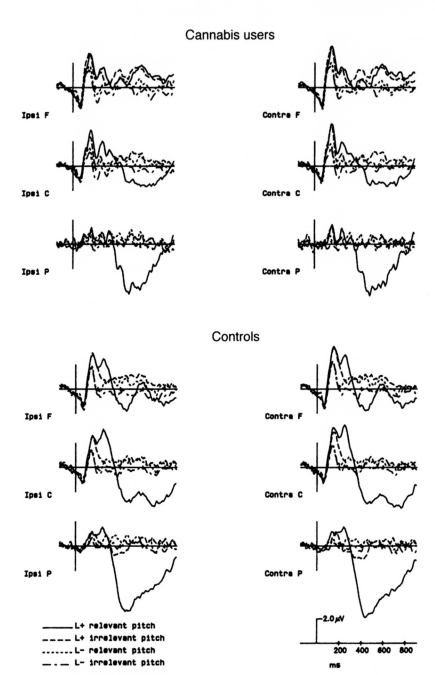

Figure 7.1 Grand average ERPs to target stimuli (long duration tones) recorded during an auditory selective attention task from cannabis users and controls. (Adapted from Solowij, N., Michie, P.T. & Fox, A.M., 1991. Reprinted by permission of Elsevier Science Inc.)

P300 in users compared to controls (F(1,16) = 3.61, $p < 0.07$), but the latency of the peak did not differ between groups ($p > 0.4$).

The other striking difference between groups was the large N200 also in the L+ relevant pitch trace in controls, which appeared greatly reduced in users. In the early part of the epoch, similar patterns of processing of the location dimension were evident in both groups, with early separation of the L+ and L− traces at frontal and central sites. By about 200 ms, the L+ relevant pitch trace separated sharply from the L+ irrelevant pitch trace in controls with a second negative peak, the N200. The L+ relevant pitch and L+ irrelevant pitch ERPs failed to separate well in the user group compared to controls.

The lack of separation between relevant and irrelevant pitch traces in users was due not only to the reduced N200 in the relevant pitch ERP, but also the appearance of an N200 in the irrelevant pitch trace in users, seen most clearly between 200 and 300 ms at frontal and central sites. There is no evidence of an N200 in the L+ irrelevant pitch trace in controls. Due to its close proximity to the N1 component and large intersubject variability in its latency, the N200 peak in both L+ relevant and irrelevant pitch traces was not measurable. Inspection of the individual subject waveforms revealed eight of the nine users to show a clear N200, while only four of the controls tended to show small negative peaks to the irrelevant pitch stimulus. Attempts to verify this difference between groups resulted in a marginally significant interaction between stimulus and group when the mean amplitude between 250 and 275 ms was analysed (F(1,16) = 4.36, $p < 0.053$), but multiple comparisons of each stimulus for each group failed to reach significance. This pattern of results is indicative of poor selection of the relevant pitch target stimulus, and unnecessary processing of the irrelevant pitch stimuli in the user group, perhaps reflecting an inability to reject pitch irrelevant stimuli at an early stage of processing.

Figure 7.2 depicts grand average ERPs to short duration standard stimuli. The importance of examining ERPs to standard stimuli is that they provide a measure of the processes involved in selective attention, uncontaminated by target detection, response preparation and response execution processes. The ERPs of the two groups appeared to be similar in the early range of the epoch. The processes of selective attention can be seen from Fig. 7.2 to commence around the beginning of the N1 peak with the separation of the two L+ and two L− ERPs. Early PN is evident around the N1 peak in both groups in the two L+ ERPs. This early enhancement of the L+ traces and positive going shift of the two L− traces indicates that cannabis users had no difficulty selecting or rejecting stimuli on the basis of location. With the processing of the pitch dimen-

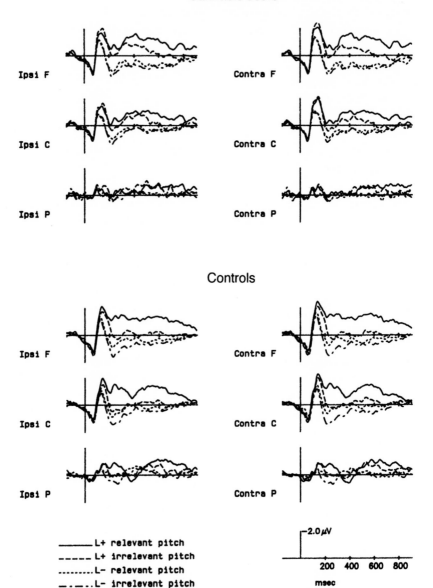

Figure 7.2 Grand average ERPs to standard stimuli (short duration tones) in an auditory selective attention task recorded from cannabis users and controls.

sion, the controls show a large PN to L+ relevant pitch stimuli, while the user group fails to sustain this negativity between 200 and 300 ms at frontal and central sites. Analysis of the mean amplitude of the L+ relevant pitch trace within this range determined a significant group difference (F(1,16) = 5.05, $p < 0.04$). This is indicative of difficulty in users in selecting relevant from irrelevant information when the selection is based on more complex stimulus attributes.

The most striking difference between the two groups apparent in Fig. 7.2 is the large PN shown by cannabis users to the irrelevant pitch stimuli in the attended ear. Relative to the L+ relevant pitch trace, the L+ irrelevant pitch ERP shows an enhanced negativity in the user group in comparison to controls. This difference between groups was evident as early as the N1 peak, where N1 appeared larger to irrelevant pitch stimuli than relevant pitch stimuli in users, but vice versa in controls. This observation was confirmed by a significant stimulus by group interaction for N1 peak amplitude measured from ERPs to the L+ stimuli ($p < 0.007$).

Mean amplitude measures over 50 ms intervals at frontal and central sites were subjected to a four-way analysis of variance with a group factor and repeated measures for stimulus type, electrode site and hemisphere. When all four stimuli were included in the analysis, the results were suggestive of interactions between stimulus and group over the range from 50 to 400 ms; however, it was apparent that large variability in the measures of the two L− stimuli may have served to obscure any group differences in PN to L+ stimuli. As a result of this observation, analyses for L+ and L− stimuli were conducted separately. Although the two L− traces appeared to show larger separation in the control group than in users, the large variability in these measures resulted in no significant differences between groups in any range measured.

Analyses of mean amplitudes of the ERPs to L+ stimuli determined a significant interaction between stimulus and group for almost every 50 ms range measured from 50 to 400 ms into the epoch ($0.001 < p < 0.09$). Low power due to the small sample size resulted in no significant effects upon multiple comparisons of the two groups for each stimulus. The trends were in the direction of larger negativity to irrelevant pitch stimuli in users over most of the range, but smaller mean amplitude in users to relevant pitch stimuli in the range from 200 to 300 ms. The mean amplitude from 50 to 400 ms was analysed and showed a significant stimulus by group interaction (F(1,16) = 4.74, $p < 0.05$); multiple comparisons suggested that this was primarily due to the large PN to irrelevant pitch stimuli in users

Difference waveforms

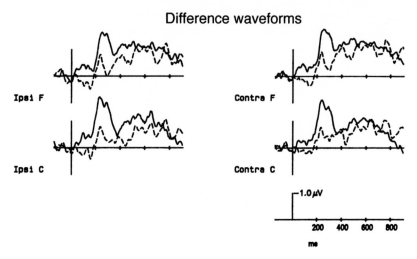

Figure 7.3 Pitch difference waveforms (L+ relevant pitch minus L+ irrelevant pitch) for cannabis users (– – –) and controls (——).

($p < 0.09$). There was also a tendency for PN to relevant pitch stimuli to be smaller in users ($p < 0.15$).

Although this negativity in the irrelevant pitch ERP appeared to persist to around 600 ms in the user group, analyses of mean amplitudes over 50 ms and 100 ms intervals failed to detect differences between groups beyond 400 ms. An analysis of the mean amplitude over 200 to 600 ms; however, did reveal a significant difference between users and controls as an interaction with hemisphere ($p < 0.04$), whereby the difference between groups was largest in the ipsilateral hemisphere. This difference is evident in Fig. 7.2. Towards the end of the epoch, there were no significant differences between the two groups on the late component of PN to pitch relevant tones and the inappropriately large PN to irrelevant pitch tones did not continue beyond 600 ms in users.

These differences between groups are also replicated in the pitch difference waveforms presented in Fig. 7.3. The difference waveforms, representing Nd, were created by subtracting the L+ irrelevant pitch ERP from the L+ relevant pitch ERP. The resulting waveforms in Fig. 7.3 emphasize the large separation between the relevant and irrelevant pitch traces in controls, whereas in users the separation is much smaller. This separation can be seen to commence with a sharp rise in Nd around 200 ms, particularly in the control group, while the earlier portion of the difference wave reflects smaller stimulus differences in the early ERP components; the lack of Nd (or positivity) prior to 200 ms in the users reflects greater negativity in the irrelevant pitch trace (as discussed for N1 above). The latency and amplitude of the largest peak in Nd within the 50–400 ms range was analysed. This indicated the point of maximum separation of the relevant and irrelevant pitch ERPs but no differences were found between groups in the latency of this point ($p > 0.15$). There was a trend toward significantly larger separation in the control group reflected in larger amplitude peak Nd ($p < 0.08$).

Visual inspection of the raw ERPs of Fig. 7.2 indicated clearly that the largest differences between groups were due to the reduced early PN to relevant pitch stimuli and the inappropriately large PN to irrelevant pitch stimuli in the user group. These observations were to an extent supported by statistical analyses, which would probably have been more robust had a larger sample been tested. Analysis of Nd measured in the difference waveforms contributed no further useful information regarding the nature of group differences. (The remainder of the studies reported in this book will therefore concentrate on analyses of PN and not Nd.) This pattern of results is indicative of an inability to select and filter out stimuli on the basis of complex stimulus attributes (e.g. pitch).

Discussion

The differences found between cannabis user and control groups in this experiment indicate that users may have some difficulty in setting up an accurate focus of attention and in filtering out complex irrelevant information. Cannabis users displayed a similar pattern to controls in the early filtering of stimuli which did not match the targets on the dimension of location, as evidenced by the separation of the L+ and L− waveforms. Both the presence of the N200 component in the ERPs to long duration irrelevant pitch tones in the attended ear and the large PN elicited by short duration irrelevant pitch stimuli in the attended ear, imply that users were unable to effectively reject stimuli on the basis of pitch attributes.

The largest differences between users and controls were apparent in the early part of the PN component. According to Näätänen (1982), this part of the PN reflects a matching process between the sensory information contained in the stimulus and an "attentional trace", an active voluntarily maintained neuronal representation of the physical features defining the stimuli which are the focus of attention. Thus, it appears to be the process of the selection and setting up of the attentional trace that is impaired, rather than its maintenance or rehearsal as would be reflected in the late component of PN according to Näätänen's theory. Furthermore, the reduced P300 amplitude suggests a dysfunction in the allocation of attentional resources and stimulus evaluation strategies (Isreal *et al.*, 1980; Pritchard, 1981).

The behavioural results of this study are important in demonstrating the value of examining the underlying mechanisms involved in processing information. Although users were no slower to respond than controls, their performance was significantly worse. It is not surprising then, that tests measuring reaction time alone may fail to detect deficits in task performance. Furthermore, performance measures alone would not reveal the nature of the attentional deficits revealed by examining the ERP measures. Taken together, both the performance and the ERP results of these studies imply that long-term cannabis use may impair the ability to efficiently process information.

At this stage it was not possible to assess to what extent this deficit may be due to a chronic build up of cannabinoids and whether functioning would return to normal upon discontinuation of use. The methodology employed precludes attribution of these results to an acute effect of cannabis: users were asked to abstain for at least 12 hours and they provided two urine samples which indicated that there had not been recent use of cannabis (see also Chapter 12 for a discussion of the users' motivation to participate in the study and to provide accurate self reports of last use of cannabis). It is possible, though, that the results might reflect a carry over effect, most likely due to cannabinoid residues remaining within the body. These may either be traces of THC and its metabolites remaining from the last exposure to cannabis, or else these residues may have accumulated as a result of many frequent exposures over a prolonged period. Presumably any effect attributable to accumulated drug residues would correlate with the frequency of cannabis use and would recover with sufficient abstinence to permit such residues to be eliminated from the body. The literature suggests that at least several weeks of abstinence would be required to eliminate accumulated cannabinoids (see Chapter 2). On the other hand, the results of this study might reflect a chronic effect of prolonged ingestion of cannabis, independent of accumulated cannabinoid residues and thus lasting beyond the period of elimination. The following experiments were designed to address these questions and to examine the quantity/frequency and duration of use at which dysfunction is first manifest. The differences found in this relatively small diverse sample warranted further investigation of cognitive functioning in long-term cannabis users.

Key findings

- *Cannabis users met strict inclusion/exclusion criteria and were matched on age, sex and education with nonuser controls*
- *All subjects required to abstain from cannabis and other drugs for 24 hours prior to testing (urinalysis confirmed at least 12 hours abstinence)*
- *Subjects performed a complex selective attention task while brain ERPs were recorded*
- *Cannabis users' task performance was poorer than that of controls*
- *Cannabis users' ERPs showed a pattern consistent with inefficient processing of information and impaired selective attention: reduced PN to relevant attended stimuli, inappropriately large PN to a source of complex irrelevant stimuli, and reduced amplitude of the P300 component to attended target stimuli compared to controls*
- *These results suggest a dysfunction in the allocation of attentional resources with an impaired ability to focus attention and ignore irrelevant information*
- *The small sample size of this study dictates caution. The findings required replication with a larger sample and an examination of the effects of frequency and duration of cannabis use, as reported in the next chapter*

8

An investigation of the effects of frequency and duration of cannabis use

Experiment 2: effects of frequency and duration of cannabis use on auditory selective attention

In Experiment 1, event-related potentials (ERPs) recorded during a complex auditory selective attention task were compared between a small and heterogeneous group of long-term cannabis users and a nonuser control group. The results indicated that compared to controls, cannabis users showed larger processing negativity (PN) to an irrelevant source of information, reflecting an inability to filter out extraneous information at an early stage of processing. Cannabis users also showed reduced P300 amplitude which was interpreted as a dysfunction in the allocation of attentional resources. The current study was designed to replicate these findings with a larger sample and to examine the effects of frequency and duration of cannabis use.

Method

Subjects

The same inclusion/exclusion criteria as those described for Experiment 1 were applied here, with the exception that regular use could be defined as at least once/month to enable the formation of a low frequency user group. The overall sample ($n = 32$) had used cannabis for a mean of 6.69 years (range 3–28 years) at a mean frequency of 12 days per month (range once/month to daily use). The characteristics of the entire sample and subgroups are presented in Table 8.1.

The user group was split at the median on both frequency (light: $\leq$ 2/week vs heavy: $\geq$ 3/week) and duration (short: 3–4 years vs long: $\geq$ 5 years) of cannabis use. Mean levels of use for each group are provided in

Table 8.1 *Sample characteristics: mean and (SD)*

Group	Sex	Age	Years of education	NART score	Alcohol consumption (standard drinks per month)	Cannabis duration (years of use)	Cannabis frequency (days per month)
Long	13M	28.9	14.1	36.8	60.9	10.1	13.7
n = 16	3F	(8.2)	(2.1)	(8.4)	(48.4)	(6.8)	(9.0)
Short	12M	19.9	13.2	35.0	47.8	3.3	10.3
n = 16	4F	(2.0)	(1.2)	(5.8)	(38.8)	(0.5)	(6.5)
Heavy	12M	23.5	13.2	34.7	68.6	6.69	17.9
n = 16	4F	(7.4)	(1.8)	(7.6)	(46.9)	(5.6)	(6.9)
Light	13M	25.3	14.2	37.0	40.1	6.69	6.0
n = 16	3F	(7.7)	(1.7)	(6.7)	(36.2)	(6.3)	(2.6)
Overall	25M	24.4	13.7	35.9	54.4	6.69	12.0
cannabis users	7F	(7.5)	(1.8)	(7.2)	(43.7)	(5.8)	(7.9)
Controls	12M	26.3	15.6	39.7	23.4	—	—
n = 16	4F	(7.0)	(2.4)	(5.2)	(17.0)	—	—

Source: Reprinted by permission of Elsevier Science Inc. See Figure 8.4 for details.

Table 8.1. Equal numbers of heavy and light users contributed to the long and short duration user groups and vice versa. A group of nonuser controls ($n = 16$) were recruited to cover the range of age, years of education and sex distribution in the user groups. No control subject had ever used cannabis on a regular basis. The mean number of lifetime experiences with cannabis in the control group was 9 ($\pm$ 11.2).

Due to the inevitable relationship between age and duration of use, long duration users were older than short duration users ($p < 0.0002$). While controls did not differ in age from cannabis users overall ($p > 0.3$), it was ensured that they did not differ in age from long duration users ($p > 0.3$). This resulted in controls being significantly older than short duration cannabis users ($p < 0.002$). Cannabis users consumed more alcohol per month than controls ($p < 0.009$) (see Table 8.1). Age and alcohol consumption were accordingly included as covariates in the analyses (where appropriate).

Seventy five percent of the sample were male and most had completed some tertiary education. Controls had slightly more years of education than users (equivalent to 1 or 2 more years at tertiary level) ($p < 0.004$). Full scale IQ, assessed by the NART (Nelson, 1982) did not differ between groups based on duration of use relative to controls ($p > 0.14$), nor between groups based on frequency of use ($p > 0.11$). A trend toward lower IQ overall in the cannabis users compared to controls ($p > 0.06$) indicated that the relation between IQ and ERP components needed to be examined in light of any group differences. The actual difference in IQ was very small at 116.3 for users compared to 119.5 for controls. These levels are in the high average to superior range for Full Scale IQ.

Cannabis users were instructed to abstain from cannabis and alcohol for 24 hours prior to testing and to provide urine samples the night before testing and during the test session to ensure that they had not consumed cannabis in the intervening period. Users were excluded if the level of metabolites detected in the second urine sample was substantially higher than that in the first. The mean level of the cannabinoid metabolite THC-COOH detected in the evening urine sample was 100.91 ng/ml (39.03 ng/ml normalized) and that on the day of testing 90.72 ng/ml (19.84 normalized). There was much variability in levels detected across subjects and approximately 60% showed zero levels of urinary cannabinoids. The control group provided a urine sample during the test session and any subject returning a positive urine for cannabis or other drugs was excluded.

Procedure and stimuli

Subjects participated in a single 3 hour test session. A detailed drug history was taken and they completed questionnaires assessing dependence on cannabis, psychiatric symptomatology and state/trait anxiety (these will be discussed in Chapter 11). Subjects were tested for normal hearing and trained on the selective attention task as described for Experiment 1.

The task and stimulus parameters were the same as that of Experiment 1, adapted from the auditory selective attention paradigm of Hansen & Hillyard (1983), with the presentation through headphones (TDH 49) of a random series of tone pips which varied in location (left ear vs right ear), pitch (high: 1319 Hz vs low: 1047 Hz) and duration (long: 102 ms vs short: 51 ms), having a rise and fall time of 10 ms. The stimuli were presented as a random sequence lasting 160 seconds per run with a random SOA of 200–500 ms (mean 350 ms). Fifty percent of the stimuli occurred in each ear with equal numbers of each pitch. Most of the tones (76%) of each type were of short duration, while a small percentage (24%) were long.

Subjects were instructed to attend to a particular ear and pitch, and respond with a button press to the infrequent long tones (the targets). The four attention conditions were left high, left low, right high and right low. Subjects completed eight runs, two of each attention condition responding with either the left or right hand. The order of attention conditions and responding hand was randomized among subjects.

ERP recording and data analysis

ERPs were recorded using an electrode cap (Electro-cap International) from midline (Fz, Cz, Pz) and lateral scalp sites (F3, F4, P3, P4) referenced to linked ears. Vertical eye movement was recorded by tin electrodes placed above and below the left eye. The data were amplified using Neomedix NT114-A amplifiers with a system bandpass of 0.016 and 50 Hz (3dB down). Data were digitized at a rate of 5.33 ms per channel. Overlapping epochs of 1350 ms including a 150 ms prestimulus baseline were extracted and epochs containing ocular artefact were rejected prior to averaging.

Separate averages were created for long and short duration stimuli, excluding those with an incorrect response, and collapsed across runs according to attention condition. Thus, ERPs were classified according to whether they matched the target on location and pitch for each run, resulting in attended (L+) and unattended ear (L−) ERPs for relevant and irrelevant pitch stimuli, as described in Chapter 7. ERPs were sorted according to whether they were recorded from the hemisphere ipsilateral or contralateral to the stimulated ear.

The processes of selective attention were assessed by comparing groups on the mean amplitude of processing negativity to short tones and the amplitude and latency of the P300 component to targets. These measures were subjected to analyses of variance (ANOVA) with frequency and duration of cannabis use as factors and repeated measures on stimulus type and electrode site. Performance data were treated as described for Experiment 1.

Results

Performance data

Performance data from the groups of cannabis users and controls are presented in Table 8.2. Analyses of variance indicated that reaction time to targets was longer ($F(1,46) = 4.56$, $p < 0.04$) and the proportion of correctly detected targets was lower ($F(1,46) = 11.26$, $p < 0.002$) in the

Table 8.2 *Performance measures of reaction time, hit rate and false alarm rate for cannabis user groups and controls: means and (SD)*

	Cannabis users (overall)	Long duration users	Short duration users	Heavy frequency users	Light frequency users	Control group (nonusers)
Reaction time (ms)	644.84 (90.56)	650.83 (98.11)	638.86 (85.13)	664.72 (81.01)	624.97 (97.68)	587.42 (81.79)
Hit rate (%)	73.71 (11.05)	74.22 (12.55)	73.21 (9.72)	70.86 (10.35)	76.56 (11.32)	84.23 (8.30)
False alarm rate (%)	0.77 (0.80)	0.83 (1.01)	0.72 (0.54)	0.80 (0.63)	0.75 (0.96)	0.50 (0.69)

Source: Reprinted by permission of Elsevier Science Inc. See Figure 8.4 for details.

cannabis user group overall by comparison with controls, with the largest difference between heavy cannabis users and controls (reaction time: heavy users vs controls ($F(1,30) = 7.21$, $p < 0.02$); hit rate: heavy users vs controls ($F(1,30) = 16.25$, $p < 0.0004$). Differences in false alarm rate did not reach significance ($p > 0.2$). Cannabis user groups did not differ significantly on any of the performance measures.

ERP data

Processing negativity

Inspection of the ERP waveforms to short tones suggested that the results of Experiment 1 had been replicated: cannabis users showed increased PN to tones which matched the target on location but not pitch. When the cannabis user group was split according to frequency and duration of use, it became apparent that PN was greatly affected by duration of use.

Long versus short duration users versus controls Grand average ERPs to short tones at frontal and central scalp sites are depicted in Figs 8.1, 8.2 and 8.3, respectively, for long duration users, short duration users and controls. Visual inspection of the waveforms suggested a difference between groups in N1 amplitude, however analyses of the peak between 50 and 250 ms at frontal and central sites revealed this not to be significant ($p > 0.2$) and groups did not differ in N1 latency, P1 or P2 amplitude or latency ($p > 0.2$).

Preliminary analyses of mean amplitude measures over 100 ms intervals at frontal and central scalp sites indicated significant differences between

Long duration users

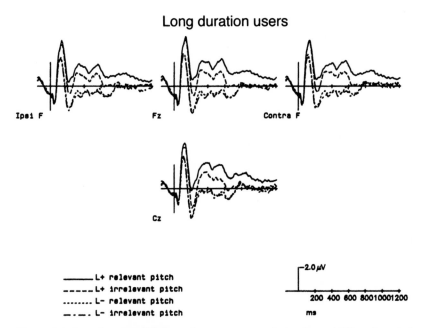

Ipsi F   Fz   Contra F

Cz

———— L+ relevant pitch
– – – – L+ irrelevant pitch
········ L- relevant pitch
— · — · L- irrelevant pitch

-2.0 μV

200 400 600 800 1000 1200
ms

Figure 8.1 Grand average ERPs to short tones recorded at frontal (F) and central (C) scalp sites from long duration cannabis users. (L+ and L− refer to attended and unattended location (ear), respectively.)

groups based on duration of use over the range from 300 to 600 ms for tones in the attended ear (L+) only, with no significant differences occurring outside this latency range. On the basis of this analysis, PN was measured as the mean amplitude over 300 to 600 ms and subjected to a repeated measures ANOVA (BMD-P2V). The results confirmed that there were no differences between groups in the processing of tones in the unattended ear (L−) ($p > 0.5$). Analysis of PN to tones of relevant and irrelevant pitch in the attended ear (L+) for groups based on duration of use (long duration users, short duration users and controls), revealed a significant effect of group (F(2,45) = 5.11, $p < 0.01$) and an interaction between group, stimulus and scalp site (F(6,135) = 3.08, $p < 0.03$). Group multiple comparisons at each scalp site were carried out using the Bonferroni procedure.

The long duration user group showed significantly larger PN to pitch irrelevant tones in the attended ear than controls at all frontal sites ($p < 0.004$) and at Cz ($p < 0.02$). Long duration users also showed significantly larger PN than short duration users at all frontal sites ($p < 0.001$), but did not differ from short users at Cz ($p > 0.3$). These results were essentially

Short duration users

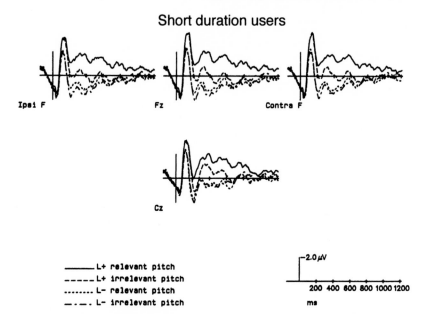

Figure 8.2 Grand average ERPs to short tones recorded at frontal (F) and central (C) scalp sites from short duration cannabis users. (L+ and L− refer to attended and unattended location (ear), respectively.)

unaltered when age and alcohol consumption were used as covariates (but see analysis of covariance for heterogeneous regression slopes, below).

Short duration users did not differ from controls at frontal sites ($p >$ 0.7), but there was a trend toward larger PN to pitch irrelevant tones in short duration users at Cz ($p < 0.072$), and this difference became significant when age was used as a covariate ($p < 0.03$). These differences between long and short duration user groups and nonuser controls are clearly apparent in Figs 8.1, 8.2 and 8.3.

Correlational analyses within the user group indicated that the ability to filter out irrelevant information, as indexed by PN, was increasingly impaired with the number of years of cannabis use (see Fig. 8.4). The relation was not initially significant in the entire sample (Fig. 8.4.A); however, it was apparent that the majority of the sample had used cannabis for up to 12 years, while the two subjects with deviant results had used cannabis for 25 and 28 years. A t test for outliers (Barnett & Lewis, 1984) determined that these two subjects were statistical outliers in terms of their duration of use compared to the rest of the sample ($t = 6.80$, $p < 0.01$). When these two outliers were excluded from the correlational analysis, the relation between PN and duration of cannabis use became highly

Controls

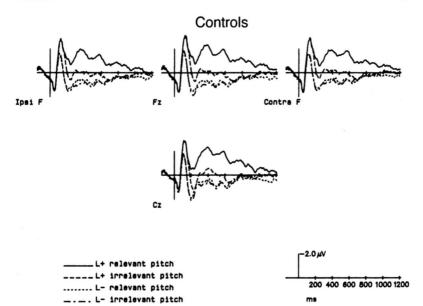

Ipsi F   Fz   Contra F

Cz

_____ L+ relevant pitch
_ _ _ _ _ L+ irrelevant pitch
.... L- relevant pitch
_ . _ . _ L- irrelevant pitch

┌─2.0 μV

200 400 600 800 1000 1200
ms

Figure 8.3 Grand average ERPs to short tones recorded at frontal (F) and central (C) scalp sites from controls. (L+ and L− refer to attended and unattended location (ear), respectively.)

significant ($r = 0.65$, $p < 0.0001$; Fig. 8.4.B). One interpretation of this result is that some kind of tolerance may develop after using for a very long number of years, producing a nonlinear relation. On the other hand, perhaps a significant linear relation would remain if more subjects with durations of use of between 12 and 30 years were tested. Nevertheless, from Figure 8.4.B it is clear that a strong relation appears to exist between the duration of cannabis use and the amplitude of processing negativity to irrelevant information.

As an inevitable relation existed between years of cannabis use and increasing age ($r = 0.77$, $p < 0.0001$), a partial correlational analysis was carried out. This indicated that the significant relationship between duration of cannabis use and PN remained after controlling for the effect of age ($r = 0.54$, $p < 0.005$), whereas there was no relation between age and PN after controlling for duration of use ($r = -0.11$). Thus, the ability to filter out irrelevant information reflected in processing negativity to pitch irrelevant tones, was progressively impaired as a function of the number of years of cannabis use.

Correlational analyses over all groups (and for each group separately) indicated that alcohol consumption was not related to PN ($r = 0.03$). A

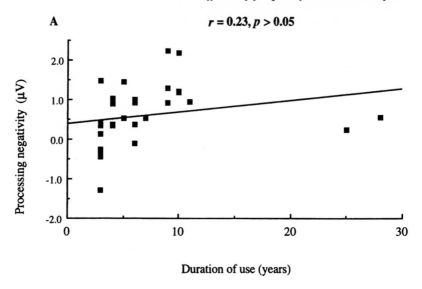

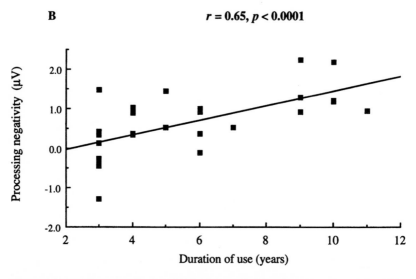

Figure 8.4 (A) Mean amplitude of PN (μV) to pitch irrelevant tones as a function of duration of cannabis use in the entire sample. (B) With two outliers excluded. (Adapted from Solowij, N., Michie, P.T. & Fox, A.M., 1995. Reprinted by permission of Elsevier Science Inc.)

relation between age and PN was found in the control group only ($r = 0.51$, $p < 0.05$), as was a relation between IQ and PN in the control group only ($r = 0.68$, $p < 0.005$), but age and IQ were also correlated in the controls ($r = 0.68$, $p < 0.005$). Partial correlational analyses revealed that the relation between IQ and PN remained significant after controlling for the effects of age ($r = 0.52$, $p < 0.05$), whereas there was no relationship between age and PN after controlling for IQ ($r = 0.10$). PN and IQ were unrelated in the cannabis user group ($r = -0.10$).

An analysis of covariance technique for heterogeneous regression slopes (Johnson-Neyman technique (Huitema, 1980)) using IQ as the covariate, determined significant PN differences between groups below a certain NART score cut off. Long duration users differed significantly from controls at frontal and central sites below a NART score of 42 (estimated Full Scale IQ 121) ($F(1,28) = 4.20$, $p < 0.05$). Short duration users were also found to differ significantly from controls below a NART score of 35 (estimated Full Scale IQ of 115). These results raise the possibility of more severe consequences from cannabis use for those of lower IQ. The cut off levels below which group differences are apparent are within the superior range of IQ for the long duration user group and the high average range for IQ for short-term users. This indicates that the effects of cannabis use are more apparent in users of low IQ when cannabis has only been used for a few years, but when cannabis has been used for many years, its effects on selective attention override any effect of IQ. This might also be interpreted to suggest that only users of superior IQ may be able to compensate and overcome subtle impairments. The positive relation between PN and IQ in controls is puzzling. One interpretation of this relation is that brighter subjects may be better able to process multiple sources of stimuli without any resultant loss of performance.

Heavy versus light users versus controls Analysis of groups based on frequency of use indicated no differences between heavy users, light users and controls on any measure derived from their ERPs to short tones. Groups did not differ in the amplitude or latency of P1, N1 or P2. PN did not differ between groups in the processing of tones in the unattended ear (L−), and analysis of PN to tones of relevant and irrelevant pitch in the attended ear (L+) also revealed no difference between heavy users, light users and controls ($p > 0.3$).

Correlational analysis showed no relationship to exist between PN to pitch irrelevant tones and frequency of cannabis use ($r = 0.19$, $p > 0.2$). A two-way analysis of variance with frequency and duration as factors found no interaction between frequency and duration of use ($p > 0.6$) and no frequency × duration × stimulus × electrode interaction ($p > 0.5$). These results imply that the large PN to pitch irrelevant tones observed in cannabis users in both this study and in Experiment 1, is not related to frequency of cannabis use but increases as a function of cumulative exposure to cannabis.

One final possibility was explored with regard to effects on PN and that was exposure to tobacco smoke. Cannabis user groups and controls were divided into cigarette smokers and nonsmokers: 15 of the cannabis users were tobacco smokers (nine long, six short-term users), while only two of the controls were smokers. An analysis of variance comparing smokers and nonsmokers in the cannabis users only, found no effect of cigarette smoking on PN ($p > 0.6$). As long-term cannabis users had differed significantly from short-term cannabis users in PN, this analysis confirmed that the large PN to irrelevant stimuli was related to exposure to cannabis smoke and not the result of smoking *per se*.

P300

The P300 component to target tones was measured as the most positive peak occurring between 200 and 1000 ms at parietal scalp sites. Subjects with poorly defined P300 components or no measurable peak were excluded from the analyses (six subjects in total were excluded: four long users and one short user (two heavy and three light) and one control subject). Inspection of the waveforms suggested that, contrary to our previous findings, there were no differences between cannabis users and controls in the amplitude of P300. This was confirmed by analysis of P300 peak amplitude for cannabis users overall compared to controls ($p > 0.2$) and for groups based on frequency ($p > 0.4$) and duration ($p > 0.2$) of use. When the cannabis user group was split according to frequency and duration of use, it became apparent that P300 latency was greatly affected by frequency of use.

Heavy versus light users versus controls The ERPs to the attended ear (L+) relevant pitch long duration (target) tone recorded at parietal scalp sites are depicted in Fig. 8.5 overlaid for heavy cannabis users, light cannabis users and controls. The P300 component appeared to be delayed by over 100 ms in the heavy user group compared to both light users and controls. The mean latency of the peak measured at parietal sites was analysed and revealed a significant group effect ($F(2,39) = 4.68$, $p < 0.02$) and an interaction between group and electrode site ($F(4,78) = 3.68$, $p < 0.01$).

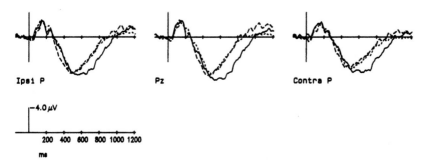

Figure 8.5 Grand average ERPs to target tones recorded at parietal scalp sites from heavy (——) and light (- - -) cannabis users and controls (- - -). (Reprinted by permission of Elsevier Science Inc. See Figure 8.4 for details.)

Group multiple comparisons at each site revealed that P300 was significantly delayed in heavy users compared to light users and controls at Pz and at the parietal site contralateral to the stimulated ear: heavy vs light users ($p < 0.04$); heavy users vs controls ($p < 0.03$). Light users did not differ from controls at any site ($p > 0.1$). These results are apparent in Figure 8.5.

There was a significant linear relation between P300 latency and frequency of cannabis use ($r = 0.50, p < 0.01$) as shown in Fig. 8.6. Age did not differ between groups ($p > 0.5$) and P300 latency was unrelated to alcohol consumption ($r = 0.23, p > 0.2$) or IQ ($r = 0.21, p > 0.3$).

Long versus short users versus controls Groups based on duration of use (long users versus short users versus controls) did not differ in the latency of P300 measured at parietal scalp sites ($p > 0.3$). Correlational analysis revealed that duration of cannabis use was unrelated to P300 latency ($r = 0.14$). There was no interaction between frequency and duration ($p > 0.17$) or between frequency, duration and electrode site ($p > 0.4$). Thus, the latency of P300, which reflects the time required to evaluate a stimulus, was delayed with increasing frequency of cannabis use, regardless of the number of years of use.

Discussion

It appears that frequency and duration of cannabis use differentially affect brain function in this selective attention task: heavy frequency use was found to prolong stimulus evaluation time, measured by P300 latency; long duration use impaired the ability to effectively focus attention and ignore irrelevant information, as evidenced by increased (PN) to irrelevant

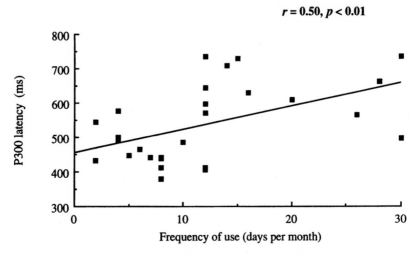

Figure 8.6 Peak latency of P300 (ms) at the contralateral parietal scalp site as a function of frequency of cannabis use. (Reprinted by permission of Elsevier Science Inc. See Figure 8.4 for details.)

stimuli. Large (PN) to pitch irrelevant tones in the long duration users indicates unnecessary processing of, and hence an inability to effectively reject pitch irrelevant information. This could be interpreted as either a failure to habituate to irrelevant stimuli (Miller & Branconnier, 1983), as faulty gating mechanisms (Hillyard & Mangun, 1987) or as the result of using inefficient information processing strategies (Hillyard & Hansen, 1986).

The increased PN to pitch irrelevant tones replicated the result of Experiment 1. But Experiment 1 also found P300 amplitude to be smaller in cannabis users, a finding which was not replicated in Experiment 2. Careful scrutiny of the ERP waveforms, however, suggests that it was the control group that differed in the two studies. The control group in the original study showed a larger P300 than did controls of the current study, as can be seen by comparing the amplitudes of controls in Figs 7.1 and 8.5. No apparent differences in the characteristics of the two samples could explain this, indicating that effects of cannabis use on P300 amplitude are less robust than effects on PN. Similarly, P300 latency was not significantly delayed in the original study (there was a nonsignificant trend), but the larger sample of this experiment provided more power to detect differences between groups. In the current study, there were no interactions between frequency and duration of use on either measure of brain function, which suggests that each affects different mechanisms or pathways in the brain.

The lack of an effect of duration of cannabis use on P300 latency suggests that the observed delay is temporary in nature and could be eliminated by reducing frequency of use. Cannabis may slow information processing by producing some (reversible) cell toxicity or disruption of brain messenger coordination. Cannabinoid compounds are lipophilic and alter membrane fluidity parameters, which may in turn alter the binding parameters of noncannabinoid receptors, inhibit adenylate cyclase and cause perturbation of mechanisms of neurotransmitter uptake or release (Martin, 1986; Makriyannis & Rapaka, 1990).

Cannabinoids accumulate in fatty tissues (and thus probably in brain) (Hollister, 1986), and may be detectable in urine for more than 2 months after use (Ellis *et al.*, 1985). While all subjects were required to abstain from cannabis for at least 24 hours (the range being 1–30 days of abstinence), the heavy users (using 3 times per week to daily) have considerably more cannabinoids continuously present in the body. Analyses confirmed that heavy cannabis users had significantly greater cannabinoid levels detected in their urines than light users (167 ng/ml vs 24 ng/ml, respectively; $p < 0.008$; long users appeared to have greater levels than short-term users, 114 ng/ml vs 77 ng/ml, but this difference was not significant, $p > 0.5$). It is possible that the continual presence of cannabinoids at these levels in heavy cannabis users may affect their performance, even when they are not acutely intoxicated.

This hypothesis is in accord with the results of a study which found aircraft pilots' simulation performance to be impaired as long as 24 hours after smoking a single moderate dose of cannabis in the absence of any awareness of the drug's influence (Leirer *et al.*, 1991; Yesavage *et al.*, 1985). Acutely, cannabis has been shown to slow complex reaction time (see Chapter 3). In this study, reaction times were significantly slower in heavy users compared to controls and there was a nonsignificant trend toward longer reaction times in the heavy users compared to light users. More importantly, the speed of information processing in the brain, P300 latency, was significantly delayed in the heavy user group compared to both light users and controls. This result emphasizes the sensitivity of ERP measures in detecting impairments in covert cognitive processes, otherwise undetected by overt measures of performance.

If the delay in P300 was due to either a carry over effect, or the result of accumulated cannabinoids, one would expect P300 latency to vary as a function of time since last use of cannabis or a measure of the level of cannabinoids present in the body. This hypothesis was tested by correlational analyses. As apparent in Fig. 8.7.A, the relation between P300 latency and self reported most recent use was nonsignificant, although the

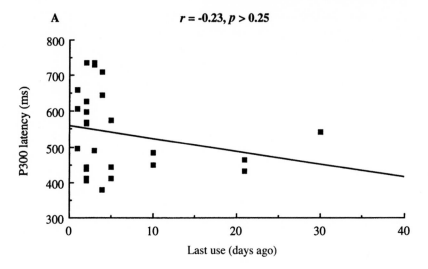

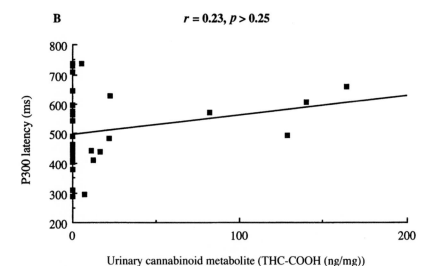

Figure 8.7 P300 latency (ms) at the contralateral parietal scalp site as a function of (A) time since last use of cannabis (days ago), and (B) normalized cannabinoid metabolite extracted from urine on the day of testing. (Reprinted by permission of Elsevier Science Inc. See Figure 8.4 for details.)

trend was in the expected direction ($r = -0.23$). It is possible that more precise measures of quantity and time since last use with controlled verification would provide evidence of a stronger relationship.

In Fig. 8.7.B, P300 latency plotted against the normalized urinary cannabinoid metabolite (THC-COOH) also showed a nonsignificant trend in the expected direction ($r = 0.23$). As mentioned above, 60% of the sample had no detectable cannabinoid metabolites in their urines. Such measures are subject to great variability (Ellis *et al.*, 1985), and while weak traces of metabolized cannabinoids may be detected, the extent of storage of THC is unknown. It has been suggested that approximately 70% of ingested THC is taken up by tissues while only 30% is converted to metabolites measurable in urine, and that particularly following chronic use there is a significant decrease in metabolites extracted in urine and a relative increase in unextracted metabolites (Hunt & Jones, 1980).

The effect of duration of cannabis use on the rejection of irrelevant information reflects a very different mechanism. Neither time since last use ($r = 0.03$) nor urinary cannabinoid metabolite levels ($r = 0.16$) correlated with increased processing negativity to pitch irrelevant stimuli, implying that increasing years of use leads to long-term changes that do not resolve with a short period of abstinence. These changes may occur at the cannabinoid receptor site.

Such an hypothesis is consistent with the high density of cannabinoid receptors in hippocampus, and the role of the hippocampus in the cognitive requirements of this task, particularly in the exclusion of extraneous information (Miller & Branconnier, 1983). Furthermore, hippocampal neurons have been shown to be sensitive to spatial, temporal and discriminatory properties of stimuli, being activated by the learned significance of relations among multiple stimuli, rather than by their particular sensory or physical properties (Eichenbaum & Cohen, 1988). Cannabinoid receptors occur in high density in other regions known to be involved in attention, such as the globus pallidus, frontal cortex, particularly anterior cingulate cortex, and the cerebellum (see Chapter 2). While much research is required to determine the functional properties of the endogenous cannabinoid like constituent anandamide, it may be that this substance plays a role in the modulation of attention.

It has recently been demonstrated that chronic administration of cannabinoids results in receptor down regulation with a reduction in the number of receptors in rat brain (Oviedo *et al.*, 1993; Rodriguez de Fonseca *et al.*, 1994; but see also Chapter 4). Previous research with animals has not established that alterations in the properties of the cannabinoid receptor are irreversible (Westlake *et al.*, 1991), although the duration of exposure in such studies has generally been for 1 year or less. The results of the present study suggest that long-term effects may only become readily apparent after 5 years of exposure, given the significant difference between the long-term users of this study and controls, in contrast to the lack of robust differences between the short-term users and controls. Nevertheless, the linear relation observed implies not only progressive impairment, but also the possibility for early detection of subtle impairments with the use of more sensitive techniques.

The precise mechanisms of cannabinoid toxicity warrant further research. Whatever the mechanisms, these data provide convincing evidence that increasing duration of cannabis use leads to a progressively impaired mode of information processing whereby complex irrelevant information is not filtered out at an early stage of processing. In the real world, this may lead to distractibility and hence impairment in any situation where concentration and focused attention are essential. The question that remained was: to what extent are these changes reversible after a longer period of abstinence? The next experiment was designed to assess the extent of reversibility in long-term cannabis users who had ceased using.

Key findings

- *Thirty-two cannabis users were split at the median according to frequency (> twice/week) and duration (≥ 5 years) of cannabis use*
- *A group of 16 nonuser controls were recruited to cover the range of age, years of education and sex distribution in the user groups*
- *Cannabis users' task performance was poorer than that of the controls, with the largest difference between heavy cannabis users and controls*
- *The results of the previous study were essentially replicated with evidence of differential impairments of the processes of selective attention due to frequency and duration of cannabis use*
- *Long duration cannabis users showed significantly larger processing negativity (PN) to complex irrelevant stimuli than short duration cannabis users or controls. PN did not differ between heavy users, light users and controls*
- *PN to complex irrelevant information, and hence the inability to filter out or ignore such information, increased progressively with the number of years of cannabis use, regardless of the frequency of use*

- *The P300 component was significantly delayed in heavy cannabis users compared to light users and controls. The latency of P300 did not differ between long or short duration users and controls. There were no group differences in the amplitude of P300*
- *The latency of P300 increased significantly with increasing frequency of cannabis use, and was unrelated to the duration of use*
- *The general slowing of information processing evidenced by a delayed P300 was interpreted as a short lasting impairment, probably attributable to cannabinoid residues or the accumulation of cannabinoids following frequent or heavy use. The lack of an effect of duration of cannabis use on this process suggested that it was probably reversible with abstinence or reduced frequency of cannabis use*
- *The ability to focus attention and reject complex irrelevant information from further processing was progressive with the number of years of cannabis use, regardless of frequency of use. This suggests an enduring impairment that may reflect gradual changes occurring in the brain as the result of prolonged and cumulative exposure to cannabis*
- *The next study was designed to examine the extent of reversibility of these effects in a group of ex-cannabis users*

9
An investigation of the reversibility of cognitive impairment in ex-cannabis users

Experiment 3: reversibility of attentional deficits in ex-cannabis users

The previous experiment established that the large processing negativity elicited by pitch irrelevant stimuli in long-term cannabis users performing a selective attention task increased with the duration of cannabis use. This was interpreted as a progressive impairment in the ability to focus attention and ignore complex irrelevant information, and suggested that long-term changes may occur as a result of cumulative exposure to cannabis.

This experiment was designed to assess the extent of reversibility of these changes with prolonged abstinence from cannabis use, and as such, examined the event-related potential (ERP) response in the same selective attention task of a group of long-term cannabis users who had ceased using cannabis. It was hypothesized that processing negativity (PN) to pitch irrelevant stimuli may gradually resolve over time as the duration of abstinence from cannabis increases.

Method

A power analysis based on the data of Experiment 2 determined an effect size greater than one standard deviation unit. With a sample of 32 ex-users there would be an 80% chance of detecting a difference between groups of 0.7 standard deviation units at an alpha level of 0.05 (two-tailed test).

Subjects

Subjects were recruited from the general community by advertising. The criteria for inclusion were to have used cannabis for at least 5 years and to have given up using cannabis within the past few years and at the very least

Table 9.1 *Sample characteristics: mean and (SD) compared with groups from Experiment 2*

Group	Sex	Age	Years of education	NART score	Alcohol consumption (standard drinks per month)	Cannabis duration (years of use	Cannabis frequency (days per month)
Ex-users	22M	27.8	14.8	34.3	39.4	9.0	19.1
n = 28	6F	(5.2)	(2.3)	(7.0)	(43.2)	(3.8)	(10.9)
Long	13M	28.9	14.1	36.8	60.9	10.1	13.7
n = 16	3F	(8.2)	(2.1)	(8.4)	(48.4)	(6.8)	(9.0)
Short	12M	19.9	13.2	35.0	47.8	3.3	10.3
n = 16	4F	(2.0)	(1.2)	(5.8)	(38.8)	(0.5)	(6.5)
Controls	12M	26.3	15.6	39.7	23.4	—	—
n = 16	4F	(7.0)	(2.4)	(5.2)	(17.0)	—	—

Source: Reprinted by permission of Elsevier Science Inc. See Figure 9.2 for details.

6 weeks prior to testing (this would allow most of the accumulated cannabinoids to be eliminated from the body). Attempts were made to select ex-users matched as closely as possible on sex, age and educational status to the long-term users and controls of Experiment 2, and to ensure that the past duration of cannabis use was equivalent among long-term users and ex-users. Thirty-two cannabis users initially met the criteria for inclusion, but after taking a detailed drug use history it became apparent that two subjects had used cannabis for less than 5 years. These two subjects were therefore excluded from comparative analyses with groups from Experiment 2, but were retained for correlational analyses. A further two subjects were excluded from all analyses due to high levels of cannabinoids detected in their urines at the time of testing. Therefore the final sample for group comparisons consisted of 28 ex-users whose characteristics are presented in Table 9.1.

Ex-users were well matched to the long-term users of Experiment 2; the groups did not differ in age ($p > 0.5$), years of education ($p > 0.3$), NART scores ($p > 0.3$) or alcohol consumption ($p > 0.1$). Furthermore, they did not differ in their mean duration of cannabis use ($p > 0.5$) which ranged from 5 to 20 years, and the two groups were equivalent in their frequency of cannabis use ($p > 0.09$). The mean frequency of use for the ex-users reflects their usage during the longest phase of their use, but many had gradually diminished their frequency of use prior to ceasing altogether. 40% had stopped "cold turkey" during the heaviest period of their use.

The ex-user group had consumed cannabis for significantly longer ($p <$ 0.0001) and at a greater frequency ($p < 0.005$) than the short-term users of Experiment 2, were older than short-term users ($p < 0.0001$), had slightly more years of education ($p < 0.02$), but did not differ from short-term users in IQ (estimated by their NART scores) ($p > 0.7$) and did not differ in monthly alcohol consumption ($p > 0.5$). Ex-users did not differ in age from controls ($p > 0.4$), alcohol consumption ($p > 0.1$) or education ($p > 0.2$), but ex-users had significantly lower NART scores than controls ($p < 0.01$). This difference in IQ was taken into consideration in analyses as described below.

The same exclusion criteria applied as for Experiment 2. The ex-users were instructed to abstain from alcohol for 24 hours prior to testing. They provided a urine sample on the day of testing and any subjects with cannabinoids (or any other drugs) detected in their urine were excluded from the sample. As stated above, two subjects were excluded on this basis. The 28 subjects of the final sample had no cannabinoids detected in their urines.

The mean duration of abstinence in the ex-user group was approximately 2 years (s.d. = 22.8 months, range 3 months to 6 years). The main reasons given by ex-users for ceasing their use of cannabis could be labelled as maturational. For example, some gave up in order to pursue further studies, some had babies, some simply stated that their lives weren't really going anywhere or that they felt they had grown out of using cannabis. Almost two-thirds of the sample claimed to have felt dependent on cannabis; for the majority this was described as a "psychological dependence", while four subjects claimed to have been both physically and psychologically dependent. Dependence, in general, was defined in various ways, encompassing the following terms: a habitual or automatic action (to smoke); a strong need to use cannabis in order to feel normal; an inability to sleep or to function without it; cannabis use as an escape from reality, an aid in the management of depression, stress, anxiety or insomnia, or an emotional or social "crutch" in navigating interpersonal relationships and social events. The 40% of subjects who claimed not to have felt dependent on cannabis when asked directly, nevertheless scored highly on a symptom checklist for dependence (see Chapter 11). One-third of the sample stated that they had no intention of ever using cannabis again, while the remainder felt that they might use occasionally at social functions in the future, but none had any desire to return to regular use.

Table 9.2 Performance measures of reaction time, hit rate and false alarm rate for ex-cannabis users compared with groups from Experiment 2: means and (SD).

	Long duration users	Short duration users	Ex-cannabis users	Controls (nonusers)
Reaction time (ms)	650.83 (98.11)	638.86 (85.13)	616.20 (92.06)	587.42 (81.79)
Hit rate (%)	74.22 (12.55)	73.21 (9.72)	75.64 (13.89)	84.23 (8.30)
False alarm rate (%)	0.83 (1.01)	0.72 (0.54)	0.72 (0.88)	0.50 (0.69)

Source: Reprinted by permission of Elsevier Science Inc. See Figure 9.2 for details.

Procedure and stimuli

This was identical to that described for Experiment 2 (see Chapter 8).

ERP recording and data analysis

This was identical to that described for Experiment 2 (see Chapter 8). The only difference in data analysis was that the main comparisons of interest in this study were between ex-users and current long-term users of Experiment 2, and between ex-users and controls of Experiment 2. The effects of past frequency of use in ex-users were also examined in correlational analyses, but with the hypothesis that past frequency of use would have no residual effect.

Results

Performance data

Performance measures for ex-users and all other groups are presented in Table 9.2. Analysis of variance showed that although ex-users appeared to have longer reaction times than controls, the difference was not significant ($p > 0.3$). Ex-users reaction times did not differ significantly from those of long ($p > 0.2$) or short duration users ($p > 0.4$); however, ex-users made significantly fewer correct detections than controls ($p < 0.03$) but did not differ from either of the cannabis using groups in terms of "hit rate" ($p > 0.5$). There were no differences between ex-users and any other group in false alarm rate ($p > 0.4$).

Ex-cannabis users

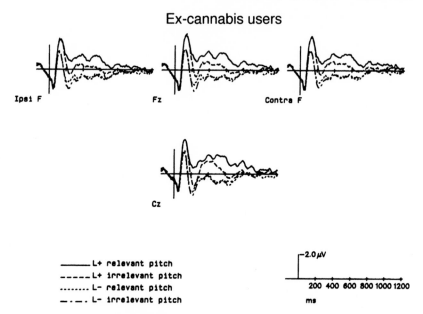

Figure 9.1 Grand average ERPs to short tones recorded from 28 ex-cannabis users depicted at frontal and central scalp sites. (L+ and L− refer to attended and unattended location (ear), respectively.)

ERP data

The grand average ERPs to short tones recorded at frontal and central scalp sites from the 28 ex-users are depicted in Fig. 9.1. Figure 9.2 depicting frontal and central midline sites only, permits direct comparison of groups. Inspection of the plots suggested that processing negativity (PN) to pitch irrelevant tones was not as large in the ex-users as that seen in the current long-term users of Experiment 2, and PN to pitch relevant tones also appeared reduced in the ex-users compared to all other groups. PN at frontal and central sites from the 28 ex-cannabis users was measured as the mean amplitude between 300 and 600 ms at frontal and central sites and subjected to an analysis of variance.

The results showed that the ex-users differed from the long duration users in the processing of both relevant and irrelevant pitch stimuli; i.e. there was a significant effect of group ($F(1,42) = 11.41$, $p < 0.002$) but no stimulus $\times$ group interaction ($p > 0.6$). PN to both relevant and irrelevant

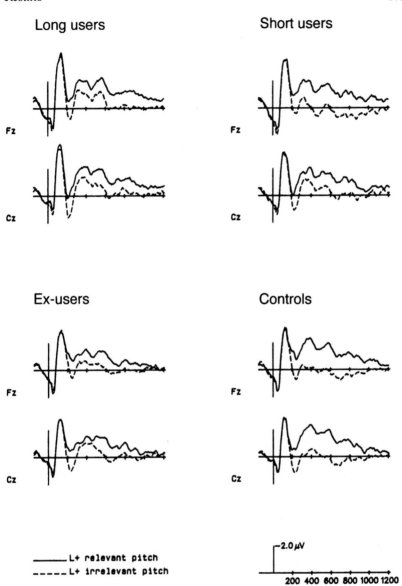

Figure 9.2 Grand average ERPs to short duration pitch relevant and pitch irrelevant tones in the attended ear recorded at frontal (Fz) and central (Cz) midline sites from long and short duration cannabis users, ex-cannabis users and controls. (Adapted from Solowij, N., 1995. Reprinted by permission of Elsevier Science Inc.)

Reversibility of cognitive impairment

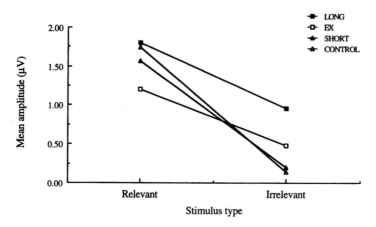

Figure 9.3 Stimulus × group interaction, depicting PN to pitch relevant and pitch irrelevant stimuli in the attended ear for long-term users, short-term users, ex-users and controls.

stimuli in the attended ear was significantly smaller in the ex-users compared to the long-term users.

The pattern of results was quite different when comparing ex-users with each of the other two groups: the main effect of group was not significant (ex vs short: $p > 0.7$; ex vs controls: $p > 0.5$) but there were significant stimulus × group interactions (ex vs short: $F(1,42) = 5.30, p < 0.03$; ex vs controls: $F(1,42) = 5.62, p < 0.03$). Multiple comparisons of each group for each stimulus revealed the following differences: ex-users vs short duration users: relevant pitch $p > 0.09$; irrelevant pitch $p > 0.1$; ex-users vs controls: relevant pitch $p > 0.05$; irrelevant pitch $p > 0.1$. While none of the comparisons reached significance the trend was in the direction of smaller PN to relevant pitch stimuli in the ex-users, but also trends toward larger PN to irrelevant pitch stimuli in the ex-user group compared to both short duration users and controls. These results are apparent in Fig. 9.3.

The slope for the ex-users in Fig. 9.3 resembles that of the long-term users, albeit reduced overall for both relevant and irrelevant pitch stimuli. This pattern is distinct from that of both short-term users and controls where a much sharper reduction is seen from PN to pitch relevant, to PN to pitch irrelevant stimuli. There was also a significant interaction between stimulus, electrode and group when comparing ex-users with short-term users ($F(3,126) = 3.45, p < 0.04$). The nature of this interaction is depicted in Fig. 9.4: ex-users have smaller PN to pitch relevant stimuli across all

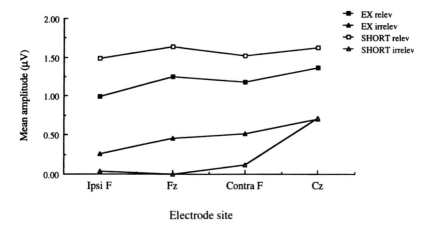

Figure 9.4 Stimulus × electrode × group interaction, depicting PN to pitch relevant and pitch irrelevant stimuli in the attended ear for ex-users and short term users across frontal and central scalp sites.

sites, but larger PN to pitch irrelevant stimuli than short-term users frontally but not at Cz, where as short-term users showed large PN to pitch irrelevant tones. Ex-users were similar to both groups of cannabis users in showing large PN at Cz (apparent in Fig. 9.2), but the interaction between stimulus, electrode and group was not significant when ex-users were compared to controls ($p > 0.4$).

As ex-users had significantly lower NART scores than controls, and therefore a lower mean IQ, the effects of IQ on PN to pitch irrelevant tones were examined by correlational analysis. There was no relation between IQ and PN in the ex-user group ($r = 0.15$); however, PN increased as a function of IQ in the control group ($r = 0.68$, $p < 0.005$) (as reported in Chapter 8). The ex-users' result essentially replicated that found in Experiment 2 with current cannabis users. Hence, the Johnson-Neyman technique for the analysis of covariance for heterogeneous regression slopes (Huitema, 1980) was applied. This determined that the groups differed significantly below a NART score of 40 (estimated Full Scale IQ of 119.7), with ex-users having significantly larger PN to pitch irrelevant tones than controls at both frontal and central sites (F(1,42) = 4.07, $p <$ 0.05). Nineteen of the ex-users (68%) had NART scores falling below 40, thus representing the majority of the sample. As discussed in Chapter 8 concerning similar results found with current cannabis users, these analyses suggest that the long-term effects of cannabis may be more apparent in

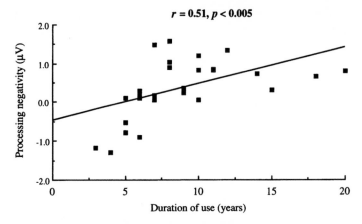

Figure 9.5 Mean amplitude of PN (μV) to pitch irrelevant tones as a function of past duration of cannabis use in the ex-user group. (Reprinted by permission of Elsevier Science Inc. See Figure 9.2 for details.)

users of lower IQ, or else, those of superior IQ compensate for the impairing effects of cannabis (given that the cut off IQ score falls in the superior to high average range). As argued in Chapter 8, the positive relation between PN and IQ in the control group may reflect the ability of brighter subjects to attend to more than one source of stimuli without concomitant impairment in performance on the task. For current and ex-cannabis users, the processing of pitch irrelevant stimuli appeared to impair their task performance. These hypotheses were tested by correlational analysis of performance data and PN. While none of the tests reached significance, there were trends in the expected direction in the relation between PN and the proportion of errors of commission (users: $r = 0.27$; ex-users: $r = 0.17$; controls: $r = -0.39$).

Correlational analysis showed a significant relation between the past duration of cannabis use in the ex-user group, and PN to pitch irrelevant tones in the attended ear ($r = 0.51$, $p < 0.005$). This is depicted in Fig. 9.5. Due to the significant relation between age and duration of use ($r = 0.84$, $p < 0.0001$), age was also related to PN ($r = 0.40$, $p < 0.03$). A partial correlational analysis revealed that a relation between duration and PN remained after removing the linear effects of age ($r = 0.34$, $p < 0.05$), whereas there was no relation between age and PN after controlling for the effects of duration of cannabis use ($r = -0.05$).

The relation between the ex-users' past duration of cannabis use and PN was examined further by reducing the sample to only those who had used for up to 12 years ($n = 26$), for better comparability with the current

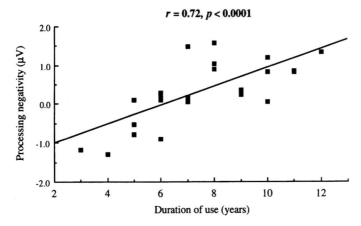

Figure 9.6 Mean amplitude of PN (μV) to pitch irrelevant tones as a function of past duration of cannabis use in a subsample of the ex-user group, those who had used for up to 12 years. (Reprinted by permission of Elsevier Science Inc. See Figure 9.2 for details.)

cannabis users of Experiment 2 (see Chapter 8, Fig. 8.4A, B). The results, depicted in Fig. 9.6, revealed a far more striking relation ($r = 0.72$, $p < 0.0001$). The relation between duration of use and age was still significant in this sample ($r = 0.69$, $p < 0.0001$), but partial correlational analysis showed that the relation between past duration of cannabis use and PN to pitch irrelevant tones remained strong after removing the linear effects of age ($r = 0.59$), whereas there was no relation between age and PN after removing the effects of duration of cannabis use ($r = 0.02$).

In Experiment 2, two subjects had used cannabis for 25 and 28 years, while the remainder of the sample had used between 3 and 12 years. When the entire sample had been included in the correlational analysis, a relation between PN and duration of cannabis use was obscured ($r = 0.23$). The two very long-term users were considered to be outliers and the correlation for the remainder of the sample became highly significant ($r = 0.65$, $p < 0.0001$). It was hypothesized that either some kind of tolerance may develop after many years exposure resulting in a nonlinear relation between duration of use and PN, or else that a linear relation between duration of use and PN would remain had more subjects using between 12 and 30 years been tested.

In this sample of ex-users the distribution of subjects having used between 3 and 20 years was reasonably even, with four of the 30 subjects having used for more than 12 years. Inclusion of these longer-term users also reduced the degree of the relation between duration of cannabis use

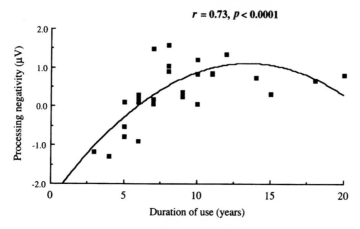

Figure 9.7 Mean amplitude of PN (μV) to pitch irrelevant tones as a two degree polynomial function of past duration of cannabis use in the ex-user group. (Reprinted by permission of Elsevier Science Inc. See Figure 9.2 for details.)

and PN. This result reinforces the hypothesis that the relation appears to be nonlinear, the turning point occurring at some point after having used cannabis for 12 years. This hypothesis was tested by fitting a second order polynomial (BMD-P5R).

As shown in Fig. 9.7, the curve appeared to fit the data very well, producing $r = 0.73$, $p < 0.0001$, with a remarkable "goodness of fit" (F(2,26) = 12.88, $p < 0.0001$). The same analysis was then applied to the data of Experiment 2 with similar results ($r = 0.64$, goodness of fit test: F(2,28) = 9.87, $p < 0.0006$).

The effects of the length of abstinence from cannabis were also explored in a correlational analysis. As shown in Fig. 9.8, there was no direct relation between the length of abstinence and PN to pitch irrelevant tones ($r = 0.09$). But abstinence cannot be examined in isolation, given the now well established effects of duration of use on PN. Nevertheless, removing the linear effects of duration of use in a partial correlational analysis had virtually no effect on the relation between abstinence and PN ($r = 0.10$). Similarly, removing any effect of abstinence did not change the relation between past duration of use and PN ($r = 0.51$, $p < 0.005$) for the entire sample.

While there was no relation between past duration of use and current length of abstinence ($r = 0.02$), a relation did exist between age and abstinence ($r = 0.36$, $p < 0.03$). Further partial correlational analyses (linear) were carried out as follows for the entire sample and for that portion of the

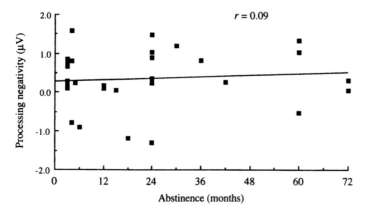

Figure 9.8 Mean amplitude of PN (μV) to pitch irrelevant tones as a function of length of abstinence from cannabis use.

sample having used for up to 12 years only ($n = 26$): the relation between duration of use and PN to pitch irrelevant tones in the attended ear remained after controlling for the effects of both abstinence and age ($r = 0.37, p < 0.02; n = 26, r = 0.60, p < 0.0005$); there was no relation between age and PN after removing the effects of duration and abstinence ($r = -0.15; n = 26, r = -0.004$); and there was no relation between abstinence and PN after removing the effects of duration and age ($r = 0.17; n = 26, r = -0.17$). PN was not related to alcohol consumption ($r = 0.11$).

The results of group multiple comparisons also showed PN to pitch relevant tones to be considerably smaller in this group of ex-users than in either current long or short-term users or controls. This was an unexpected finding as PN to relevant stimuli was not affected by cannabis use in the sample of current users of Experiment 2. In Experiment 1, early PN to relevant pitch stimuli was reduced in users between 200 and 300 ms only. The measure of PN from 300 to 600 ms in this experiment was for the purpose of comparing ex-cannabis users with groups from Experiment 2 on the processing of pitch irrelevant tones in the attended ear, since no differences between groups in Experiment 2 had occurred outside this range, nor had there been any group differences in PN to pitch relevant tones. In order to further explore the reduction in PN to pitch relevant tones in ex-users, mean amplitude measures over 100 ms intervals were analysed for ERPs to both relevant and irrelevant pitch tones in the attended ear.

When ex-users were compared with current long-term users, there was a trend toward greater negativity in the long-term users to both relevant and irrelevant pitch tones across almost the entire epoch ($p < 0.1$ for all but one 100 ms range from 200 to 300 ms). Differences between groups were significant over three ranges only: from 100 to 200 ms ($p < 0.05$), 300 to 400 ms ($p < 0.004$) and 500 to 600 ms ($p < 0.004$). The difference between groups in the 100–200 ms range suggests that N1 was smaller in ex-users than current long-term users. There were no interactions between stimulus and group, indicating that both PN to relevant and PN to irrelevant pitch tones were larger in current long-term users than in the ex-users.

In contrast, when ex-users were compared with controls, the only differences between groups appeared as stimulus by group interactions over three ranges: 300–400 ms ($p < 0.007$), 400–500 ms ($p < 0.04$) and 700–800 ms ($p < 0.03$). Multiple comparisons of each group for each stimulus revealed ex-users to have smaller PN to pitch relevant stimuli than controls only in the 300–400 ms range ($p < 0.03$), with nonsignificant trends in the same direction for the other two ranges, but also nonsignificant trends towards larger PN to pitch irrelevant stimuli in ex-users compared with controls.

Differences between ex-users and short-term cannabis users commenced at 300 ms and continued to the end of the epoch. From 300 to 400 ms there was a significant stimulus by group interaction ($p < 0.03$). From 500 ms onwards, there were significant interactions between stimulus, electrode and group for each 100 ms range to 1000 ms ($p < 0.04$). Group multiple comparisons for each stimulus at each scalp site revealed a multitude of effects.

From 300 to 400 ms, PN to pitch relevant tones was smaller for ex-users than short-term users ($p < 0.03$), but groups did not differ in PN to pitch irrelevant tones ($p > 0.7$). However, from 400 to 500 ms, ex-users showed significantly larger PN to the pitch irrelevant tones than short-term users at all frontal sites ($p < 0.02$), but not at Cz ($p > 0.1$). These effects are apparent in Fig. 9.2 where it can be seen that short-term users show a positive shift in the trace for irrelevant pitch stimuli at about 400 ms, while ex-users continue to process pitch irrelevant stimuli for longer, with continued negativity to 600 ms. From 500 to 600 ms there is a negative deflection in the irrelevant pitch trace in short-term users; there was a resultant lack of significant differences between groups in multiple comparisons for that range. In Fig. 9.2 it is clear that both long- and short-term cannabis users show a double negative peak in the PN to pitch irrelevant tones between 300 and 600 ms, with a positive shift occurring around 400 ms and then a negative deflection peaking between 500 and 600 ms. The ex-cannabis users show no evidence of such a double-peaked negativity, merely a prolonged negativity that appears to be smaller than that seen in current long-term users, but larger than that of controls. The finding that at least within a small range ex-users showed greater negativity to pitch irrelevant stimuli than short-term users but not controls is surprising, but probably reflects large variability in the results of both ex-users and controls. Beyond 600 ms, there were no significant effects from multiple comparisons, but there were trends toward smaller PN to pitch relevant tones in ex-users than short-term users, as well as greater negativity to pitch irrelevant tones in ex-users compared with current short-term users, at frontal sites continuing to 900 ms.

In summary, these results indicate that ex-users showed significantly smaller PN to relevant pitch stimuli than every other group (current long- and short-term users and controls) from 300 to 400 ms. From 400 to 500 ms, ex-users appeared to be more similar to current cannabis users in PN to irrelevant pitch stimuli than to controls.

PN to pitch relevant tones in the ex-user group was also investigated by correlational analysis. An inverse relation was found to exist between past duration of use and PN to relevant pitch stimuli ($r = -0.43$, $p < 0.02$), even though no such relation was found in the current user sample of Experiment 2 ($r = 0.24$). The relation observed here did not remain after controlling for the effects of age and abstinence ($r = 0.02$). Age was also inversely related to PN to pitch relevant tones ($r = -0.39$, $p < 0.04$), although the association weakened after removing the effects of duration and abstinence ($r = -0.26$, $p > 0.1$). Age and PN to pitch relevant tones were unrelated in the control group ($r = -0.04$). A relation was not initially apparent between the length of abstinence from cannabis and PN to relevant pitch tones ($r = 0.17$), but increased in strength after removing the effects of duration and age ($r = 0.32$, $p < 0.05$). The greater the duration of abstinence from cannabis, the larger the PN to relevant pitch tones (thus approaching normality). IQ was unrelated to PN to relevant pitch tones for either ex-users ($r = -0.09$) or controls ($r = 0.16$), and PN was unrelated to alcohol consumption ($r = 0.18$). There were no grounds for suspecting that any of these relations may be nonlinear.

Finally, the ex-users were compared with the groups of current users in Experiment 2 in their processing of long target tones by analysing the P300 component. P300 was measured as the most positive peak between 200 and 1000 ms at parietal scalp sites and was measurable in every subject in the ex-user group (no peak was detected in a number of subjects of Experiment 2 as described in Chapter 8). The ex-users did not differ from long-term cannabis users or controls in the amplitude or latency of the P300 component to targets ($p > 0.2$). Ex-users had a significantly smaller

P300 component over all parietal scalp sites than short-term cannabis users ($p < 0.04$) but they did not differ in latency from short-term users ($p > 0.3$). The possibility that the sample of controls may have had unrepresentatively small P300 components has been discussed in Chapter 8.

For thoroughness, the ex-users were also compared with the heavy user group of Experiment 2 as the latter had shown a marked delay in P300 latency. It was hypothesized that the observed delay was only temporary in nature and this was substantiated by a significant difference between ex-users and current heavy cannabis users of Experiment 2 ($p < 0.03$), and further by the analysis reported above where ex-users did not differ from controls in P300 latency.

Discussion

A number of factors arising from the statistical analyses of the ERP data from this sample of ex-users imply that the effects of long-term exposure to cannabis are similar to those established in the prior two experiments. The strong relationship between PN to pitch irrelevant tones and the past duration of cannabis use of this sample reflects that seen in Experiment 2 with current users. There is no evidence from correlational analysis that the length of abstinence has contributed to a resolution of large PN to pitch irrelevant stimuli. It is clear from the ERP plots of Fig. 9.2 and the graph of Fig. 9.3, and supported by the results of analyses of variance, that PN to the pitch irrelevant tones is smaller in this sample of ex-users than in the current long-term users of Experiment 2. This suggests that the cessation of cannabis use did in fact result in a reduction of the unusually large PN to irrelevant stimuli, even though no analysis was able to identify any relation between the length of abstinence and the degree of attenuation. It may be argued, therefore, that the attenuation occurs fairly rapidly, possibly within the same period of time that it takes to eliminate stored cannabinoids from the body, about 6–12 weeks. If this were the case, one would expect to see a dramatic improvement in the ERP signature of the processing of irrelevant information within the first 6–12 weeks following cessation of use, with no further slow or gradual improvements with increasing abstinence as was hypothesized.

Nevertheless, the reduction in PN observed here has not returned the ERP signature to the level of that in nonuser controls. Initial analyses prior to controlling for IQ, suggested that there was no difference in PN between ex-users and either short-term users or controls: this may be due to large variability in the ex-cannabis user group. In a report based on preliminary analyses of a subsample of the ex-cannabis users (the first 12 to volunteer for the experiment) (Solowij *et al.*, 1995c), the results showed the opposite effect: ex-users did not differ from long-term users in PN to pitch irrelevant tones ($F(1,22) = 0.19$, $p > 0.6$), but differed significantly from both short-term users ($F(1,22) = 5.59$, $p < 0.03$) and controls ($F(1,22) = 5.13$, $p < 0.03$). The reverse of these results with the larger sample emphasises the large variability within the sample of ex-users, and the need to investigate further the possibility that individual differences contribute to an increased susceptibility to cognitive impairment associated with long-term cannabis use. Clearly, for a portion of the sample studied here, there was no resolution of the inappropriately large PN to pitch irrelevant stimuli.

In an attempt to investigate possible contributory factors in an exploratory way, the ex-user sample was split at the median according to their PN response to pitch irrelevant stimuli and high responders were compared with low responders on all possible variables pertaining to subject characteristics, i.e. age, sex, education, IQ, duration and frequency of cannabis use, alcohol consumption, and a variety of test measures of anxiety and psychopathology as discussed in Chapter 11. The only variable which distinguished between the two groups was duration of cannabis use [11.0 vs 7.1 years: $F(1,26) = 9.59$, $p < 0.005$], as would be expected, and there was a trend for the high PN group to be older than the low PN group [29.6 vs 25.9, $p < 0.064$]. As age itself does not correlate with PN to pitch irrelevant tones, this result probably reflects the fact that older subjects are more likely to have used cannabis for a longer period than younger subjects. It is also possible that the large PN may be more likely to resolve with cessation of use in younger subjects. This analysis did not identify IQ as a factor distinguishing the high from the low responders, but the analysis of covariance for heterogeneous regression slopes (with IQ as the covariate) reported earlier showed that the majority of the sample did have significantly larger PN to complex irrelevant stimuli than the controls and suggested that those of higher IQ may be better able to compensate for the impairing effects of cannabis.

The finding that PN to relevant pitch stimuli was reduced in the ex-user group was unexpected; such a reduction was not previously found to be associated with the long-term use of cannabis. A small reduction in PN to relevant stimuli was seen in the cannabis users of Experiment 1 but had not replicated in Experiment 2. In this study, not only did ex-users show smaller PN to relevant pitch stimuli than controls, but also smaller PN than current cannabis users. It may be posited, therefore, that the *cessation* of cannabis use resulted not only in partial resolution of PN to irrelevant pitch stimuli for the majority of ex-users, but also a reduction in PN to stimuli of relevant pitch. The relation between PN to pitch relevant tones and length of abstinence implies a slow and gradual improvement with PN becoming increasingly larger over time. This interpretation hinges on the assumption that PN to pitch relevant stimuli in this sample of ex-users was as large prior to their having ceased using cannabis as that seen in all other groups studied. With cessation of cannabis use, PN to relevant tones may decrease dramatically, perhaps as a reaction to the withdrawal from cannabis.

Knight *et al.* (1981) reported that patients with dorsolateral frontal lesions showed less attention related negativity in a simple auditory selective attention task. It is possible that the observed reduction in PN to relevant attended stimuli here reflects some frontal dysfunction. Reduced PN to relevant pitch stimuli has also been demonstrated in schizophrenics (Michie *et al.*, 1990b; Ward *et al.*, 1991). These studies found PN to relevant pitch stimuli to be smaller in the early part of the epoch (100–200 ms), but primarily PN was smaller in the later part from 400 to 1000 ms, representing what they termed "late PN". The early PN reduction was correlated with both positive and negative schizophrenic symptom scores. These findings were interpreted as evidence of a number of deficiencies in the information processing strategies of schizophrenics, with an inability to set up an accurate attentional trace and then a failure to maintain it.

While the reduction found in PN to pitch relevant stimuli in the ex-cannabis user sample reported here is not entirely within the same range as that found in schizophrenics the pattern is similar. It is interesting to speculate on the possibility that similar to claims made about the use of cannabis by schizophrenics (e.g. Dixon *et al.*, 1990), cannabis users may be "self-medicating". It is possible that cannabis users experience certain psychopathological symptoms which they try to correct by using cannabis (or else their symptoms lead them to use cannabis). In doing so, they bring their attentional trace, represented by PN to relevant stimuli, up to "normality", perhaps by enhancing attentional mechanisms to all stimuli. This results not only in increased PN to relevant, but also increased PN to complex irrelevant stimuli, and as such does not enhance their ability to *selectively* attend, but merely to attend, to an extent, indiscriminately. When cannabis use is stopped, they return to their predrug level of less efficient attentional processing of relevant information, but also more efficient rejection, or lack of processing, of irrelevant information. Whether this is the case, it is interesting to speculate on these hypotheses.

An alternative explanation may be one based simply on withdrawal symptomatology: the abrupt, or even weaned, cessation of a psychoactive substance that has been used on a regular basis for many years, may result in disruption of various chemical systems in the brain with resultant impaired cognitive functioning. Any such withdrawal symptoms should not, however, be expected to endure for a very long time. The mean level of abstinence in the group was around 2 years; any withdrawal-like symptoms should well have dissipated by such time.

Yet another explanation similar to the withdrawal hypothesis may be based on learning theory. It may be that being under the influence of a psychoactive substance for many years, i.e. being chronically "stoned", enforces a learned compensation for the effects of the chronic intoxication. In this sense, the cannabis user has to put more resources into attending to complex stimuli. These extra resources may not be distributed in an appropriate manner and hence irrelevant stimuli are also accorded more resources, evident in their increased PN. This hypothesis cannot explain the reduction in PN to relevant pitch stimuli. Clearly, further research is required to replicate and elucidate these findings. The ideal study would be one that examined the same group of cannabis users before, immediately after stopping cannabis use and at various times thereafter but the practice effects of repeated testing sessions would need to be taken into account.

The other interesting finding from this study, which corroborated an hypothesis formed in Experiment 2, was that of a nonlinear relation between duration of cannabis use and PN to pitch irrelevant stimuli, as seen in Fig. 9.7. In both this sample of ex-users and in the sample of current cannabis users of Experiment 2, PN to pitch irrelevant tones appeared to increase in a linear manner with duration of cannabis use, up to approximately 12 years of use. Beyond 12 years use, the curve flattens asymptotically or may even revert to greater positivity with very long duration use. It is not possible to be certain about the nature of the relation beyond 12 years use given the small number of subjects contributing to that portion of the curve.

It is likely that there is a ceiling beyond which PN would not increase any further, particularly given the fact that PN is a measure of an electrophysiological response reflecting a cognitive process. This suggests that the curve would become asymptotic. If further research with more subjects confirmed a positive shift beyond 12 years' use, this may reflect a complex interaction between duration of cannabis use and increasing age. Although PN to pitch irrelevant tones appeared to increase with age in the control group of Experiment 2, others have reported PN to decrease with age in older samples, for example those above 50 years of age (e.g. Karayanidis *et al.*, 1995). This hypothesis of a complex relation between prolonged cannabis use and increasing age is consistent with other studies examining the interactions between cannabis and the glucocorticoid system of the brain, which suggests that cannabis use may accelerate brain aging (Landfield *et al.*, 1988; Eldridge *et al.*, 1992).

A further possibility to consider is that there may be something particular associated with use of cannabis beyond 12 years that contributes to this levelling of PN to pitch irrelevant stimuli. For example, if it is considered that the most common age for commencing regular use of cannabis is somewhere between 16 and 20 years of age, after 12 years use, one would be approximately 30 years of age. It is interesting to speculate on various factors associated with reaching that age, perhaps factors such as maturity and "settling down". There is evidence that most cannabis users discontinue their use in their mid to late twenties (Kandel & Logan, 1984; Kandel and Raveis, 1989). There may be something qualitatively different about those who continue to use through their thirties and later. Factors such as psychopathology and anxiety, while discussed to some extent in Chapter 11, may be worthy of further research in this regard. It is not known whether any of these factors would have the observed effects on PN.

Perhaps the simplest explanation of the reduction or stability of PN beyond 12 years use may be in the operation of an effect of natural selection: those who do not experience cognitive and other impairments would be those more likely to continue to use. Those who are consciously aware of experiencing problems associated with their use of cannabis are more likely to discontinue their use. Thus, the very long-term cannabis users who continue to use through their thirties and into their forties and beyond, may be those for whom cannabis use has either none or few adverse consequences. This group would be worthy of further investigation, as indeed are the individual differences that might lead to such stratification.

The finding of a relation between IQ and PN to irrelevant pitch stimuli in the control group but not in users or ex-users is also puzzling. Such a relationship has not previously been reported. It is possible that brighter subjects may find the task relatively easy and may allocate "spare" resources to processing other stimuli within the task purely to maintain some interest in the task, without compromising their performance in any way. Clearly, for the ex-users of this experiment and all cannabis users studied in previous experiments, large PN to pitch irrelevant stimuli accompanied poorer performance on the task and was therefore interpreted as reflecting an inefficient way of processing information, with unnecessary allocation of attentional resources to pitch irrelevant information. Furthermore, it is important to note that both current cannabis users of Experiment 2 and the ex-users studied here tended to have a lower mean IQ than the controls, but also showed larger PN to pitch irrelevant tones. If the effects were solely due to IQ differences, one would have expected the reverse, i.e. cannabis users should have showed smaller PN to pitch irrelevant tones than controls.

A further interpretation of these data may be in terms of a broadening of the attentional "spotlight" (Woods, 1989). It is possible that the use of a particular strategy broadens the attentional spotlight to include stimuli irrelevant to the task but sharing one or more close attributes with the relevant attended stimulus. It may be that the use of such a strategy varies as a function of IQ in the control group, but as a function of cumulative exposure to cannabis in the users. The use of such a strategy could reflect greater cognitive flexibility, which is exercised by bright controls with no resultant impairment in performance. For cannabis users and ex-users, such a cognitive style may be learned from the intoxicating experiences with cannabis or may come about following changes that occur in the brain as a result of cumulative exposure to cannabinoids. The altered cognitive style may indeed be a reason for using cannabis, i.e. for the experience of noticing more things (or being distractable). Whatever the reason, clearly for cannabis users and ex-users, unlike controls, the broadening of the attentional spotlight is accompanied by poorer performance.

A further finding corroborated in this experiment was that of possibly greater consequences of long-term cannabis use in users of low IQ. Although this may appear to be contrary to Soueif's (1976b) hypothesis that performance decrement is more marked in the best educated subjects, Soueif's hypothesis was formulated on the basis of comparing illiterate, rural subjects with educated urban dwellers. The subjects of this study were well educated, and those of lower IQ still within the high average range of IQ. This suggests, as argued above, that this finding should be interpreted in terms of the better ability of subjects of superior IQ to compensate for the impairing effects of cannabis on cognitive function.

In summary, the results of this experiment suggest that the long-term effects of cannabis on the ability to selectively focus attention and reject irrelevant information may *partially* recover with cessation of use for the majority of users (although, a subset of users appeared to show no recovery of function). There was sufficient evidence from this investigation that the past duration of cannabis use continued to have an adverse effect upon electrophysiology and cognition well after discontinuing use. The length of abstinence had no effect upon PN to pitch irrelevant tones or performance, and hence there was no gradual improvement over time. This suggests that partial recovery may occur rapidly following cessation of cannabis use. The relation between cumulative exposure to cannabis and PN to pitch irrelevant tones is robust. In Experiment 2, this relation was interpreted as being suggestive of gradual changes occurring in the brain as a result of prolonged exposure to cannabis. The fairly rapid partial recovery that is suggested to occur here following cessation of use, raises questions regarding the hypothesis that gradual changes occur in the brain, unless the nature of such changes permits rapid recovery. The apparent "partial recovery" may in fact simply be a function of the mean when a group of unrecovered ex-users are combined with a group of recovered ex-users. The mechanisms underlying the relationship between PN to irrelevant information and duration of cannabis use require further investigation, as do the individual differences that may contribute to recovery of cognitive function following cessation of cannabis use.

We have recently reported that verbal learning as measured by the RAVLT improved within weeks of cessation of cannabis use, but retention following interference remained significantly impaired 6 weeks after quitting (Solowij *et al.*, 1997). Impaired frontal lobe function, indicated by perseveration on the WCST, appeared to persist beyond the period of elimination of cannabinoids from the body and all measures were impaired more by the duration of cannabis use than by quantity/frequency measures.

Key findings

- *Thirty ex-cannabis users with a mean abstinence of 2 years (range 3 months to 6 years) performed the selective attention task while ERPs were recorded. Their results were compared with those of the current cannabis users and controls of the previous study*
- *The task performance of the ex-users appeared to fall between that of current users and controls. They made significantly fewer correct detections than controls*
- *There appeared to be a reduction in the inappropriately large PN to complex irrelevant stimuli such that the ex-users' response fell between that of current long-term users and controls. Initial analyses indicated no difference in PN between ex-users and controls, however, after controlling*

for IQ, 68% of the ex-users showed significantly larger PN to complex irrelevant stimuli than controls. This suggested that only those of higher IQ were able to compensate for the impairing effects of cannabis. Furthermore, a subsample of the ex-users (those who had the longest past history of use) did not differ in PN from current long-term users

- *PN to complex irrelevant information increased significantly as a function of the past duration of cannabis use, but was unrelated to the length of abstinence, indicating that recovery was not gradual*
- *These results suggest that a partial recovery may rapidly follow the cessation of cannabis use and that there are individual differences contributing to the long-term consequences of cannabis use and indeed to their recovery*
- *An exploration of a variety of personal and psychological variables found no relation with this ERP measure other than the number of years of past use of cannabis*
- *The P300 component to attended target stimuli did not differ from controls, supporting the hypothesis generated in the last study, that the slowing effect on the speed of information processing was indeed reversible following the elimination of cannabinoids from the body*
- *The enduring effects on PN imply that the cognitive consequences of cannabis use may not be entirely reversible*

10

A single case study of cessation of cannabis use

The question of whether cognitive impairments associated with long-term use of cannabis are reversible on cessation of use has not been entirely resolved. The previous experiment assessed event-related potential (ERP) measures of selective attention in a group of ex-cannabis users, examining the effects of past duration of use and the length of abstinence. The group result suggested partial recovery of function, but there was also evidence for individual differences in the extent of reversibility of impairment. A subset of the sample (those who had used for the greatest number of years) did not differ from the current long-term cannabis users of Experiment 2 in their ERP signature reflecting unnecessary processing of complex irrelevant information. The impairment was progressive with the number of years of use in both current users and ex-users, and ex-users showed no indication of gradual improvement with increasing abstinence. It was hypothesized that if partial recovery did occur, it must occur fairly rapidly upon cessation of use.

The previous study did not assess subjects before and after the cessation of cannabis use and therefore it is not known to what extent individual subjects showed the deficit in selective attention prior to giving up, or indeed what other factors might contribute to the manifestation or resolution of such an impairment. The present study therefore was designed to investigate in detail changes in cognitive functioning following cessation of cannabis use in an individual subject.

Experiment 4: a single case study of the effects of acute and chronic cannabis use and cessation of use on selective attention

A volunteer subject who had approached the research team for assistance in quitting his long-term use of cannabis was tested on the selective attention paradigm over multiple sessions prior to and for several weeks following the cessation of cannabis use. Previous normative research investigated the effect of repeat test sessions on ERPs using the same selective attention paradigm and showed that practice effects are apparent in the second test session but stabilize by the third, and that ERPs then remain essentially unchanged over 6 weeks of testing (Shelley *et al.*, 1991). Minor changes were confined mostly to ERPs to tones at the unattended location (becoming more positive) and there was some loss of late PN to the attended relevant pitch stimuli. No changes were seen in the irrelevant pitch ERP, which was the crucial one for this research. Prior to cessation, the individual's response to an acute dose of cannabis was examined. The acute effects of cannabis intoxication on the specific cognitive processes involved in this paradigm and their ERP signatures have never been investigated. It may be that the individual response to acute intoxication could predict both success at quitting and possibly the extent of recovery of functioning.

In order to facilitate the cessation of drug use, the subject was provided treatment in the form of supportive-expressive psychotherapy (Grenyer *et al.*, 1995). The treatment programme and outcome measures have been described elsewhere (Grenyer *et al.*, 1995; Solowij *et al.*, 1995a). The primary aims of the study reported here were to conduct a longitudinal investigation into whether cessation of cannabis use leads to a recovery in known deficits in selective attention and to investigate the effects of acute intoxication on ERP measures of selective attention.

Method

Subject

A 35 year old male with an 18 year history of daily cannabis use requested assistance in ceasing his drug use and volunteered to participate in research. He had commenced using cannabis at the age of 17 years, progressing immediately to regular use of approximately 6 g of cannabis per day (mostly potent "heads") on a near to daily basis up to the age of 28 years. He then went through a period of irregular use with an attempt at giving up but by the age of 30 had resumed heavy daily use. He claimed not to feel physically dependent on cannabis but defined a psychological dependence as a strong "urge to smoke" and irritability when unable to smoke. The subject gave the following reasons for his current desire to cease using cannabis: (1) he felt he had simply "had enough", as he knew that he was using cannabis in order to avoid dealing with life's problems and at this age he felt he should be doing better things with his life, and (2) he was concerned about the long-term effects of cannabis on mental functioning, having himself noticed difficulties with concentration, memory and motivation.

The subject had a minimal history of alcohol use, drinking at the level of two cans of beer per month for the past 15 years, and he currently smoked tobacco at approximately 10 cigarettes per day. He had dabbled in some experimental drug use between the ages of 18 to 21 years (e.g. amphetamines, cocaine, LSD) but had not used any drugs on a regular basis since that time. He met all the inclusion criteria for participation described for the previous experiments. He had completed 11 years of formal schooling and a trade certificate and was currently employed in a managerial position in the field of marketing. His full scale IQ as estimated by the NART was 120.

Procedure

The subject was required to attend three experimental test sessions prior to the date of intended cessation of cannabis use and a further three sessions after quitting at 1, 3 and 6 weeks post-cessation. The parameters of the selective attention task and ERP recording techniques were identical to those of Experiments 2 and 3. Three baseline test sessions were conducted in order to achieve a stable baseline eliminating practice effects. Daily urine samples were collected throughout the course of the study and analysed for the presence of cannabinoids in order to provide verification of abstinence, examine elimination curves and to correlate the levels of cannabinoid metabolites with ERP measures over time. A number of questionnaires monitoring psychopathology and withdrawal sequelae were administered over the course of the study. The results of these have been described elsewhere (Solowij *et al.*, 1995a). Changes in anxiety, depression and global severity of symptoms as assessed by the State-Trait Anxiety Inventory (Spielberger *et al.*, 1970), the Beck Depression Inventory (BDI) (Beck, 1987) and the Symptom Checklist 90-R (Derogatis, 1983), respectively, will be briefly reported here as some of these measures are discussed further in association with cannabis use in Chapter 11.

Following the second pre-quit test session, the subject returned to the laboratory after having smoked two "joints" and was then tested in the acutely intoxicated state. The subject provided a sample of the cannabis he

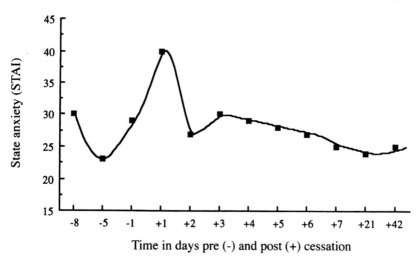

Time in days pre (-) and post (+) cessation

Figure 10.1 State anxiety (STAI-1) scores over time. (Adapted from Solowij, N., Grenyer, B.F.S., Chesher, G. & Lewis, J., 1995. Reprinted by permission of Elsevier Science Inc.)

had smoked for analysis which revealed a high potency of 17% tetrahydrocannabinol (THC). It is estimated from the subject's description of the two joints, that he had consumed approximately 1.5 g of cannabis prior to this acute test session.

Results

Clinical assessments

At intake the subject scored 0.57 on the SCL-90-R global severity index (GSI) (63rd percentile) indicating a level of functioning non-significantly worse than the mean of the normal adult male population (0.33). On the BDI his depression score was 18, indicating significant clinical depression, well above the accepted cut off of 13. His anxiety was also elevated with trait anxiety at 42 (68th percentile). His state anxiety at the time of initial consultation, however, was relatively low at 30 (28th percentile), indicating that he felt comfortable in the clinical setting.

The subject was successful in quitting his use of cannabis with the help of psychotherapy. By 6 weeks post-cessation, his SCL-90-R GSI score was 0.14 (48th percentile) which indicates low distress from symptoms. Changes in state anxiety and depression over the course of the study are depicted in Figs 10.1 and 10.2. State anxiety reached a peak on the day

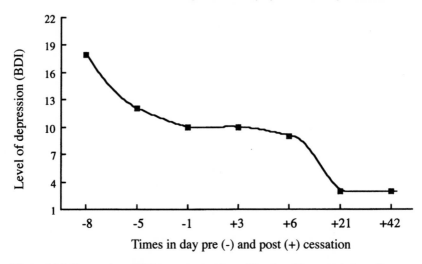

Figure 10.2 Depression (BDI) scores over time. (Reprinted by permission of Elsevier Science Inc. See Figure 10.1 for details.)

following cessation of cannabis use, which coincided with a major argument in his relationship (score of 40, 70th percentile). The particular psychotherapy employed in this study, supportive-expressive dynamic psychotherapy (see Grenyer *et al.*, 1995) was very useful for helping the subject through this period as it focuses on interpersonal conflicts and the way these relate to the use of drugs. Anxiety fell off in slow decrements over the week following cessation and was continuing to decline 3 weeks later. The subject clearly responded quickly to the onset of treatment with his depression score falling into the mild range (above 7) at the time of cessation, and dropping further to a nonsignificant level at 3 weeks post-cessation. Although these improvements in psychological state are inextricably tied with the provision of treatment, their relation to cannabis use is further discussed in Chapter 11.

Performance data

The subject's performance on the selective attention task is depicted in Figs 10.3 and 10.4. From Fig. 10.3, a general practice effect can be seen to operate independently of cannabis use or its cessation. The number of correct detections or "hit rate" was quite high over the course of the study and showed general improvement over time, ranging from 79.6% in the first test session to 95.4% in the third test session post-quitting. The lowest hit rate was obtained in the acute test session, but at 78.2% performance

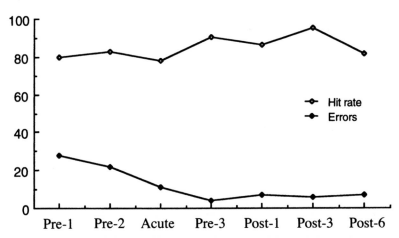

Figure 10.3 Task performance over time, depicting the percentage correct detections (hit rate) and the number of errors of commission. (Reprinted by permission of Elsevier Science Inc. See Figure 10.1 for details.)

was not very impaired by intoxication. This is also clear from the number of errors of commission which was quite low at 11 for the acute test session, and showed a gradual decline over time from the first test session through the course of the study. This trend toward improved performance on the task cannot be attributed to the cessation of cannabis use but only to a general practice effect. The reaction time data depicted in Fig. 10.4 also reflect a practice effect with no change as a result of cessation of cannabis use, but reaction time was markedly delayed in the acute test session (by about 140 ms). Taken together with the other performance data, this suggests greater caution in responding while intoxicated rather than any marked impairment on the task.

ERP data

Figure 10.5 depicts ERPs to short tones of relevant and irrelevant pitch in the attended ear (L+) and unattended ear (L−) recorded from the frontal midline electrode (Fz) for each of the baseline pre-quit test sessions, the acute test session and the three post-quit test sessions. The ERP pattern shown by this subject in the three pre-quit test sessions is typical of that seen in long-term cannabis users: a negative shift of the ERP to L+ irrelevant pitch tones is indicative of unnecessary processing of, or an inability to reject, these complex irrelevant stimuli.

Inspection of the plots suggests that neither the L+ irrelevant pitch

Single case study of cessation of cannabis use

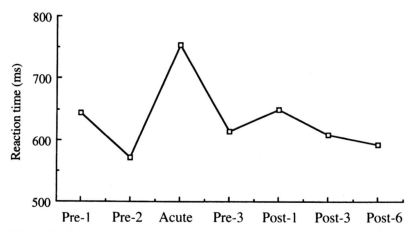

Figure 10.4 Reaction time (ms) to correctly detected target tones depicted for each test session. (Reprinted by permission of Elsevier Science Inc. See Figure 10.1 for details.)

ERP nor the L+ relevant pitch ERP appeared to change in any substantial manner over the course of the study, either prior to quitting or after cessation of cannabis use. Processing negativity (PN) was evident in the L+ irrelevant pitch ERP, ie. it remained negatively shifted toward the L+ relevant pitch ERP, in every post-quitting test session without any indication of resolution with increasing abstinence. PN in the L+ irrelevant pitch trace was most prominent within the range from 300 to 600 ms, consistent with that seen in the previous experiments with current long-term and ex-cannabis users.

The two L− ERPs showed the greatest change over time, shifting negatively toward baseline. Clearly not associated with cessation from cannabis use (as it was apparent already from pre-quit session two), this shift could be interpreted as reflecting less effortful rejection of tones in the unattended ear due to practice. This, together with the increasingly large positive P2 component observed around 200 ms, is consistent with normative research (Shelley *et al.*, 1991). The development of the P2 component can be seen also in the L+ irrelevant pitch ERP, particularly in the post-cessation sessions, but the trace quickly becomes negative again with large PN evident from 300 to 600 ms. There was no evidence in this trace of a positive shift towards baseline over time which would reflect more efficient rejection of irrelevant pitch tones. The time course of effects is most clearly seen in Fig. 10.6 which depicts the mean amplitude measure from 300 to 600 ms for each ERP trace in each test session. The lack of changes

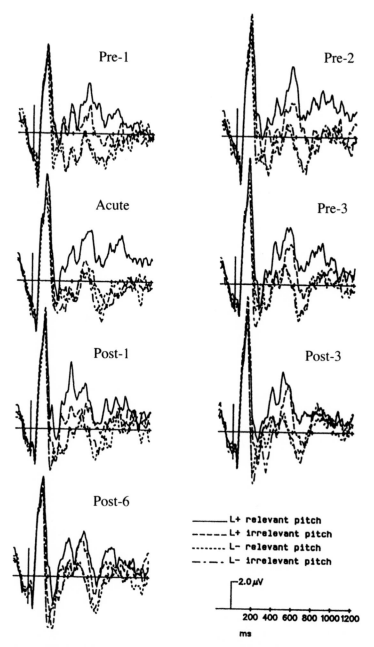

Figure 10.5 Brain event-related potentials (ERPs) to short tones of relevant and irrelevant pitch in the attended ear (L+) and unattended ear (L−) recorded from a frontal midline electrode (Fz) during three pre-quit test sessions, a test session under acute cannabis intoxication, and three post-quit test sessions at 1, 3 and 6 weeks post-cessation of cannabis use. (Reprinted by permission of Elsevier Science Inc. See Figure 10.1 for details.)

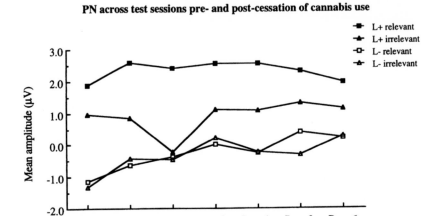

Figure 10.6 Processing negativity (μV) measured over time as the mean amplitude from 300 to 600 ms in ERPs to relevant and irrelevant pitch tones in the attended (L+) and unattended ear (L−). (Reprinted by permission of Elsevier Science Inc. See Figure 10.1 for details.)

pre- and post-cessation in the two L+ ERPs is evident from this figure, as is the gradual negative shift of the two L− ERPs. The figure also depicts the dramatic effect observed under acute intoxication, discussed below. Figure 10.7 shows the elimination curve for cannabinoid metabolites in urine. By 3 weeks of abstinence the level of the THC-COOH metabolite fell below 20 ng/ml and remained at this low level to the end of the study. Correlational analysis confirmed no relation between PN to L+ irrelevant pitch tones across time and the level of metabolite in urine ($r = -0.13$).

The ERPs recorded in the acute test session showed a striking result. As mentioned above, the acute effects of cannabis on ERPs in a complex selective attention task have not previously been examined. From Figs 10.5 and 10.6 it can be seen that there was a dramatic positive shift toward baseline in the L+ irrelevant pitch ERP. The negativity of the L+ relevant pitch ERP appeared enhanced. This pattern showing large separation between the relevant and irrelevant pitch ERPs, is typical of that seen in nonuser controls. Thus, the acute intoxication may have served to "normalize" the processing of complex information in this selective attention task for this individual. Contrary to what might have been expected, there was no indication of any abnormality or impaired processing observed in the ERPs recorded in the acutely intoxicated state and this was consistent with the performance data showing greater caution with a high hit rate and few errors.

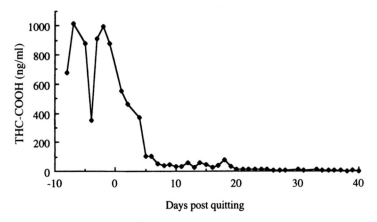

Figure 10.7 Elimination curve for the cannabinoid metabolite THC-COOH (ng/ml) measured in daily urine samples before ($-$) and after ($+$) cessation of cannabis users. (Reprinted by permission of Elsevier Science Inc. See Figure 10.1 for details.)

Unfortunately, any effects on the P300 component to targets were not examinable as this component was absent from the ERP signature of this individual in both intoxicated and unintoxicated states and hence unmeasurable.

Discussion

The first aim of this study was to investigate whether cessation of cannabis use leads to a recovery in known deficits in selective attention. No recovery of function was apparent in this individual over 6 weeks of abstinence. The second aim was to investigate the effects of acute intoxication on selective attention. It appeared that intoxication actually "normalized" information processing in this individual. While caution should be observed when making conclusions based on data from a single case study, these results are nevertheless interesting.

Contrary to the partial recovery of cognitive functioning suggested by the overall group result of the ex-cannabis users of Experiment 3, the individual studied here showed no trend toward resolution of the large negativity in the ERP to irrelevant pitch tones in the attended ear. In Experiment 3 it was hypothesized that if partial recovery does occur, it must occur fairly rapidly on cessation of use. There was no evidence of this in the current study, thus favouring the hypothesis that there are individual differences in predisposition toward cognitive impairments associated with cannabis use and indeed their recovery. The data from the individual studied here were in accord with the subsample of ex-cannabis users of Experiment 3, who had a long history of use and showed no recovery of function. A current replication study with a large sample is monitoring ERPs over a period longer than 6 weeks post-cessation to see if there is indeed any recovery of function beyond this time (N. Solowij *et al.*, unpublished results).

The finding of an apparent correction of the ERP pattern following an acute dose of cannabis was surprising. This suggests that cannabis may serve to normalize information processing in highly dependent individuals. Indeed, anecdotally, many such individuals report smoking cannabis in order "to feel normal again". It may be that long-term cannabis users gradually develop the pattern of large PN to complex irrelevant information, observed here and in all previous studies, over many years of exposure to cannabis and that perhaps this becomes the "norm" in their style of information processing in the unintoxicated state. Whether this reflects a learned or compensatory phenomenon, or a physiological or biochemical alteration is open to speculation. One very speculative hypothesis regarding the mechanisms involved is that prolonged exposure to cannabis may either deplete levels of anandamide in the brain or disrupt their normal function, but a single dose of cannabis temporarily restores the deficit by binding to the receptor. Whatever the mechanism, a single acute dose of cannabis in this individual reversed the large and inappropriate PN to pitch irrelevant tones, resulting in greater caution in responding, more focused attention and the facilitation of rejection of complex irrelevant information in the demanding auditory selective attention task utilized in this research.

As reviewed in Chapter 6, some early research in the 1970s reported that cannabis may facilitate "tuning out" of environmental input (e.g. Roth *et al.*, 1973) and some even suggested that brain mechanisms subserving attention may be enhanced by cannabis at low doses (e.g. Kopell *et al.*, 1972; Low *et al.*, 1973). The effects of cannabis on CNV amplitude were reported to be dose-dependent or subjective "high"-dependent (Kopell *et al.*, 1972; Low *et al.*, 1973; Braden *et al.*, 1974), but also to interact with task difficulty (Herning *et al.*, 1979). The effect of orally ingested THC or smoked cannabis on CNV amplitude was in the form of an inverted U; this was interpreted as low dose THC (or below average subjective high) improving interest in a simple, yet boring task or perhaps producing a compensatory effort to concentrate, neither of which could be sustained at high dose or above average subjective high, or in more complex or demanding tasks. The specific effect observed here on ERPs to the pitch irrelevant tones in the attended ear, with no effect on ERPs to other tones, suggests that THC was not reducing attention to the environment in general but did appear to be facilitating the selectivity of attention. The task employed in the studies reported throughout this book was a complex and demanding one, and the dose contained in the cannabis cigarettes smoked by the subject was estimated to be approximately 255 mg, substantially higher than the high doses used in the acute studies of the 1970s (generally 10 mg). The subject's history of cannabis use would have made him more tolerant to the effects of cannabis than the subjects of the early research, but the estimated dose consumed was proportionally far greater, and he nevertheless reported an average to slightly above average high. Other studies have reported generally decreased amplitudes of visual, auditory and somatosensory evoked potential components and reduced CNV amplitudes following low and high doses of THC (e.g. Lewis *et al.*, 1973; Roth *et al.*, 1973; Herning *et al.*, 1979), but this general reduction cannot explain the selectivity of the effect observed here: PN to relevant pitch stimuli was not reduced in amplitude. Clearly further research is required to replicate and clarify the effect and its underlying mechanisms.

A specific effect on selective attention similar to that observed here was reported to occur following the administration of naloxone, an opiate antagonist (Arnsten *et al.*, 1983; 1984). Arnsten and colleagues found that naloxone augmented selective attention by positively shifting unattended ERP waveforms to easily discriminable stimuli. As here, this was interpreted as more effective rejection of irrelevant stimuli, either through a narrowing of the focus of attention or through a decrease in distractibility. In contrast to the effect on PN to difficult to discriminate (complex irrelevant pitch) stimuli reported here, Arnsten's facilitatory effect was limited to easily discriminable stimuli in a somewhat more simplistic auditory selective attention task. The authors discussed an endogenous opioid role in the regulation of selective attention, citing the density of naloxone binding sites in prefrontal cortex and an involvement of the noradrenergic system. It is likely that ingested cannabinoids interact with these systems (see Chapter 4), but it is also probable, as proposed in Chapters 8 and 12 that the endogenous cannabinoid system is itself involved in the modulation of attention.

This hypothesis is supported by an elegant series of recent animal studies which demonstrated uncoupling of the cannabinoid receptor from G proteins following prolonged administration of THC (Sim *et al.*, 1996), and investigated cannabinoid effects on hippocampal function in short-term memory tasks (Heyser *et al.*, 1993; Hampson *et al.*, 1996; see Chapter 4). From this research it is proposed that endogenous cannabinoids may be selectively associated with blockade of hippocampal cell activation during the encoding phase of certain memory tasks (Sim *et al.*, 1996; S.A. Deadwyler, personal communication). Endogenous cannabinoids may participate in the process of selective elimination of information when it no longer is of value, or at the encoding stage by ensuring that information is encoded "weakly" and therefore would decay or become inaccessible in a shorter period of time (S.A. Deadwyler, personal communication). Hampson & Deadwyler (1996a) reported a hippocampal mechanism of this kind, which would be vulnerable to exogenous cannabinoid mediated interference as demonstrated in the delayed match to sample tasks of their earlier research (Heyser *et al.*, 1993). If information such as that presented on a single trial of a delayed match to sample task were encoded too strongly, it would persist for a longer period of time and hence be at greater risk to proactively interfere (S.A. Deadwyler, personal communication). Thus, in a nontolerant animal or human, endogenous or exogenous cannabinoid agonists would serve to facilitate performance on such a task by removing the tendency to remember information for too long, i.e. they might clear the buffer so that residual information would not contaminate the new sample information on the next trial (S.A. Deadwyler, personal communication). Terranova *et al.* (1996) had shown facilitation of performance on a short-term memory task by administration of an antagonist (SR141716A). The task used (not a delayed match to sample task) had a high degree of proactive or retroactively useful information, and thus the presence of endogenous (or exogenous) cannabinoids under normal conditions might have prevented the full benefit of information carried over from one trial to the next being realized (S.A. Deadwyler, personal communication).

As an agonist, THC activates the cannabinoid receptor to produce an effect similar to but more exaggerated and distorted than that of the endogenous cannabinoids, with selective elimination of information occurring at an inappropriate time (see Chapter 4). THC activates cannabinoid receptors constantly in a nondynamic fashion which ultimately leads to a pharmacological disconnection of the hippocampus. In a tolerant individual, a much greater dose is required to achieve essentially the same result. Thus, the acute effect of high dose THC on the ERPs of the subject reported here may reflect the greater facilitation of selective elimination of information (rejection of complex irrelevant information from further processing). In this particular selective attention task, as in delayed match to sample tasks, a mechanism of this sort may well be adaptive, in contrast to the continued rehearsal and consolidation of information crucial to so many other memory tasks. This may also explain why over the years there have been so many equivocal findings in human cognitive studies of long-term cannabis users which have all used a vast array of cognitive tasks.

In not just a tolerant user, but a regular user of 18 years, it is difficult to predict the long-term impact of the uncoupling of the cannabinoid receptor from G proteins and the changes in its downstream effectors. No doubt future research will aim to elucidate this. Clearly, however, the function of the endogenous cannabinoid system would be severely compromised, with possible loss of regulation of transmitter release being manifested as if there were less endogenous cannabinoids available to perform their normal functions. This would explain the inability to selectively reject complex irrelevant information in the unintoxicated state in the (tolerant) long-term cannabis users observed in this series of studies. Thus, a single acute dose of cannabis administered to a long-term cannabis user (both tolerant and dependent) may still be interpreted as "normalizing" this state of dysfunction. However, a final caveat to this interpretation of the ERP pattern under acute intoxication rests with inspection of acute effects of THC on the P300 component to targets. This component reflects the allocation of attentional resources and stimulus evaluation strategies and may well be affected by the acute administration of cannabis to chronic users in ways that might also be contrary to expectation. Any such effects were unexaminable in the individual reported here due to the complete absence of a definable P300 component in his waveforms in every recording session. A current replication study using a cohort of long-term cannabis users wanting to quit and a nondependent control group of limited experience with cannabis aims to further investigate these phenomena (N. Solowij *et al.*, unpublished results). Information gained from this research may contribute toward a general theory of drug use, particularly if the drug does serve to normalize functioning once dependent on it. It is also interesting to speculate on whether the acute effect observed here and the proposed role of endogenous cannabinoids may be consistent with anecdotal evidence that cannabis users often play computer games and engage in other focused or repetitive activities for extended periods while intoxicated. These phenomena have appeared to be at odds with other well known acute effects of cannabis, such as distractibility and lack of concentration, but are worthy now of further investigation incorporating the models described above (the performance of many computer games would no doubt be facilitated by selective forgetting of events that might proactively interfere with progress on a fast moving game).

Key findings

• *The ERPs of an individual long-term cannabis user were examined over repeated test sessions prior to and for 6 weeks following the cessation of long-term cannabis use*

• *The subject was given supportive-expressive dynamic psychotherapy to facilitate quitting cannabis use, and depression, anxiety and psychological symptomatic distress were monitored over time*

• *Prior to quitting the subject showed the characteristic ERP pattern of inappropriately large PN to complex irrelevant stimuli. The P300 component was totally absent from this subject's ERP signature and therefore unmeasurable*

• *There was no change in PN to complex irrelevant stimuli in the 6 weeks following cessation of cannabis use and thus no indication of any recovery of function in this individual*

• *These results support the hypothesis that there are large individual differences in predisposition to recovery from the long-term cognitive effects of cannabis*

• *Prior to quitting, the subject performed the selective attention task while acutely intoxicated. Intoxication with cannabis resulted in an apparent dramatic normalization of the large PN to complex irrelevant stimuli*

• *Caution must be observed when interpreting data from a single subject but these interesting results warrant further investigation in a larger sample*

11
Anxiety, psychopathology and the qualitative experience of long-term use of cannabis

The cannabis users and ex-users studied in each experiment reported here completed a number of questionnaires. These assessed levels of anxiety, symptoms of psychopathology and dependence on cannabis and provided an opportunity for the self report of any problems associated with long-term cannabis use. A qualitative description of the experience of long-term cannabis use was obtained through structured and open-ended questionnaires.

The inclusion of these assessments was important for two reasons: (1) to exclude the possibility that the event-related potential (ERP) findings might reflect some psychological differences between users and nonusers rather than being the result of cannabis use, with anxiety and psychopathology judged to be the most likely candidates, and (2) to examine the consistency between self reported symptoms of dependence, subjective effects and cognitive failure and the results obtained from assessment of cognitive functioning by means of ERP measures of selective attention.

This chapter will present descriptive summaries of the results of all questionnaires administered, provide results of quantitative analyses where appropriate and discuss the qualitative experience of long-term cannabis use. The results from each sample from each experiment will be discussed separately but also combined across studies where appropriate. Correlations between test measures and the ERP results of each study will be presented where appropriate. The ERP measures used in correlational analysis were PN to pitch irrelevant tones measured over 300 to 600 ms at frontal and central sites, which reflects the unnecessary processing of complex irrelevant information, and P300 latency measured at the contralateral parietal scalp site, as a measure of stimulus evaluation time, or the speed of information processing. Wherever possible, the results were considered in terms of frequency and duration of cannabis use.

Anxiety

Many drug using populations have been reported to show higher levels of anxiety than the general population (e.g. Meyer, 1986; Ross *et al.*, 1988; Rounsaville, 1989; Rounsaville *et al.*, 1991; Grenyer *et al.*, 1992). Also, high anxiety levels are known to influence cognitive test performance in an adverse manner. For example, high levels of anxiety have been shown to reduce both the storage and processing capacity of working memory (Darke, 1988). High anxiety may be reflected in an inability to maintain attentional focus on a particular stimulus or task in the presence of extraneous stimuli. Eysenck (1982, 1988) argued that highly anxious subjects engage in significantly more task-irrelevant processing than their low anxiety counterparts. Task irrelevant thoughts, which are thought to characterize highly test anxious individuals, may be symptomatic of an underlying distractibility to various sources of interference, both internal and external. Therefore, it was considered essential to assess anxiety levels in these cannabis using samples.

The State-Trait Anxiety Inventory (STAI) (Spielberger *et al.*, 1970) was selected as the assessment tool as it has been widely used for research purposes, has demonstrated reliability and validity, and provides two measures of anxiety pertinent to the purposes of this assessment. First, it provides a measure of the current state of the individual in terms of the level of transitory anxiety at the time the questionnaire was completed. This enables an assessment of whether subjects may have been anxious as a result of the testing procedure. If it were found that cannabis users' state anxiety was significantly higher than that of controls, it could be conjectured that users were significantly more anxious than controls as a result of the testing procedure and hence may have performed more poorly than controls as a result of this anxiety. Second, a measure of trait anxiety provides an assessment of the general level of background anxiety with which an individual operates in normal life, and their disposition toward being anxiety prone, regardless of the current state of the subject or the testing procedure. This measure enables a comparison of resting levels of anxiety in cannabis using samples versus controls to determine whether users may be generally more anxious than controls. A further measure of trait anxiety, useful for reliability purposes, was provided by the Anxiety subscale of the Symptom Checklist 90-Revised (SCL-90-R) (Derogatis, 1983). Composed of nine subscales, the SCL-90-R was administered as a measure of psychopathology and is discussed further below.

Mean STAI scores for subjects of Experiments 1, 2 and 3 are presented

Table 11.1 *Mean state–trait anxiety scores (and SD) for cannabis users, ex-users and controls*

	n	State	Trait
Experiment 1			
Cannabis users	10	35.20 (7.18)	40.10 (8.37)
Controls	10	27.90 (3.73)	29.60 (6.40)
Experiment 2			
Cannabis users overall	32	34.56 (6.48)	36.91 (7.66)
Long-term users	16	33.31 (5.45)	38.88 (9.29)
Short-term users	16	35.81 (7.32)	34.94 (5.16)
Heavy users	16	37.00 (5.96)	40.44 (7.77)
Light users	16	32.13 (6.21)	33.38 (5.85)
Controls	16	33.94 (9.45)	34.94 (5.27)
Experiment 3			
Ex-cannabis users	28	33.54 (6.71)	38.39 (9.53)

in Table 11.1. All scores obtained were comparable to the normative data of undergraduate students (Spielberger *et al.*, 1970), with the exception perhaps of the control group of Experiment 1 whose scores fell within the lower range, at around the 20th percentile for both state and trait measures.

Scores were subjected to an analysis of variance with factors of group and anxiety type (state or trait). For the samples of Experiment 1, there was a significant main effect of group ($F(1,18) = 12.54$, $p < 0.003$) and a near significant main effect of anxiety type ($F(1,18) = 4.35$, $p < 0.0515$), but no group by anxiety type interaction ($p > 0.3$). Thus, cannabis users were significantly more anxious than controls on both state and trait levels of anxiety. The near significant main effect of anxiety type indicated that trait levels tended to be higher than state levels for both groups. When the groups were analysed separately, state–trait anxiety did not differ in controls ($p > 0.4$), but trait levels in cannabis users were significantly higher than their state levels ($F(1,9) = 5.36$, $p < 0.05$). This indicates that the cannabis users were generally more anxious than controls, but their lower state scores suggest that they were not more anxious than controls as a result of the testing procedure. Due to the relatively small sample size of Experiment 1, any relations between anxiety and ERP measures were not examined.

The cannabis users of Experiment 2 showed a similar pattern of results to those of Experiment 1, although overall group differences diminished due to the higher scores of the control group. Overall, cannabis users did not differ from controls ($p > 0.4$), mean levels of state and trait anxiety over both groups did not differ ($p > 0.1$), and there was no group by anxiety type interaction ($p > 0.5$). Similarly groups based on duration of use did not differ overall ($p > 0.7$) and there was no main effect of anxiety type ($p > 0.1$), but there was a trend toward a group by anxiety type interaction ($p < 0.07$), suggestive of higher trait than state anxiety in both long-term users and controls, but nonsignificantly higher state than trait anxiety in short-term users. There were no differences between these groups when state and trait anxiety were analysed separately [state $p > 0.6$; trait $p > 0.1$].

A significant group difference emerged when groups were compared on the basis of frequency of use (F(2,45) = 4.98, $p < 0.02$). Group multiple comparisons determined that heavy users had significantly greater anxiety levels overall than both light users ($p < 0.001$) and controls ($p < 0.05$). Light users did not differ from controls ($p > 0.4$). There was no main effect of anxiety type ($p > 0.1$) and no group by anxiety type interaction ($p > 0.6$). However, analyses of state and trait anxiety separately confirmed that the group differences were significant only for trait anxiety (F(2,45) = 5.39, $p < 0.008$), whereas groups did not differ in terms of state anxiety (F(2,45) = 1.79, $p > 0.1$).

These results were corroborated by analysis of the anxiety subscale of the SCL-90-R (see below), where heavy users scored significantly higher than both light users (F(1,30) = 8.04, $p < 0.008$) and controls (F(1,30) = 5.56, $p < 0.03$), and light users did not differ from controls ($p > 0.4$). Overall, cannabis users did not score significantly higher than controls ($p > 0.3$) and groups did not differ in anxiety on the basis of duration of use ($p > 0.5$).

The ex-cannabis users of Experiment 3 were compared with long and short-term users and controls of Experiment 2. The ex-users did not differ from any group on either state or trait anxiety scores (state $p > 0.3$; trait $p > 0.1$).

Correlational analyses found no relation to exist between duration of cannabis use in the current users of Experiment 2 and either state ($r = -0.12$) or trait anxiety ($r = -0.12$) as measured by the STAI. Similarly, past duration of cannabis use in the ex-user sample did not correlate with state ($r = -0.22$) or trait anxiety ($r = -0.15$). As might be expected on the basis of the results reported above, the frequency of cannabis use in current users was significantly related to trait anxiety ($r = 0.44$, $p < 0.01$)

but not state anxiety ($r = 0.29$). A similar relation was evident in the sample of ex-users (trait: $r = 0.31$, $p < 0.05$; state: $r = 0.17$). Interestingly, while state and trait anxiety were highly correlated in the control group ($r = 0.78$, $p < 0.0001$) and in the ex-user group ($r = 0.55$, $p < 0.005$), the relation was nonexistent in current cannabis users ($r = 0.19$). This finding is difficult to interpret but may reflect either inconsistencies in self reported anxiety levels in cannabis users, or a different mode of operation of anxiety in cannabis using populations. The latter hypothesis is given credence by the some of the differential relations found between anxiety levels and performance measures for cannabis using and nonusing groups, as reported below.

An unexpected finding was that both measures of anxiety were inversely related to PN to pitch irrelevant tones in the control group (state: $r = -0.56$, $p < 0.005$; trait: $r = -0.49$, $p < 0.01$). Thus, PN to pitch irrelevant tones was smaller with higher levels of anxiety. This finding suggests that increased anxiety may have actually improved the ability to focus attention by tuning in to the relevant stimuli and rejecting irrelevant stimuli more efficiently. This is contrary to Eysenck's hypothesis that highly anxious subjects engage in significantly more task irrelevant processing; however, it may be that there is an optimum level of anxiety which boosts performance, beyond which performance deteriorates, i.e. it is reasonable to assume that a certain amount of anxiety generated by motivation to do well on any given task and not reflect badly upon the self would be useful and advantageous as opposed to a lack of concern with one's performance (similar to the Yerkes-Dodson law). If anxiety levels were to exceed these hypothetical optimal levels, this might result in significant processing of task irrelevant thoughts and stimuli. There is no reason to suspect that the levels of anxiety measured in any group of this series of studies were excessive and as such would not be expected to affect their performance. Thus, the finding of large PN to pitch irrelevant tones in long-term cannabis users cannot be explained by increased anxiety levels. In fact, users also showed a marginally significant inverse relation between PN to pitch irrelevant tones and state anxiety ($r = -0.33$, $p < 0.06$) but no relation with trait anxiety ($r = 0.02$), and PN in ex-users showed no relation with either state ($r = -0.21$) or trait ($r = -0.05$) levels of anxiety. The reduced PN to pitch relevant tones in the ex-users could not be explained by anxiety levels either as there was no relationship with either state ($r = 0.17$) or trait ($r = 0.16$) anxiety.

P300 latency, which increased as a function of frequency of cannabis use in current users was also found not to be significantly related to levels of state anxiety ($r = 0.10$), and a nonsignificant trend toward longer latency P300 with greater trait anxiety ($r = 0.25$) disappeared after controlling for the effect of frequency of cannabis use ($r = 0.06$). In controls there was a trend toward a reduction in P300 latency with increasing levels of state anxiety ($r = -0.34$, $p > 0.05$) but no relation with trait anxiety ($r = 0.02$). P300 amplitude did not vary as a function of anxiety in any group (range $r = -0.23$ to 0.12).

Reaction time in the current cannabis users increased as a function of state anxiety ($r = 0.40$, $p < 0.05$) but not trait anxiety ($r = 0.26$), whereas for ex-users and controls there were trends in the opposite direction (ex: state $r = -0.23$, trait $r = -0.21$; controls: $r = -0.26$, trait $r = -0.35$). There was no relation between anxiety and number of correct detections in the cannabis users (state: $r = 0.01$; trait: $r = -0.16$) or ex-users (state: $r = 0.04$; trait: $r = -0.16$), although for controls there was a trend toward poorer performance with increasing anxiety (state: $r = -0.32$; trait: $r = -0.31$). The most striking difference between groups was in the relation between anxiety and the number of errors of commission (false alarms). Neither state nor trait anxiety correlated with false alarm rate in the cannabis users (state: $r = 0.08$; trait: $r = -0.01$) or ex-users (state: $r = 0.04$; trait: $r = -0.07$), but in controls the number of false alarms increased dramatically as a function of state anxiety ($r = 0.76$, $p < 0.0001$), and to a lesser degree with trait anxiety ($r = 0.58$, $p < 0.01$). These results are difficult to interpret and suggest that anxiety may operate in different ways in cannabis users and controls. Nevertheless, the finding that the false alarm rate is correlated with state anxiety in controls but not in ex-users or current users lends credence to the ERP interpretation of a long-term effect due to past use of cannabis.

The results of these investigations suggest that cannabis users were not more anxious than controls as a result of the testing procedure. Therefore, the differences found between groups on measures of test performance and efficiency of information processing are more likely to reflect the effects of long-term cannabis use and not be due to higher levels of anxiety in the cannabis users. The results do suggest that cannabis users may have generally higher resting levels of trait anxiety than controls, particularly if they are frequent or heavy users of cannabis. It is possible that individuals with high anxiety choose to use cannabis to "self medicate". The other possibility is that heavy cannabis use might lead to the development of greater anxiety; to what extent this may occur is difficult to determine without prospective studies. Some support for this hypothesis was provided by the ex-cannabis users' descriptions of increasing paranoia and anxiety with prolonged heavy use, as prime factors for ceasing cannabis use (see below).

Psychopathology

Many studies have also established that drug using populations show significantly more signs and symptoms of psychopathology than seen in the general population (e.g. Meyer, 1986; Ross *et al.*, 1988; Rounsaville, 1989; Swift *et al.*, 1990; Anthony & Helzer, 1991; Rounsaville *et al.*, 1991; Darke *et al.*, 1992). There has been extensive debate over the possible causal significance of this psychopathology: does an underlying psychopathology induce a person to seek out and use drugs, either as an attempt to self medicate the symptoms of the pathology, or is drug use itself a symptom? Some claim there is sufficient evidence that cannabis use is causal in the development of psychotic disorders. Hall *et al.* (1994) reviewed the literature pertinent to this issue and found little support for the hypothesis that cannabis use can cause either an acute or a chronic functional psychosis which persists beyond the period of intoxication. There is suggestive evidence that heavy use may produce an acute toxic psychosis and that long-term use may precipitate a latent psychosis in vulnerable or predisposed individuals, but the estimated attributable risk is small. There is no doubt, however, that cannabis use may exacerbate symptoms of schizophrenia (Negrete *et al.*, 1986; Hall *et al.*, 1994). Others have argued that drug use is merely an expression of deviance without any negative connotation, and that deviant persons are more likely to show deviant scores in measures of psychiatric symptomatology (e.g. Mugford & Cohen, 1989). Regardless of the true causality, psychopathology was considered worthy of investigation, and given that various psychiatric groups are known to have different ERP signatures to the normal population, it was deemed essential to determine the relation between cannabis use, psychopathology and the ERP effects found in this course of study.

The Symptom Checklist 90-R (SCL-90-R) (Derogatis, 1983) was selected to assess psychopathology in cannabis users and controls in the studies reported here. This is a 90 item checklist of symptoms that the subject rates on a five point scale ranging from "not at all" (0) to "extremely" (4), to indicate the level of distress caused by each symptom within the past week. The 90 symptoms are subdivided into nine categories of primary symptom dimensions: (1) Somatization, (2) Obsessive-Compulsiveness, (3) Interpersonal Sensitivity, (4) Depression, (5) Anxiety, (6) Hostility, (7) Phobic Anxiety, (8) Paranoid Ideation, (9) Psychoticism.

In addition, three global measures of psychopathology indexing distress are calculated: the Global Severity Index (GSI), the Positive Symptom Distress Index (PSDI) and the Positive Symptom Total (PST). The GSI is the mean value of all 90 raw scores, the PSDI is the average value of all items scored from 1 to 4, and the PST is the total number of items scored between 1 and 4. Although there have been numerous studies that demonstrate adequate reliability and validity for the SCL-90-R, there has been criticism that the subscales are not well differentiated and that its primary value may be as a measure of global symptomatology (Riskind *et al.*, 1987). The test manual itself recommends the GSI as the most meaningful overall measure of global symptom distress (Derogatis, 1983). It states that the GSI is the single best indicator of depth of disorder or psychopathological distress as it combines information on the number of symptoms and the intensity of perceived distress.

Mean scores for cannabis users, ex-users and controls of Experiments 2 and 3 are presented in Table 11.2. When cannabis users overall were compared with controls, they differed significantly only on one subscale, that of Hostility (F(1,46) = 4.77, $p < 0.04$), with cannabis users scoring significantly higher than controls. There were trends toward higher scores in cannabis users on a number of other subscales: Paranoid Ideation ($p < 0.07$), Phobic Anxiety ($p < 0.096$), and Psychoticism ($p < 0.097$). Cannabis users had a significantly greater Positive Symptom Total (PST) than controls (F(1,46) = 5.13, $p < 0.03$), indicating that users reported experiencing distress on a greater number of symptoms overall than did controls. There were trends toward a higher total score ($p < 0.09$), and a higher Global Severity Index (GSI) ($p < 0.08$) in cannabis users than in controls. The normative data provided in the test manual gave a score of 0.31 (s.d. = 0.31) on the GSI for an adult population, or 0.76 (s.d. = 0.54) for adolescents. It is clear that the sample of controls of the studies reported here were very close to the normal adult GSI score, whereas cannabis users scores fell between the scores for adults and adolescents. This may be a reflection of delayed maturation in the cannabis users.

When groups were compared on the basis of duration or frequency of cannabis use, there were few differences between long-term users, short-term users and controls, but heavy frequency use resulted in higher scores on many subscales and global measures of distress. Comparison of heavy users, light users and controls resulted in significant group differences on the following measures: Total score ($p < 0.005$), Depression ($p < 0.02$), Anxiety ($p < 0.008$), Hostility ($p < 0.002$), Psychoticism ($p < 0.02$), GSI ($p < 0.005$) and PST ($p < 0.006$).

Group multiple comparisons indicated that for every measure above,

Table 11.2 Mean scores (SD) from subscales of the SCL-90-R for cannabis users, ex-users and controls

	Cannabis users overall	Long term users	Short term users	Heavy users	Light users	Ex-cannabis users	Controls
TOTAL	48.06 *(33.49)*	47.38 *(38.32)*	48.75 *(29.12)*	63.00 *(38.06)*	33.13 *(19.83)*	58.29 *(38.46)*	30.75 *(27.64)*
SOM	0.457 *(0.396)*	0.376 *(0.225)*	0.537 *(0.509)*	0.527 *(0.512)*	0.386 *(0.227)*	0.476 *(0.432)*	0.444 *(0.577)*
O-C	0.753 *(0.483)*	0.688 *(0.429)*	0.819 *(0.538)*	0.906 *(0.537)*	0.600 *(0.380)*	1.018 *(0.653)*	0.563 *(0.486)*
IPS	0.732 *(0.624)*	0.826 *(0.818)*	0.639 *(0.340)*	0.916 *(0.777)*	0.548 *(0.358)*	0.845 *(0.555)*	0.443 *(0.569)*
DEP	0.646 *(0.646)*	0.678 *(0.714)*	0.614 *(0.369)*	0.875 *(0.675)*	0.418 *(0.284)*	0.767 *(0.565)*	0.428 *(0.464)*
ANX	0.378 *(0.380)*	0.344 *(0.403)*	0.413 *(0.365)*	0.550 *(0.408)*	0.206 *(0.262)*	0.582 *(0.640)*	0.269 *(0.247)*
HOS	0.594 *(0.566)*	0.636 *(0.667)*	0.552 *(0.462)*	0.833 *(0.650)*	0.355 *(0.343)*	0.530 *(0.499)*	0.261 *(0.311)*
PHOB	0.218 *(0.372)*	0.231 *(0.442)*	0.204 *(0.299)*	0.303 *(0.448)*	0.133 *(0.263)*	0.260 *(0.383)*	0.053 *(0.146)*
PAR	0.558 *(0.527)*	0.501 *(0.533)*	0.614 *(0.532)*	0.667 *(0.640)*	0.448 *(0.374)*	0.691 *(0.517)*	0.271 *(0.416)*
PSY	0.381 *(0.453)*	0.388 *(0.480)*	0.375 *(0.440)*	0.544 *(0.462)*	0.219 *(0.394)*	0.432 *(0.477)*	0.169 *(0.303)*
GSI	0.535 *(0.372)*	0.526 *(0.426)*	0.543 *(0.323)*	0.701 *(0.422)*	0.369 *(0.222)*	0.647 *(0.428)*	0.342 *(0.307)*
PSDI	1.458 *(0.332)*	1.449 *(0.378)*	1.468 *(0.290)*	1.579 *(0.334)*	1.337 *(0.290)*	1.487 *(0.359)*	1.363 *(0.393)*
PST	31.00 *(16.25)*	29.69 *(16.44)*	32.31 *(16.49)*	37.44 *(16.73)*	24.56 *(13.33)*	36.11 *(19.44)*	20.19 *(14.13)*

Notes:
TOT: Total score; SOM: Somatization; O-C: Obsessive-Compulsiveness; IPS: Interpersonal Sensitivity; DEP: Depression; ANX: Anxiety; HOS: Hostility; PHOB: Phobic Anxiety; PAR: Paranoid Ideation; PSY: Psychoticism; GSI: Global Severity Index; PSDI: Positive Symptom Distress Index; PST: Positive Symptom Total.

heavy users scored significantly higher than light users and controls, while the latter two groups did not differ. Trends toward greater distress reported by heavy cannabis users were also apparent for Obsessive-Compulsiveness ($p < 0.089$), Interpersonal Sensitivity ($p < 0.07$), Phobic Anxiety ($p < 0.08$), Paranoid Ideation ($p < 0.085$) and on the global measure of PSDI

($p < 0.099$). Thus, the subscale of Somatization was the only measure where there was no tendency toward an effect of frequency of cannabis use. The only indication of some effect due to duration of use appeared as trends toward group differences for Hostility ($p < 0.097$) and the PST ($p < 0.083$).

The cannabis users of Experiment 1 showed similar results to the heavy users of Experiment 2. They differed significantly (or marginally) from their nonuser controls on every measure except Somatization. The control group of Experiment 1, however, may have been somewhat atypical: not only did they fall within a low percentile with their STAI scores (as reported above), but their SCL-90-R scores were lower than those of the control group of Experiment 2. Caution must be observed when analysing and interpreting data from small samples. For this reason, correlational analyses between SCL-90-R scores and ERP and performance measures were not conducted for Experiment 1.

Ex-cannabis users did not differ significantly from long-term or short-term current cannabis users on any measure from the SCL-90-R. There was a trend toward higher scores for ex-users than long-term users on Obsessive-Compulsiveness ($p < 0.077$). In contrast, when ex-users were compared with controls, they differed significantly (or near to significantly) on every measure except Somatization and the PSDI: Total score $p < 0.02$; Obsessive-Compulsiveness $p < 0.02$; Interpersonal Sensitivity $p < 0.03$; Depression $p < 0.05$; Anxiety $p < 0.07$; Hostility $p < 0.06$; Phobic Anxiety $p < 0.05$; Paranoid Ideation $p < 0.008$; Psychoticism $p < 0.06$; GSI $p < 0.02$; and PST $p < 0.007$.

The higher scores for ex-users compared to controls may be interpreted in a number of ways. It is possible that their long-term use of cannabis resulted in an increase in the kind of symptoms assessed by the SCL-90-R. Most of the measures on the SCL-90-R appear to be affected by frequency of cannabis use and the ex-user group had used cannabis heavily in the past. While current heavy users scored significantly higher on most SCL-90-R measures compared to both light users and controls, frequency of use did not correlate significantly with the GSI in current cannabis users ($r = 0.27$) nor in ex-users ($r = 0.24$), nor did a relation exist between GSI and duration of cannabis use in current users ($r = -0.20$) or ex-users ($r = -0.15$). Nevertheless, it may be that the sample of ex-cannabis users represent those more vulnerable to the harmful effects of cannabis and this is precisely the reason why they ceased their use of cannabis. Another possible interpretation is that the ex-users had used cannabis to self medicate underlying psychopathological symptoms which have resurfaced since the cessation of use. Given the self reports of the ex-users experiences with cannabis, this explanation seems unlikely and also the duration of abstinence in the ex-users did not correlate significantly with the GSI ($r = 0.22$).

PN to pitch irrelevant tones was unrelated to the GSI in any group (current users: $r = -0.19$; ex-users $r = -0.05$; controls $r = -0.09$). P300 latency did not vary as a function of GSI in current cannabis users ($r = -0.05$) or ex-users ($r = 0.29$), although a striking inverse relation was found to exist in the control group ($r = -0.73$, $p < 0.001$). Thus, in controls only, it appeared that the greater the global symptoms of distress, the earlier P300 occurred. This was initially considered puzzling, possibly reflecting a spurious association due to small sample size ($N = 15$ controls for this analysis). A search of the literature on P300 latency and psychiatric symptomatology found one recent report of shorter latency P300 in obsessive compulsive patients (Towey *et al.*, 1990), which was suggested to be the result of hyperactive perceptual systems. The nonuser controls studied here scored more highly on obsessive-compulsiveness than the normative sample published in the test manual (mean 0.39, s.d. $= 0.45$). In fact, the controls scored higher on obsessive-compulsiveness than on any other subscale, but in most instances so did the cannabis user groups. This suggests that once again there are underlying differences in the modus operandi of cannabis users and controls.

In the current cannabis user group, the relation between their frequency of cannabis use and P300 latency ($r = 0.50$) was only strengthened by removing any effects of GSI ($r = 0.69$). GSI was unrelated to any of the performance measures from cannabis users (RT: $r = 0.11$; hit rate: $r = -0.12$; false alarm rate: $r = 0.15$) whereas in controls there were nonsignificant trends toward a lower hit rate ($r = -0.43$, $p > 0.09$) and greater false alarm rate ($r = 0.35$) with increasing GSI, but no relation with reaction time ($r = -0.20$).

Cannabis dependence

The Diagnostic and Statistical Manual of Mental Disorders (DSM-III-R) (American Psychiatric Association, 1987) defines cannabis dependence as daily or almost daily use of the substance, while cannabis abuse is defined as episodic use with evidence of maladaptive behaviour, such as driving while intoxicated. Both develop over a substantial period of time with repeated use; typically it is the frequency of use that increases over time rather than the absolute amount, often with concomitant loss of pleasurable effects and an increase in dysphoric effects. It is stated that impairment in social and occupational functioning, and the development of physical disorders, are less than those typically seen with other psychoactive substances. The more recent edition, DSM-IV (American Psychiatric Association, 1994) refers to its general criteria for substance abuse and dependence, but additionally defines cannabis dependence as compulsive use with or without physiological dependence, and states that individuals with cannabis dependence "may use very potent cannabis throughout the day over a period of months or years". Cannabis abuse is defined as periodic use and intoxication which can interfere with performance at work or school and lead to a variety of legal and personal problems. By either of these definitions, most of the cannabis users participating in the studies reported here could be labelled "cannabis dependent" or "cannabis abusers".

Despite these definitions, there has been debate over the years about the existence of a dependence syndrome, with claims that the concept remains poorly defined and its existence questionable. Hall *et al.* (1994) reviewed the literature pertaining to evidence for the existence of cannabis dependence and concluded that the syndrome as defined by DSM-III-R probably does exist in chronic heavy users and that the general diagnostic criteria for psychoactive substance abuse disorders provided by DSM-III-R are probably appropriate. Nevertheless, unlike alcohol and other drugs such as opiates, for which many scales and assessment tools for dependence have been formulated, there is no internationally accepted measure of dependence on cannabis. One scale developed by Hannifin (1987), the Cannabis Abuse Severity Screening Test (CASST), was piloted but has not been widely applied. As a short scale consisting of 11 yes/no questions each worth one point (Appendix A), this provided for the purposes of this study an assessment of "cannabis dependence" that was quick to administer, with a maximum score of 11. The questions were paraphrased retrospectively for the ex-users of Experiment 3. The CASST was only added to the experimental protocol from Experiment 2 onwards. Hence, no data is available for the small sample of cannabis users of Experiment 1, although six of the 10 users claimed to have felt dependent on cannabis.

Mean scores on the CASST for each of the cannabis using groups of Experiment 2 and the ex-users of Experiment 3 are presented in Table 11.3. The ex-users scored significantly higher than either the current long-term ($p < 0.04$) or short-term users ($p < 0.0009$). Ex-users did not differ from current heavy users ($p > 0.1$) but scored significantly higher than light users ($p < 0.0001$). Of the current user groups, long-term users did

Table 11.3 *Mean "cannabis dependence" scores (and SD) from the CASST for cannabis user groups and ex-users*

Long-term users	Short-term users	Heavy users	Light users	Ex-users
4.44	3.50	5.13	2.81	6.14
(2.63)	(2.10)	(2.00)	(2.23)	(2.51)

not differ from short-term users ($p > 0.2$) and heavy users scored significantly higher than light users ($p < 0.005$).

These results reinforce the concept of cannabis dependence, as measured by the CASST, as being related to frequency of use. This was supported also by a significant correlation between CASST scores and frequency of cannabis use ($r = 0.51$, $p < 0.005$) in the current user group, whereas there was no relation between CASST score and duration of cannabis use ($r = -0.21$). Interestingly, CASST scores did not correlate with monthly alcohol consumption ($r = 0.02$), which suggests a dissociation between dependence on alcohol and cannabis. Caution with such interpretations is warranted as eight of the 11 questions of the CASST are specific to cannabis, and also it is not well established that the CASST is indeed measuring "dependence". Only two questions specifically address frequency of use, whereas the other items address possible problems associated with cannabis use.

The CASST did not correlate with past reported frequency of use in the ex-user group ($r = 0.10$), but tended toward a stronger inverse relation with their past duration of use ($r = -0.27$). It is possible that ex-users over report symptoms of dependence as a justification for giving up and as a source of motivation to remain abstinent and not give in to their perceived "addiction". Similarly, current long-term users may be less likely to report symptoms of dependence, perhaps to justify their continued use of the drug, than those who have successfully given up.

Perhaps for the ex-users, the perception of cannabis related problems was unrelated to their frequency of use, but was related to use in general. Thus, for many ex-users the idea of cutting down was not feasible and they saw a "cold turkey" approach as the only way of succeeding in "beating the addiction". Indeed, one ex-user reported regular weekly attendance at both Narcotics Anonymous and Alcoholics Anonymous meetings since his cessation of cannabis use 2 years ago. This particular subject claimed never to have used any other drug on a regular basis or to have ever had a problem with his alcohol consumption. He complained of feeling embarrassed at the meetings if others found out that his problem drug was cannabis and not narcotics or alcohol, and tried to conceal this fact whenever possible. He lamented the lack of support groups for "cannabis dependent" individuals and had felt a need himself to resort to the above organizations for assistance. This came in the way of constant reinforcement of the notion of addiction, which for him was a method of justifying and coping with abstinence.

Ex-users' self reports of dependence and definitions of the concept of dependence, have already been discussed in Chapter 9 (60% of the sample claimed to have felt dependent on cannabis). The remaining 40% of the sample of ex-users denied ever having felt dependent on cannabis, but nevertheless scored between 3 and 9 on the CASST with a mean score of 5.17. In the sample of current users of Experiment 2, the figures were reversed, with 40% reporting having felt dependent and 60% claiming never to have felt dependent. The CASST scores of the latter group were lower than in the ex-users who had denied feeling dependent, ranging from 0 to 6 with a mean of 2.84. Some clarified this denial of dependence by stating that they had experienced a strong desire to smoke cannabis but not a need to. Some said they had felt strong cravings but would not label this as dependence, whereas for others the experience of strong cravings or even just the frequent desire to get "high" defined the concept of dependence. Dependence was seen as primarily emotional and psychological, not physical, with descriptions of cannabis being an integral part of daily life, a crutch used to assist in the completion of routine activities, a habitual cure for boredom and stress, an escape from depression. A number of subjects described dependence on the ritualistic cues associated with the actual smoking of cannabis, and the enormous amounts of time and energy involved in going out to "score" and the feelings of stress and "hanging out" (strong craving) when unable to obtain any cannabis.

Withdrawal symptoms were described by 47% of the ex-cannabis users, the remainder claiming not to have experienced any, or reporting that these could be minimized by gradual cutting down as opposed to sudden "cold turkey" cessation of use. The types of symptoms experienced included both physical and psychological effects: headaches, palpitations, flushes, tingles and shakiness, sweating, suppression of appetite, weight loss, tension, irritability, depression, insomnia, nightmares and strong cravings for cannabis. Most reported that these symptoms diminished within a few weeks of cessation of use. These withdrawal sequelae are consistent with those reported in the literature (Hall *et al.*, 1994).

Correlational analyses between CASST scores and performance measures on the selective attention task found marginally significant longer reaction times and a smaller number of correct detections as a function of CASST score in the ex-cannabis user group (RT: $r = 0.34$; hit rate: $r = -0.32$, $p = 0.05$), but these effects were not apparent in current users (RT: $r = 0.11$; hit rate: $r = -0.13$). Errors of commission did not correlate with CASST score in either sample (current users: $r = 0.19$; ex-users: $r = 0.21$). CASST scores were unrelated to PN to pitch irrelevant tones in current users ($r = 0.03$) or ex-users ($r = -0.02$), and no relation was apparent with P300 latency (users: $r = 0.03$; ex-users: $r = 0.11$). None of these relations was altered by controlling for the effects of frequency of cannabis use.

Qualitative experience of long-term cannabis use: effects and problems by self report

It has often been assumed that because cannabis does not evince a well defined physical dependence and is not lethal, extensive use by adults must by definition be less problematic than that of alcohol and most other drugs (Roffman & George, 1988). Unfortunately, there has been little systematic effort to assess and understand chronic or problematic cannabis use. The literature devoted to the assessment of cannabis users and the perceived effects of cannabis use has been scant, and there have been no standardized instruments for research purposes. The questionnaires administered to the cannabis users studied here were designed in an attempt to incorporate suggestions for consistency in the assessment of self reported problems and effects. Thus, ideas and items were adapted from Roffman & George's (1988) discussion of cannabis abuse assessment, Rittenhouse's (1979) pool of questionnaire items developed to tap users' perceptions concerning the effects of marijuana use on their lives, and Huba *et al.*'s (1981) examples of questionnaire items for both positive and negative marijuana consequences. The final questionnaire items selected are presented in the Appendix.

The purpose of this assessment was to provide an opportunity for cannabis users to self report perceived effects and problems associated with their use. It was hoped to ascertain to what extent users themselves are aware of the types of cognitive deficits generally attributed to the chronic use of cannabis (Chapter 5), and the deficits in selective attention detected in the research reported here.

First, why do humans like to smoke cannabis? The most frequent reasons given by the users across all experiments fell into two categories:

therapeutic/self-medicating reasons (e.g. in order to relax, relieve stress or boredom, elevate mood, escape depression or the reality of the outside world, enhance appetite, facilitate sleep, dispel aggression, and for its analgesic effects in curing headaches, stomach aches, nausea, etc.); and general pleasurable effects (e.g. for fun, mental stimulation, creativity, enhancement of the senses, enhanced enjoyment of music and films, alteration of perception and consciousness, sociability). Some noteworthy reasons provided by a few subjects were that they like to smoke in order to cure the cravings, to feel normal again, and because they genuinely like the actual ritual of smoking cannabis.

In response to a short checklist of perceived acute effects of cannabis, 70% of current users reported their ability to relax was enhanced by the use of cannabis (47% of ex-users agreed). Just over two thirds of the sample of users reported enhanced sexual experience under acute intoxication (corroborated by 53% of ex-users). Although many reported using cannabis to enhance creativity and the flow of ideas, one third of the sample reported diminished ability to think clearly under the influence of cannabis (43% of ex-users) and 48% reported variation in the acute effect of cannabis sometimes enhancing, sometimes diminishing the ability to think clearly (50% of ex-users). While many acknowledged an impaired ability to drive a motor vehicle while under the influence of cannabis (47% of users and 50% of ex-users), a substantial proportion believed cannabis to sometimes enhance and sometimes diminish their driving ability (35% of users, 23% of ex-users). The small number of subjects who believed that cannabis consistently improved their driving performance were offset by the small number of subjects who claimed never to drive while under the influence of cannabis.

Subjects reported the following as most disliked about cannabis: its cost, its illegal status, the lack of availability, the development of tolerance and cannabis's addictive qualities, the development of paranoia, lethargy, depression and tiredness, loss of motivation, and the detrimental effects on memory, concentration, study and communication. Some subjects claimed there was nothing they disliked about cannabis.

In response to an open ended question about any problems associated with the use of cannabis, memory and in particular short-term memory, was the most frequently reported problem, nominated by approximately 50% of the sample. This was closely followed by problems with concentration, and third in order of frequency was a loss of motivation and general lethargy. Depression and paranoia were reported by a small percentage of

Table 11.4 *Percent reporting impairment as a long-term consequence of cannabis use and the percent of ex-users reporting improvement following cessation of use*

	Current users	Ex-users	Percent improved
Memory	52	77	70
Physical health	50	53	94
General level of energy	36	70	76
Ability to think clearly	29	80	79
Ability to concentrate on complex tasks	26	80	75
Work performance and studies	24	70	95
Ability to cope and solve life's problems	21	60	89
Ability to communicate	14	57	88
Relations with employers/seniors	14	43	69
General confidence	14	60	83
General coordination	12	40	92
Excitement and enthusiasm for lfie	5	43	54

the samples studied, and a few reported the addictive qualities of cannabis as problematic. One third of the current user sample claimed never to have experienced any problems associated with their use of cannabis. Some subjects claimed to be aware of problems with memory and concentration during only the acute phase of intoxication. In general, few of the current users believed there to be any persistent adverse effects on cognition, but some were concerned that they themselves may not perceive or be aware of the deficits.

These general results were also apparent in current cannabis users' responses to a checklist of the perceived consequences of use. The percentages reporting impairment on a variety of items in the checklist are presented in Table 11.4, listed in rank order for current users. The item judged by the largest proportion of users and ex-users combined as a long-term consequence of cannabis use was that of impaired memory. Interestingly, the abilities to think clearly and concentrate on complex tasks were judged as being impaired by slightly more ex-users than judged memory to be impaired. Thus, the rank order of perceived impairments was slightly different in the ex-cannabis user group, and impairment was perceived by a vastly larger percent of the sample in ex-users compared with current users. The reasons for this have already been discussed above with regard to dependence and it is not surprising that those who choose to cease their use of cannabis would be those who experience greater problems with their use. Otherwise, there would be no good reason to stop.

When cannabis is used regularly over a prolonged period of time, a state of chronic intoxication is believed to develop (e.g. Lundqvist, 1995a, b, c). This state of chronic intoxication is characterized by "cloudy", "foggy" or "muddy" thought processes as described by users themselves. It is likely, therefore, that during such a state of continued use, the user is unable to perceive the long-term consequences of his or her use. As argued by Lundqvist (personal communication), this is because the user has nothing to compare against, has no drug free reference point. The "normal" state of being becomes the state of chronic intoxication and hence the user can only contrast the state of being acutely intoxicated with that of being chronically intoxicated, but cannot be aware of the differences between chronic intoxication and drug free "normality". This is particularly because the chronic state of intoxication develops gradually over time. According to this hypothesis, when the use of cannabis is stopped and the accumulated cannabinoids given sufficient time to flush out of the body, the ex-user will notice differences between the new drug free state and the past state of functioning as a cannabis user and will be more aware of the effects that cannabis use was having on their general state of functioning. Such an explanation is also consistent with the reports of ex-users versus current users in this study.

Clearly, from Table 11.4, the majority of those who reported experiencing long-term consequences of cannabis use, also reported an improvement upon cessation of use. Perhaps the area most resilient to improvement was that of excitement and enthusiasm for life, possibly reflecting difficulties with general motivation. While most report improvement on each item, it is nevertheless of concern that some do not. For example, 30% of those who perceived impaired memory function reported that it had not improved following cessation of cannabis use. Similar figures can be seen for concentration, energy levels, clear thinking and relations with seniors.

The course of studies reported here established subtle impairments in focusing attention and rejecting irrelevant information as being associated with the long-term use of cannabis. It is possible that such specific processes and mechanisms involved in selective attention are not amenable to conscious awareness by users themselves. On the other hand, it is possible as argued above, that current long-term users may be unable to perceive such deficits, but ex-users certainly reported difficulties in concentration on complex tasks. The finding that the ability to reject irrelevant information may partially resolve upon cessation of use is in accord with the report of 70% of ex-users of an improvement in the general functions associated with performance on such a task. It is difficult to ascertain to what extent the recovery is partial, and to what extent the apparent partial recovery may be due to the 30% of subjects who claim not to have improved functioning after stopping cannabis use. It appears that, for some reason, some individuals may recover from the cognitive impairments while others may not.

It is likely that numerous individual differences in response to cannabis lurk beneath the findings of this series of studies. A variety of variables were examined to explore possible individual differences. It is possible that the younger the age at which cannabis use is commenced, the more severe long-term consequences will be experienced. The age at which cannabis was first tried was similar across all samples studied, generally around 15 years (s.d. = 2.3), and the age at which regular use commenced was around 17 (s.d. = 3.0). Neither age first tried nor earliest age of regular use correlated with PN to pitch irrelevant tones ($r = 0.02$ and $r = 0.08$, respectively). A recent study has reported an early age of onset of cannabis use to be a potent predictor of reduced speed of information processing (Kunert *et al.*, 1997). Further research on this issue is clearly warranted.

The types of cannabis preparation nominated as usually smoked by users were heads and hashish, both far more potent than leaf material. Thus, regular users specifically sought to purchase stronger varieties. On a scale from 0 to 10 representing potency, users rated the strength of what they usually smoked as about 7.5, and on a scale from 0 to 10 representing degree of intoxication, the usual mean level reached was reported to be 6.6. These cannabis users were smoking to this level of intoxication, highly potent forms of cannabis at quantities of between 15 to 300 mg per day, 3 days per week on average. A combination of high potency, large quantity, heavy frequency and long duration use may interact with other factors specific to the individual, and may contribute to the exacerbation of long-term adverse consequences. It is beyond the scope of this book to examine further possibilities or propose more hypotheses in this regard, but this is an important area for future research.

To summarize the findings of this chapter, there is no reason to suspect that the ERP and performance differences between cannabis users and controls were related to greater levels of anxiety or psychopathology, and the self reported cognitive consequences of long-term use are mostly in accord with those found in the research reported here.

Key findings

- *Anxiety, symptoms of psychopathology and dependence on cannabis were assessed in all subjects who participated in the studies reported in this monograph. Self report of any problems associated with cannabis use and a qualitative description of the experience of long-term cannabis use were obtained through structured and open ended questionnaires*
- *Heavy cannabis users showed significantly greater trait anxiety levels than light users and controls and frequency of cannabis use was significantly related to trait anxiety. Neither P300 latency nor PN to complex irrelevant stimuli were related to anxiety levels in cannabis users*
- *Cannabis users scored higher than controls on a measure of hostility and reported experiencing distress on a greater number of psychological symptoms than did controls. Heavy users and ex-users reported significantly more symptoms of depression, anxiety, hostility and psychoticism than light users or controls and a greater severity of symptoms overall. Neither PN nor P300 latency were related to any symptoms of psychological distress*
- *Heavy users and ex-users scored significantly higher on a measure of dependence on cannabis than light users. Long-term users did not differ from short-term users and this measure of dependence on cannabis did not correlate with any of the ERP measures*
- *Subjects reported the addictive nature of cannabis, the development of paranoia, lethargy, depression and tiredness, loss of motivation, and the detrimental effects on memory, concentration, study and communication as the most disliked aspects of cannabis use*
- *Problems with memory, concentration and motivation were most frequently self reported in association with cannabis use and the majority of ex-users reported a subjective improvement in these functions upon cessation of use. However, one third of the sample reported no improvement in cognitive functioning with abstinence*
- *The self reported cognitive consequences of long-term use were mostly in accord with those found in the original research reported here*

12
Summary, synthesis and conclusions

This concluding chapter integrates the findings of the original research reported here with the cumulative results of the research reviewed in Chapters 2 to 6. The synthesis of neuropsychological test data and event-related potential (ERP) indices of cognitive functioning with the results of other investigations of brain function and structure, enables the formulation of a preliminary model of neuropsychological function in long-term cannabis users. The evidence for long-term use of cannabis leading to subtle cognitive impairments is discussed together with the role of other possible confounds. The nature of the cognitive impairments is discussed in terms of proposed attentional / neuropsychological and neurophysiological / biochemical mechanisms. The implications of these findings for future research is discussed, as are implications for long-term cannabis users.

Summary and synthesis

Is the cognitive functioning of long-term regular cannabis users impaired in comparison to nonusers ? What is the nature of this impairment ?

Previous reviewers have generally concluded that there is insufficient evidence to conclude that cannabis produces any long-term cognitive deficits (e.g. Wert & Raulin, 1986a, b). This is probably a reasonable conclusion when gross deficits are considered: the weight of evidence suggests that the long-term use of cannabis does not result in any severe or grossly debilitating impairment of cognitive function. Recent reviewers agree, however, that there is now sufficient evidence that the long-term use of cannabis leads to a more subtle and selective impairment of cognitive functioning (Hall *et al.*, 1994; Pope *et al.*, 1995; Block, 1996). The findings of the original research reported in this monograph, together with the other recent methodologically rigorous research reviewed here, provide evidence for complex but subtle impairments which include the organization and integration of complex information involving various mechanisms of attention and memory processes. These cognitive impairments are either associated with the frequency of cannabis use or increase with duration of cannabis use. There is evidence that impairment on some standard neuropsychological tests may become apparent only after 10–15 years of use (e.g. Leavitt *et al.*, 1993). But as demonstrated in the ERP studies reported here, very sensitive measures of brain function are capable of detecting specific attentional impairments after 5 years of use and cannabis users of only 3–4 years showed early signs of impairment. Consistent with these findings, other recent well-controlled research has demonstrated impaired executive / attentional function and learning in relatively short-term but heavy users of cannabis by means of specific and sensitive neuropsychological tests (Pope & Yurgelun-Todd, 1996).

The original research presented in this monograph evolved from an identification of selective attention as a specific aspect of cognitive functioning worthy of assessment in long-term cannabis users. Attentional mechanisms underly most of the functions where impairments have been observed or reported in the literature: a particular susceptibility to distraction, loosening of associations and intrusion errors in memory tasks, all point to a problem with the focusing of attention. Brain ERP recording techniques provided a sensitive means of examining the processes of selective attention and the results demonstrated the relative insensitivity of some performance measures to cannabinoid effects on otherwise inaccessible, covert cognitive processes. This research elucidated the mechanisms underlying distractibility in long-term cannabis users by showing that such subjects are unable to reject complex irrelevant information at an early stage of processing. They continue to unnecessarily process distractor stimuli (as evidenced by inappropriately large processing negativity (PN) to complex irrelevant stimuli), and hence are unable to effectively focus their attention. This impairment was found to be progressive with the number of years of cannabis use and possibly only partially reversible with abstinence (or else, reversible in some individuals but not others). Increasing frequency of use contributed to a general slowing of information processing, specifically with a delay in the detection, evaluation and recognition of relevant (target) stimuli requiring a decision and a response (evidenced by a delayed P300). These specific information processing deficits might explain the various impairments that have been reported in the literature, which collectively could be indicative of impaired executive function.

The ERP results are consistent with the findings of recent neuropsychological research, reviewed in Chapter 5. Pope & Yurgelun-Todd's (1996) study found that regular heavy use of cannabis compromized the ability to learn and remember information primarily by impairing the ability to focus, sustain and shift attention. The ERP studies described here confirmed a deficit in the ability to selectively attend and identified the brain processes involved in this deficit. The continued processing of complex irrelevant information would most likely affect the ability to rapidly shift one's focus of attention when required from one source (or mental set) to another. Pope & Yurgelun-Todd (1996) argued that such deficits in turn affect the ability to register, organize and manipulate information, as shown in decreased word list learning, errors in card sorting, and perseveration when required to shift mental set. Yet they found that recall of learned information was relatively unaffected.

Pope's study was important as it suggested that heavy use of cannabis for even a relatively short period of time (2 years +) can impair performance on a number of neuropsychological tests. Heavy (almost daily) users differed significantly from light ($\leq$ 3 days per month) users, but it is not known to what extent their performance was significantly impaired compared with published normative data on these tests. The ERP studies in this monograph also found an impairment associated with frequency of cannabis use – a general slowing of information processing. It is likely that such a slowing of information processing and delay in the recognition and evaluation of stimuli might affect a number of aspects of cognitive processes and hence performance on a number of neuropsychological tests. The ERP research extended these findings by showing that any such effects associated with frequency of cannabis use appear to be reversible. This supports the notion that effects related to frequency of cannabis use are probably due to the accumulation of cannabinoids, possibly reflecting a state of chronic intoxication. When sufficient time is allowed for such accumulated cannabinoids to eliminate from the body, the effects dissipate. On the other hand, the ERP results demonstrated that the primary effects on attention were associated with the duration of cannabis use and not frequency. That these effects were consistently replicated, were progressive with the number of years of cannabis use, and were still apparent, albeit to a lesser degree, in ex-cannabis users, suggests an enduring alteration of brain function that is slow to recover. It is important to recognize that frequency and duration of cannabis use may indeed have differential effects on cognitive function.

The ERP data reported here demonstrate that long-term cannabis users have no difficulty in filtering out irrelevant information when the discrimination between to be attended and to be ignored stimuli is large and therefore relatively easy (e.g. ignoring all stimuli presented to one ear). An impairment becomes apparent when the task involves greater complexity, such as the detection of difficult to discriminate targets from a set of frequent stimuli which in turn must be discriminated from another source of competing distractor stimuli. These findings are also entirely consistent with Leavitt's conclusions from neuropsychological test results (Leavitt *et al.*, 1992, 1993) that: (1) while basic attentional processes appear to be intact, long-term cannabis users are less efficient when performing complex cognitive tasks or attempting to resist distraction, (2) long-term users' ability to efficiently process information declines more rapidly under a moderate cognitive load compared with short duration users or controls, and (3) long-term users show increased susceptibility to interference, consistent with difficulty in resisting distraction (J. Leavitt, personal communication). These researchers also found that the impairments they detected on specific neuropsychological tests were progressive with the number of years of cannabis use.

The results of the ERP research are also in accord with the electroencephalogram (EEG) findings of Struve *et al.* (1992, 1993, 1994) discussed in Chapter 4. While the functional significance of the alterations in EEG observed by Struve *et al.* is difficult to interpret, the EEG changes were most apparent in frontal regions of the brain. The major differences between the groups studied here occurred in frontal ERP components reflecting processes thought to be subserved by the frontal lobes. Furthermore, the EEG alterations observed by Struve's group were progressive with the duration of cannabis use, as were the neuropsychological impairments reported by the same team (Leavitt *et al.*, 1992, 1993), but the relations between these measures have not been examined. Struve and coworkers suggested that the quantitative EEG changes they observed in association with increases in cumulative exposure to cannabis may reflect organic change. In Chapter 8 it was suggested on the basis of the ERP evidence of altered cognitive processing that there may be gradual changes occurring in the brain, possibly at the cannabinoid receptor site.

Hypotheses regarding the possible mechanisms involved in such changes are discussed further below. The results of the study of ex-cannabis users reported here (Chapter 9) lend some support to the hypothesis that any long-term changes associated with chronic cannabis use are likely to be reversible, although perhaps not entirely, or at least not for everyone. The single case study reported in Chapter 10 is a prime example, although it is possible that recovery of function may have been more apparent if the subject had been tested again following a longer period of abstinence.

Pope *et al.* (1995) reviewed the literature on cannabis and cognitive functioning and concluded that while there is evidence for impaired attention, short-term memory and psychomotor function in long-term cannabis users, there is insufficient evidence to explain this impairment as being of a more enduring nature than simply the result of drug residues remaining in the body. The original research reported in this monograph indicates a more enduring effect for the following reasons. There was a strong and replicable relation between increased processing of irrelevant information and the number of years of cannabis use. This relation was independent of the frequency of cannabis use. Thus, long-term cannabis users who used only infrequently (e.g. once/month) were just as likely to show the impairment in rejecting distracting information as were those using on a daily basis. Infrequent use of that nature would permit most drug residues to eliminate from the body between successive uses. All subjects abstained from cannabis for at least 12 hours prior to testing, and most had abstained for the requested 24 hours before testing. The less frequent users had abstained for even longer, between 2 and 4 weeks in some cases. Also, the fact that these effects were still apparent in the *ex*-cannabis user group, with a significant relation between the processing of irrelevant information and the number of years of past use of cannabis, and the lack of effect of the duration of abstinence, suggest that the observed effects in current long-term users were neither due to withdrawal nor to drug residues remaining in the body, but to an enduring effect that suggests an alteration of brain function.

Is this impairment due to some confounding factor other than cannabis use, or does it merely reflect a simple difference in motivation, strategy or style ?

A slim possibility remains that the dysfunction in information processing observed here, and the cognitive impairments reported more generally in the literature, could be due to some factor other than cumulative exposure to cannabis use. It is hard to imagine what such a factor might be, as it would have to correlate highly with duration or extent of cannabis use. One of the obvious candidates, age, was examined here in specific analyses conducted to disentangle the relation between duration of cannabis use and age. The results indicated that age did not correlate with PN to complex irrelevant stimuli, although the study with ex-users suggested that recovery of function may occur more readily in younger subjects. Impairments were found here to be greater in cannabis users and ex-users of lower IQ. As the cut off below which impairments were manifest was a Full Scale IQ of 119–121, the latter finding might indicate that only subjects of high average to superior intelligence are able to compensate for the detrimental effects of long-term cannabis use.

Another possible candidate could be personality or some other qualitative differences between cannabis users and nonusers. For this reason, Pope & Yurgelun-Todd (1996) used a group of infrequent cannabis users, rather than nonusers, as the comparison group for their study of the effects of heavy cannabis use. They argued that light users might be expected to differ less from heavy users on a variety of confounding variables than would control subjects who had never used cannabis at all (see also Kouri et al., 1995). In terms of duration of cannabis use, it is possible that those who are prone to using cannabis for a prolonged period may possess particular characteristics associated with a different style of information processing (see below). Many short-term cannabis users are on their way to becoming long-term users, and are arguably therefore of the same personality type, yet short-term users did not demonstrate the same degree of cognitive impairment as that found in long-term users in the studies reported here. They did, however, show early signs of such impairment, supporting the notion that the impairment is progressive with years of cannabis use. No personality typologies have been shown to affect ERP components and selective attentional processing in the way demonstrated in long-term cannabis users. While anxiety and certain aspects of psychopathology were found to be related to heavy frequency use of cannabis in the sample studied here, none of these variables correlated with duration of cannabis use or with PN to complex irrelevant stimuli. Nevertheless, the possibility of differing cognitive styles does exist, and the possibility that personality changes are effected by long-term use of cannabis must be considered also. The phenomenological experience of acute intoxication has been shown to vary as a function of personality characteristics (e.g. Musty, 1988), and cannabis use has been shown to be significantly associated with psychological distress in highly introspective individuals (Zablocki et al., 1991). Future research might attempt to better characterize such influences.

One psychological variable that has not been assessed routinely in cognitive research on cannabis is motivation. It could, for example, be argued that cannabis users may have been less motivated than controls to do well on the selective attention task reported here, and that any differences found between groups could have been due to these motivational differences. There is no reason to suspect that the long-term users would have been any less motivated than the short-term users, unless one believes that an "amotivational syndrome" occurs only in long-term cannabis users. In fact, there is no evidence that an amotivational syndrome exists (Hall *et al.*, 1994), and the loss of motivation and achievement in some heavy users has been shown to be associated more with depression than with cannabis use *per se* (Musty & Kaback, 1995). Furthermore, it is worthy to note that participants of the studies reported here were observed to fall into two broad categories. One group of users believed that their long-term use of cannabis had had no severe long-term consequences. As such, they almost challenged the experimenter to perform whatever test they like and they would "prove" that cannabis had no long-term adverse effect. Some participants, particularly those who belonged to the organization NORML (National Organization for the Reform of Marijuana Laws), were actively involved in lobbying for legalization. The other broad category of participants were those who were genuinely interested in contributing to scientific knowledge regarding their drug of choice, and some of these subjects were concerned that their use of cannabis had adversely affected their cognitive functioning. Some hoped that their involvement in this research might provide them with a personal assessment. Not all subjects belonged to one of these categories, but in general terms the categories describe a majority of participants. In each case, the motivating factor to participate in this research was one that suggests both categories of subjects were motivated to do well. It could be argued that even those who were motivated more by payment for research participation, rather than any personal or political concerns about cannabis, would nevertheless be unlikely to perform in such a way as to jeopardize the future availability of their drug of choice by providing evidence that cannabis may indeed be harmful. Future research might nevertheless aim to tease apart effects associated with motivation, depression, or indeed other psychological factors.

Some might wish to argue that the ERP findings of the original research reported here, along with EEG and cerebral blood flow (CBF) alterations reported by others (Chapter 4), do not necessarily indicate a cognitive deficit or an impairment, but merely a difference. This hypothesis is not sustained when the performance data from the ERP task are examined: these indicate generally slower reaction times, lower correct hit rates and a greater number of errors of commission in cannabis users and ex-users compared with controls. Thus, the ERP pattern must be interpreted as reflecting a less efficient mode of information processing. The hypothesis is not sustained by the fact that there was some evidence in ex-users of improved information processing following abstinence. Importantly, the ERP findings and their interpretation are consistent with the findings of neuropsychological research and the growing consensus regarding the long-term cognitive effects of cannabis. It is possible, nevertheless, that the neuropsychological and ERP results reflect not so much a physical alteration within the central nervous system, as a difference in cognitive style or the adoption of alternative cognitive strategies in cannabis users. This type of approach is less efficient than that of nonusers, clearly results in poorer task performance and appears to increase with the duration of cannabis use (see further below).

What are the mechanisms of the impairment ?

As discussed in Chapter 9, from the perspective of cognitive models, it may be that cannabis acts to broaden the attentional "spotlight" to include irrelevant stimuli that share some of the attributes of the relevant attended stimuli (Woods, 1989). This may be the result of a direct neurophysiological effect of prolonged exposure to cannabinoids, or it may reflect the use of different strategies in performing cognitive tasks, influenced by having experienced the intoxicating effects of cannabis. This is a question for future research (although a new model being developed by Deadwyler and colleagues (see below) may go a long way toward explaining and integrating both of these possibilities). Even if the large PN to complex irrelevant stimuli found here is a consequence of a strategy difference between groups, it is still a less than optimal strategy to adopt for the cannabis users. The processing of irrelevant information, reflecting perhaps a wider distribution of attentional resources, need not necessarily be disruptive; it does not appear to be detrimental in high IQ nonuser controls (Chapter 8). If the strategy employed by cannabis users is no different to that utilized by nonusers, users are less able to utilize that strategy to maximize efficiency in information processing. This indicates an underlying impairment which, given our knowledge of the pharmacodynamics of cannabis, is probably most easily explainable by some kind of physiological alteration of brain function. It is also now fairly universally accepted that all forms of mental activity have a neurophysiological substrate. It is possible also that cannabis use camouflages the relations between electrophysiological measures and intellectual functioning and personality; this hypothesis would explain the contrasting direction of correlations between ERP measures and the numerous other variables tested throughout the studies reported here, and particularly in Chapter 11; the direction of the relations, even when not significant, was consistent between cannabis users and ex-users, but usually in the reverse direction to that found in controls. Further research might elucidate these discrepancies.

There is good theory to support a neurophysiological mechanism for the broadening of the attentional spotlight. Woods (1989) proposed that neurons in higher order sensory association cortex have large receptive fields and that their selective priming would result in a broad attentional spotlight. Further, he suggested that attentional selection may begin in higher order association cortex and proceed, when necessary to narrow the focus of attention, backward "through a reafferent modulation of lower order sensory cortex and koniocortex, to modulate neurons with narrower receptive fields" (Woods, 1989). It is possible that cannabinoid receptors reside along the pathways involved in the narrowing of the attentional spotlight, and that cumulative exposure to cannabinoids disrupts these mechanisms. Recent animal research has identified a more precise neurophysiological mechanism involving changes in cannabinoid receptor function in the hippocampus and various inhibitory processes governed by endogenous cannabinoids (which might explain the adoption of different strategies), which is being developed by Deadwyler and colleagues into a very elegant model (see below).

The involvement of anandamide or other endogenous cannabinoids was proposed in Chapter 8. Naturally, as an endogenous cannabinoid like substance in the brain, anandamide (or other members of its family) would be involved in the interactions between ingested cannabinoids, and the cannabinoid receptors and pathways. What is proposed here is that anandamide may itself play a role in the modulation of attention. As a newly discovered neurotransmitter, there is much speculation about its role in the nervous system.

The distribution of receptors in the brain, as discussed in Chapter 2, provides clues as to the various functions in which anandamide may be involved. It is likely that it plays some role in movement or motor control (Mechoulam *et al.*, 1994), and as proposed here, in the modulation of attention. The cannabinoid receptor dense cerebellum in particular, traditionally viewed as being responsible for motor coordination, has now been shown to play a role in selective attention, and particularly in switching attention (Akshoomoff & Courchesne, 1992; also Garmezy, 1977). The globus pallidus and anterior cingulate cortex, both rich in cannabinoid receptors, have been shown to respectively be activated under selective and divided attention (Corbetta *et al.*, 1991). Just as there are times when it is essential to focus attention and concentrate solely on the task at hand, there are other times when it is important to be able to switch attention between the monitoring of a number of sources of information (e.g. in the work of flight controllers or in driving a motor vehicle). It is not unreasonable to presume that the switching of attentional requirements may be regulated by neurotransmitter systems, and that anandamide may well perform such a function. It is possible that ingestion of cannabinoids over a long-term period displaces the normal levels of anandamide or modifies its normal functioning, resulting in impaired modulation of the switching of attention and a wider distribution of resources over irrelevant sources of information. This is in stark contrast to the selective and focused attention required in tasks such as that utilized in the ERP research reported here, and in the performance of many neuropsychological tests. The theories of attention which link attention to response activation and incorporate the activation of automatic motor schemata (e.g. Norman & Shallice, 1980, 1986; Houghton & Tipper, 1994) may fit well with the proposed roles of anandamide in both attention / executive function and motor coordination. Activation of such a dual role might primarily occur within frontal cortex, although reciprocal connections with posterior regions, thalamus and hippocampus are likely to be involved in integrating perceptual information to guide nonroutine behaviours (ie. those requiring attention) and in regulating cortical activity (Houghton & Tipper, 1994). Support for such a dual role is suggested by the anatomical connections between the cerebellum and prefrontal cortex and hippocampus (Harper & Heath, 1973; Heath & Harper, 1974; Middleton & Strick, 1994; Schmahmann, 1996).

Support for this hypothesis of endogenous cannabinoids being involved in the processes of modulating attention comes from recent animal research. Sim *et al.* (1996) demonstrated profound desensitization of cannabinoid activated signal transduction mechanisms (uncoupling of the receptor from G-proteins) following chronic administration of THC, while Deadwyler *et al.* (1995) showed that the same regimen of administration of THC produced tolerance to the initially impairing effects on a delayed match to sample task, and other studies by this group confirmed that the disruption in memory processes occurs via cannabinoid receptor mediated effects on hippocampal neural activity (Hampson & Deadwyler, 1996a; Hampson *et al.*, 1996). This research was described in Chapter 4 and the role of the endogenous cannabinoids suggested by these findings and others was discussed in Chapter 10. Essentially, it is proposed that endogenous cannabinoids are involved in the selective forgetting or elimination of certain information at the encoding stage of short-term memory (S.A.

Deadwyler, personal communication). Exogenous cannabinoids (e.g. THC) override the normal function of the endogenous cannabinoids by disrupting the encoding of information when it is not appropriate nor advantageous to do so, yet they produce an effect not altogether unlike that of the latter. Whereas the function of the endogenous cannabinoids is an adaptive one, the result of the actions of THC and other exogenous cannabinoids in a nontolerant individual are generally impairing. As stated above with regard to the switching of attentional requirements, there are times also when it is of greater benefit to eliminate certain information before it is consolidated within memory (e.g. in situations where proactive interference would be of detriment). In the model presented here, endogenous cannabinoids facilitate the rejection of irrelevant information in the complex selective attention task. Once the user becomes tolerant to the effects of cannabis, after frequent use over a relatively short period, brain cannabinoid receptors become uncoupled from G-proteins and this may have a profound effect on a variety of other processes. It is not known what becomes of this state over the long-term in chronic cannabis users; however, it can be stated with relative confidence that it is likely that the normal functioning of the endogenous cannabinoid system would be compromised. In the model presented here, this manifested as an inability to effectively focus attention and ignore or reject complex irrelevant information from further processing (long-term users continued to unnecessarily process distractor stimuli).

There is increasing evidence that the types of impairments associated with long-term use of cannabis may also reflect a disturbance of executive function, and hence a dysfunction in the frontal lobes, particularly of prefrontal cortex. Efficient executive / frontal lobe function is important for organizing, manipulating and integrating a variety of information, and in structuring and segregating events in memory. One of the functions of the frontal lobes is the temporal organization of behaviour which is important not only for memory function, but for self awareness and planning. The frontal lobe hypothesis of impairments due to long-term use of cannabis is consistent with the altered perception of time demonstrated in cannabis users (e.g. Webb *et al.*, 1993), with PET studies of glucose metabolism (Volkow *et al.*, 1996), CBF studies (Mathew & Wilson, 1992) and EEG studies (Struve *et al.*, 1992, 1993, 1994) which demonstrate alterations in the region of the frontal lobes. The original studies reported here also found electrophysiological evidence of altered brain functioning in frontal regions, and the kinds of cognitive processes and executive functions examined here and elsewhere (e.g. Fletcher *et al.*, 1996; Pope & Yurgelun-Todd, 1996) are thought to be subserved by the prefrontal lobes. Further research to investigate the effects of cannabis use on these processes is clearly indicated.

There have been vast differences in the functional significance assigned to the frontal lobes, with some authors regarding them as the seat of all thinking and abstraction, and yet others observing no evidence for a disruption of function following frontal lobe damage (see Shallice, 1982, 1988; Baddeley, 1986; Stuss & Benson, 1986). Similar discrepancies have plagued the cognitive literature with regard to the long-term effects of cannabis. Patients with known frontal lobe lesions do not differ from controls on a variety of neuropsychological tests (Stuss, 1991), and yet show many similarities to cannabis users in the kinds of subtle impairments they exhibit. These include short-term memory deficits, increased susceptibility to interference, lack of impairment on general tests of intelligence or IQ, perseveration and lack of mental flexibility. If cannabis and endogenous cannabinoids exert their influence on frontal lobe/executive function this, together with the use of insensitive tests, might have contributed to the equivocal research findings of past studies. As Baddeley (1986) observed, one source of difficulty in this area stems from a contrast between striking results from individual cases, coupled with weaker and more variable findings when groups of patients (e.g. cannabis users) are studied. Baddeley argued that this is due to the complexity of functions subserved by the frontal lobes and also the complex relations that exist with other brain structures. Theoretical development in the area of frontal lobe research is at a very elementary level with adequate measurement or identification of frontal lobe functions dependent on adequate conceptualization of such functions: a similar observation can be made with regard to understanding the effects of cannabis on cognitive function. Baddeley suggested that a dysfunction of the supervisory attentional system or the central executive is particularly difficult to measure by means of traditional experimental psychology because it involves problems of will – voluntary action and the ability to evaluate situations. Rydlander (1939) described the characteristic dysfunction of the frontal lobes as "disturbed attention, increased distractability, a difficulty in grasping the whole of a complicated state of affairs . . . well able to work along old routine lines . . . cannot learn to master new types of task, in new situations". The syndrome is also characterized by a lack of flexibility and a tendency to perseverate, and difficulty in initiating activity. Some of these characteristics were evident in Pope & Yurgelun-Todd's (1996) study of heavy cannabis users, particularly in such tasks as the Wisconsin Card Sort, the FAS verbal fluency test and the California Verbal Learning Test.

The supervisory attentional system (SAS) of Norman & Shallice's (1980, 1986) model is involved in monitoring and controlling behaviour and in the planning of future activities. Problems occur when the subject is required to initiate new behaviour or to discontinue or modify ongoing activity. An apparent paradox with cannabis users, which is also readily apparent in frontal lobe patients, is that they are on the one hand highly distractable, and on the other inclined to perseverate. According to Shallice (1982) this is because the patient remains engaged within currently active or dominant schemata because the SAS is not functioning properly and thus conscious attentional control is compromised. If a number of competing schemata of approximately equal strength emerge, with no direction from the SAS, there will be a tendency for control to switch from one schema to another on the basis of relatively minimal changes in the environmental context. Models of attention and action such as those of Norman & Shallice (1980, 1986) and Houghton & Tipper (1994) hold much promise for explaining the impairments of attention and of executive function associated with long-term or heavy cannabis use.

Cannabis users are relatively unimpaired on simple tests of short-term memory, including recency and digit span (although backward span may be more susceptible). As Baddeley (1986) argued in the case of aging, these tasks place the least demand on the central executive. Tasks that require active organization of material (such as complex manipulation of learned items, or time sharing between information from two sources) are most impaired and sensitive to the effects of cannabis. As Pope & Yurgelun-Todd (1996) and others have found, retrieval processes *per se* are often unaffected in cannabis using populations. This may be because the actual process of retrieval may involve the running off of largely automatic schemata rather than directly involving the central executive (Baddeley, 1986). This may also be due to the primary effect of cannabinoids on the encoding phase of memory processes, as discussed above.

Until further research may be conducted to examine executive function in cannabis users in greater depth, the evidence that attentional processing is progressively impaired as a function of cumulative exposure to cannabis remains convincing, although the mechanism behind such a relation has not been entirely elucidated.

Implications for future research

The demonstration in the original research reported here of differential impairments due to frequency and duration of cannabis use is important in terms of distinguishing short-term effects that may be due to drug residues, from more long lasting impairments that are related to the number of years of cannabis use. The mechanisms involved in such differential impairments, however, remain obscure. If a given effect is strongly correlated with cumulative exposure to cannabis in terms of the number of years that it is used, this implies a progressive impairment that reflects gradual long-term changes in brain function. Future research might aim to determine whether such effects are related to cumulative exposure to cannabis in terms of the total amount of cannabis consumed, although such a lifetime measure is very difficult to estimate with any degree of accuracy. Knowledge of the general pharmacology of drugs suggests that there should be an interaction between frequency and duration of use (and the model of Deadwyler and colleagues depends upon both parameters), yet nowhere in the course of studies reported here was such an interaction observed: effects due to frequency and duration of use were entirely separable; nor has an interactive effect of frequency and duration of cannabis use been reported in the literature, but the relative contributions of these use variables have not been routinely examined. Future research should address these issues and aim to elucidate the mechanisms involved.

Most of the recent research described in this monograph has attempted to identify specific cannabis effects by using strict exclusion criteria and matching control groups on numerous variables to ensure that any deficits observed are attributable to cannabis. Nevertheless, interactions between the effects of long-term cannabis use concurrently with other substances need to be further explored, particularly as many regular cannabis users also use alcohol and other substances to a greater degree than the rest of the population, and the cumulative effects of polydrug use may be additive. Furthermore, subjects have tended to be excluded if they have had a history of childhood illness, learning disabilities, brain trauma or other neurological or psychiatric illness. The effects of long-term cannabis use on such individuals may be worthy of further investigation, especially as evidence suggests that such individuals are more likely to use cannabis (Hall *et al.*, 1994).

When comparisons are made between groups of users versus nonusers, differences may not always reach statistical significance due to large individual variability, particularly when small sample sizes are used. Carlin (1986) proposed that "studies that rely upon analysis of central tendency are likely to overlook impairment by averaging away the differences among subjects who have very different patterns of disability". Individual differences in vulnerability to the acute effects of cannabis are well recognized and are likely to be a factor in determining susceptibility to cognitive dysfunctions associated with prolonged use of cannabis.

Cognitive deficits may not be an inevitable consequence of cannabis use. The long-term effects of cannabis on healthy individuals may differ from those in individuals with coexisting mental illness or pre-existing cognitive impairments. As a clinical example, cannabis may trigger psychotic episodes in those already predisposed to psychiatric disturbances. On the other hand, some individuals can maintain sufficient work performance even in high ranking professions despite their long-term use. To what extent their mental proficiency would improve further if possible subtle cognitive deficits were resolved by discontinuing cannabis use is unknown. Wert and Raulin suggested that some individuals may adapt and overcome some forms of cognitive impairment by a process of relearning: "it is well known that a chronic or slow developing lesion will often be masked by the adaptation of the patient to the deficits produced by the lesion" (Wert & Raulin, 1986b).

There has been very little research designed specifically to identify individual differences, predispositions or susceptibilities to the adverse effects of cannabis. A predisposition may be due to structural, biochemical or psychological factors, or as Wert & Raulin (1986b) suggested, to lack of the "cerebral reserve that most of us call on when we experience mild cerebral damage", for example, after a night of heavy drinking. They propose that "that functional reserve can mask very real cerebral damage". As Wert and Raulin suggested, prospective studies are the ideal way to identify those subjects who show real impairment in functioning by comparing pre- and post-cannabis performance scores.

Virtually all of the studies investigating cognitive functioning in long-term cannabis users have been retrospective studies of naturally occurring groups (users vs nonusers). Although the matching of control groups has become more stringent, and attempts to obtain estimates of premorbid functioning have increased, prospective studies where each subject is used as his/her own control would eliminate the possibility that cannabis using subjects may have demonstrated poorer performance before commencing their use of cannabis. A longitudinal study in which several cohorts at risk for drug abuse are followed over time would certainly be an excellent approach to assessing the detrimental effects of long-term cannabis use on cognition and behaviour. Recommendations that prospective studies be carried out using measures of greater sensitivity and specificity have been made in almost every review of the topic since the early 1970s.

Unfortunately, actual research has been slow to adopt this design and incorporate such measures, or else has been hindered by a lack of commitment of research funds to such long-term ventures.

Carlin (1986) has suggested as an alternative approach, that a meta-analysis be conducted of the studies to date. Such an analysis would "estimate effect size in order to cumulate research findings across studies", perhaps allowing the apparently conflicting findings of the studies to be reconciled. The adequacy of control groups, entry criteria, health factors and other possible contaminating variables could be coded and entered into the analysis. Carlin states that "an overall determination can be made of the extent of the relationship between consumption of a substance and measures of impairment which is relatively independent of traditional statistical significance". Such an analysis would be of particular importance if the impact of the drug on neuropsychological function is modest, as is likely to be the case with cannabis. A modest or even small effect size may have major public health implications. To date, no such research has been applied to the cannabis literature, and perhaps the limited number of studies utilizing similar methodology and outcome measures would preclude the application of a meta-analytic approach. Nevertheless, the substantial advances that have been made in recent years justify the continuation of retrospective studies.

In a carefully controlled retrospective design it is possible to retrospectively compare the characteristics of subjects who show impairment with those who do not, thereby identifying possible risk factors. Insufficient consideration has been given to gender, age, IQ and personality differences in the long-term consequences of cannabis use. Gender differences may be important given that such differences have become apparent in differential responses to alcohol. Pope & Yurgelun-Todd (1996) found some evidence of gender differences in the performance of heavy cannabis users on a number of neuropsychological tests with males being more impaired than females. Further research examining the impact of the age of onset of cannabis use is warranted. Kunert *et al.* (1997) report an association between early onset of use and later impairment in speed of information processing in adult users.

The equivocal results of past studies of cognitive functioning in long-term cannabis users appear to be due primarily to poor methodology and insensitive test measures. Wert & Raulin (1986b) had rejected the possibility that tests used previously were not sensitive enough to detect impairments on the grounds that the same tests had demonstrated impairment in alcoholics and heavy social drinkers; however, the cognitive deficits produced by chronic alcohol consumption may be very different to those produced by cannabis. The mechanisms of action of the two substances are different with cannabis acting on its own specific receptor. As demonstrated in Chapter 8, the attentional impairment evidenced by brain ERP alterations in long-term cannabis users was not related to their alcohol consumption. Pope & Yurgelun-Todd (1996) were also able to show that the cognitive impairments of their heavy cannabis users were not attributable to their use of alcohol or other substances. Thus not only have tests used previously not been sensitive enough, they have probably not been specific enough to detect impairments peculiar to cannabis.

Furthermore, tests may have been selected inappropriately because they were previously shown to be affected by acute intoxication, when the consequences of chronic use may be very different. Block and colleagues (Block *et al.*, 1992; Block & Ghoneim, 1993) showed reasonable, albeit imperfect agreement between acute and chronic effects of cannabis on cognition and the authors emphasized that such effects can be markedly different. The patterns of cognitive deficit associated with long-term cannabis use have still not been entirely characterized. A priority for future research would be the identification of mechanisms of impairment with greater specificity, perhaps by making direct comparisons with the acute effects of cannabis and the long-term effects of alcohol and a variety of other substances. Until such comparisons can be properly made it is not possible to conclusively classify cannabis as a lower level threat to cognitive function than alcohol or other psychoactive substances.

Future research must adhere to rigorous methodology. This should include the use of the best available techniques for detecting the presence of cannabinoids in the body to provide greater precision in the investigation of the influence of length of abstinence on performance. This would permit a distinction to be made between those impairments which may be due to drug residues remaining in the body, and likely to resolve with abstinence over time, from those of a more enduring or chronic nature, which would be associated with the duration of use. The original research reported here has identified cognitive impairments that are associated with the duration of cumulative exposure to cannabis and has suggested that there may be partial reversibility of these impairments with cessation of use. It is therefore a priority to investigate further the recovery of function following cessation of cannabis use.

There is clearly a need to examine the time course of improvement in cognitive functioning and its association with the elimination of accumulated cannabinoids from the body. Subjects should be monitored before and for at least 3 months after stopping regular, long-term cannabis use. A strong association would provide evidence that cognitive impairments are due to the chronic state of intoxication produced by accumulated cannabinoids. If the association proved to be weak, the mechanisms of more lasting changes in brain function should be explored further. In addition to research on naturalistic cognitive recovery following cessation of cannabis use, the utility of incorporating specially designed cognitive rehabilitation programmes, such as the Attention Process Training exercises developed by Sohlberg & Mateer (1989), into treatment protocols for long-term cannabis users is worthy of evaluation and further investigation.

The existence of naturally occurring cannabinoids in the human brain (e.g. anandamide) signifies that these substances play some role in our normal functioning. It has been suggested that anandamide may play a role in movement or motor control (Mechoulam *et al.*, 1994), in the induction of sleep (Mechoulam *et al.*, 1997), in cognition, and as proposed by this author, in the modulation of attention. The neurotransmitters and peptides that govern our behaviour are finely balanced and any major surplus or depletion generally results in dysfunction. With long-term use of cannabis, prolonged or continual binding to the cannabinoid receptor may alter its functional properties and/or the levels of endogenous cannabinoids in the brain. There is a need to further elucidate these physiological mechanisms and the interactions between ingested cannabis, anandamide and the cannabinoid receptor. The use of brain imaging techniques such as PET and functional MRI hold promise for elucidating some of these interactions.

The parameters of drug use require careful scrutiny in terms of evaluating how much cannabis must be smoked and for how long before impairments are manifest in what kinds of individuals. One of the problems in assessing the cannabis literature is the arbitrariness with which various groups of users have been described as "heavy", "moderate" or "light", "long-term", or "short-term". Is a light user someone who uses once, twice or ten times per month? Is a heavy user one who uses daily or at least 10 times per day?

Further measures of executive function, such as strategy formation, self monitoring and cognitive flexibility, might be included in future research and the data examined in relation to ERP indices of attention and to different levels of cannabis use. The use of very sensitive measures of cognitive function, such as ERP measures or specific, sensitive neuropsychological tests (as opposed to general test batteries), is important for the detection of early signs of impairment which may permit a harm minimization approach to be applied to cannabis use. With further research, it may be possible to specify levels of cannabis use that are "safe", "hazardous" and "harmful" levels from the perspective of cognitive impairment. These could be used in health education in the same way similar guidelines have been used in advising people about safe levels of alcohol consumption.

Implications for long-term cannabis users

There is now sufficient clinical and experimental evidence that long-term or heavy use of cannabis leads to subtle impairment of various aspects of attention, memory, and the organization and integration of complex information. While these impairments may be subtle, they could potentially affect functioning in daily life. The evidence suggests that increasing duration of use leads to progressively greater impairment. To what extent such impairment recovers with abstinence is still uncertain, although the evidence from this course of study suggests that there is at least partial recovery for some, if not most, individuals.

Attention underlies many cognitive functions. The ability to focus attention, ignore irrelevant stimuli and efficiently process and manipulate complex information is essential in the execution of many everyday tasks. The consequences of the attentional impairments observed in this and other research may be apparent in high levels of distractibility, for example when driving, operating complex machinery, learning in the classroom situation, and may interfere with memory function. The typical age range of most intense cannabis use occurs between 15 and 25 years, precisely the age during which educational and intellectual achievements are at their most crucial stage, and emotional and maturational development is coming to fruition. Indeed the heavy cannabis users of Pope & Yurgelun-Todd's (1996) study came from a college student population, and many of the subjects who participated in the ERP studies reported here were also university students. It is difficult to gauge the degree to which their educational performance might have been compromised by the cognitive impairments they demonstrated within each of the respective studies; it can only be surmised that had they not used cannabis, they would most likely have made greater academic achievements. Other research suggests that the early commencement of cannabis use (e.g. prior to the age of 16) contributes to a greater risk of generally poor psychosocial adjustment in young adulthood (Fergusson & Horwood, 1997) and may predict delayed speed of information processing with continued use (Kunert *et al.*, 1997).

The evidence from the research reviewed and reported here suggests that the use of cannabis three times per week or more frequently results in a state of chronic intoxication, probably due to the accumulation of cannabinoids. This results in a general slowing of information processing with sluggish mental performance in a variety of tasks. Near daily use for at least 2 years has been shown to impair executive function, which involves the integration of a variety of cognitive processes involving attention and memory. Not only might scholastic achievement be adversely affected by such impairments, but the integration of thoughts and experiences so crucial to personal development may be disrupted. Continued use at or above these levels may lead to the experience of high levels of anxiety, and greater signs and symptoms of psychological distress or overt psychopathological symptomatology, such as paranoid ideation, depression and hostility. Recent reviews suggest that cannabis is not as benign a drug as has been thought in terms of its effects on the mental health of users (Hall & Solowij, 1997).

If the use of cannabis is prolonged, for more than 3 years for example, the user may incur gradual long-term changes in brain function. In particular, the ability to focus attention and ignore irrelevant information may be progressively impaired. Some users may become aware of this impairment, primarily in the form of memory problems, difficulties with concentration, or distractibility, others may be aware of general decline in cognitive abilities but unable to specify where the problem lies, while others may be totally unaware of any such impairment. Nevertheless, it is likely that their general level of performance abilities will be below that of their optimum level of functioning.

If the user continues to use cannabis for many years and then decides to cut down or cease using, it is likely that their mental proficiency will improve somewhat, and probably noticeably so, but perhaps not entirely. The evidence so far suggests that partial impairment in attentional processes may remain, regardless of the duration of abstinence. As with all of the above implications, these predictions are not hard and fast. There clearly are individual differences in response to cannabis; certain individuals may be more predisposed to adverse cognitive consequences and there has been insufficient research devoted to examining such predispositions. The original research presented in this monograph suggests that users of lower IQ may be more vulnerable to adverse cognitive consequences, and that younger users may be more likely to improve with abstinence. Insufficient research has been conducted to examine the recovery of function following cessation of cannabis use.

In general, the message to cannabis users is one of common sense, applicable to almost all substances: experimental use or use in moderation is unlikely to lead to problems in most individuals, but prolonged or excessive use can result in adverse physical, psychological and cognitive consequences. The parameters of cannabis use that result in cognitive impairments are still uncertain, particularly in terms of absolute quantities of THC exposure. Little is known about even infrequent consumption of large quantities of high potency cannabis, and given the known harmful effects of binge drinking of alcohol for example, caution must be observed. Nevertheless, on the basis of research to date, users might be advised that use of more often than twice per week for even a short period of time, or use for 5 years or more at the level of even once per month, may each lead to a compromised ability to function to their full mental capacity, and could possibly result in lasting impairments. (This does not imply that use below these levels may be considered safe.) It is important to present such information to the user in an informed and realistic manner to avoid the misperception of yet more sensationalized antidrug propaganda. In spite of its illegal status, use of cannabis is widespread. We therefore have a continuing responsibility to minimize drug related harm by identifying potential risks, subtle though they may be, and communicating the necessary information to the community.

Implications for society

Given the growing prevalence of cannabis use, and proposals to reduce legal restrictions on cannabis use, it is essential that research into the cognitive functioning of long-term cannabis users continues. According to American survey data (Deahl, 1991), more than 29 million people in the United States may be using cannabis, and more than seven million of these use on a daily basis. While there is some controversy surrounding the issue, it seems likely that the potency of cannabis has increased over the years as more potent strains have been developed. Increased THC potency combined with decreased age of onset of use may result in the longer term in more marked cognitive impairments in larger numbers of individuals.

While it may be true that "real and substantial inconsistencies in the literature have been magnified by those who tend to cite selected pieces of evidence in support of their own ideological beliefs" (Fehr & Kalant, 1983b), it is essential that "any new evidence implicating cannabis with persistent harmful effects is subject to critical scrutiny and careful replication if accusations of prejudice and moral bias are to be avoided" (Deahl, 1991). It appears that the onus of proof is on researchers to prove impairment rather than on the proponents of cannabis use to prove safety. In the case of cognitive impairments in young people, "safe until proven unsafe" may be a dangerous stance to take. It is well accepted that cannabis impairs cognitive and psychomotor functioning while intoxicated and that cannabis smoke is damaging to the respiratory tract (Tashkin, 1993). There is now sufficient evidence for subtle long-term cognitive impairments associated with cannabis use. Further research is clearly warranted to determine the parameters of use that lead to impairment considering the relative contributions of frequency and duration of cannabis use, to elucidate further the nature of the cognitive deficits and assess their recovery, and to compare the cognitive consequences of cannabis use to those of other substances. The dissemination of research findings in a realistic and less sensational manner would provide users with the ability to make an informed decision about whether to use the drug and, if they use, how long, how much and how often to use.

Appendix*: Screening and drug use questionnaire

Name: —————————————————————————————
Date of birth: ——————————————

General health and education

1. Are you on any prescription medication or receiving treatment for any medical condition?
2. Have you ever been hospitalized for any condition?
3. Have you ever had any of the following:
   Serious illnesses
   Fits, convulsions or epileptic seizures
   Serious head injuries or periods of unconsciousness
4. Have you ever been in treatment for drug or alcohol problems?
5. Have you ever consulted a psychologist, psychiatrist or counsellor or undergone therapy for any reason?
6. Is there any psychiatric illness in your family?
7. What is the highest level of education that you have completed or are currently completing?
8. What is your usual occupation?

Now I would like to ask you some questions about your drug and alcohol use.

Alcohol

1. Do you drink alcohol?
2. On how many days would you drink alcohol in a typical week?
3. On a day when you drink, how many drinks would you have (per occasion)?
4. How long have you been drinking at that level?
5. Has there ever been a period in your life when you drank much more heavily?
6. When did you have your last drink of alcohol? How much did you drink?
7. How much did you drink last week? (go through each day of the week). Was this a typical week in terms of drinking habits?

---

* Portions of this questionnaire have been adapted from Rittenhouse (1979); Huba *et al.* (1981); Hannifin (1987); Roffman & George (1988).

Selection criteria:

- Males: Preferably no more than 42 drinks / week on average
- Females: Preferably no more than 28 drinks / week on average
- (No significant history of heavy consumption of alcohol, never been in treatment for alcohol dependence)

Other drugs

1. Do you or have you ever used any of the following substances?
   If so, how frequently, and when was the last time you used each particular substance.

Drug	Quantity / frequency	Last use
Tobacco		
Amphetamines		
Cocaine		
Barbiturates (downers)		
Tranquilizers		
LSD, Mushrooms, Ecstasy		
Opiates (heroin, methadone)		
Inhalents (amyl, aerosols)		
Anything else?		

2. Have you ever had any problems associated with the use of any of these drugs?
   e.g. been arrested, involved in a car accident, felt you were dependent, etc.

Selection criteria: Reject anyone with a history of use ≥ 1 / month or use in the month prior to testing.

(Controls only)

1. Have you ever tried marijuana?
2. Have you ever used marijuana on a regular basis?
3. When was the last time you used marijuana?
4. How many times have you had marijuana in total, over what time period?

Selection criteria: Reject anyone who has used cannabis recently or more often than once/month.

(Users only)

Now I'd like to ask you some detailed questions about your use of cannabis.

1. How old were you when you first tried marijuana?
2. How old were you when you first started using regularly?
3. How often are you currently smoking marijuana? e.g. on how many days would you smoke marijuana in a typical month?
4. What do you usually smoke? i.e. leaf, heads, hash?
5. How would you rate the strength of the marijuana you usually smoke on a scale from 0 (mild) to 10 (strong)?

6. Do you mix your marijuana with tobacco?
7. Do you smoke joints, bongs or pipes?
8. How many would you smoke in a typical session?
9. On a day when you are smoking marijuana, how many sessions would you have?
10. On a scale from 0 to 10, where 0 = totally straight, and 10 = the most stoned you've ever been, what level of intoxication do you usually like to reach?
11. How long have you been smoking at this level?
12. Has your pattern of use changed over time?
13. Has there ever been a period in your life when you smoked much more heavily?
14. Have you ever used on a daily basis? When was the last time you were using on a daily basis and for how long?
15. Altogether, if you added up every month that you have ever used DAILY, for about how much of your life would you estimate that you have used daily or almost daily? e.g. < 3 months, 3–9 months, 1 year, 2–3 years, 5–9 years, >10 years.
16. Have you ever felt dependent on cannabis? How would you define that?
17. Have you ever had any problems associated with your use of cannabis? (e.g. arrests, problems with concentration or memory, etc., anything)
18. In the last 3 years, what is the longest period you've gone without marijuana?
19. When did you have your last smoke? How much did you smoke at that time?
20. How much did you smoke last week? Was this a typical week in terms of marijuana use? (If not last week, think back to the last time you smoked)

Effects of cannabis

1. Sometimes the effects you experience when you take drugs are the ones you want; sometimes they are not. Sometimes drugs improve things for you; sometimes they make matters worse. This section asks about the short-term effects you get just after smoking marijuana. Tick one answer for each question.

The SHORT-TERM or immediate effects of marijuana on your:

	Usually made better	Usually made worse	Sometimes better sometimes worse	Usually no effect
Ability to think clearly	____	____	____	____
Excitement and enthusiasm for life	____	____	____	____
Enjoyment of sex	____	____	____	____
Ability to relax	____	____	____	____
Driving ability	____	____	____	____

2. Using marijuana sometimes leads to changes in people's lives. For each question listed below, indicate whether you think marijuana has improved, impaired or had no effect on your life. What we are asking about here are long-term effects, not the effects you experience just after taking the drug.

The LONG-TERM effect of marijuana on your:

	Improved	Impaired	No effect
Ability to think clearly	——	——	——
Ability to cope and solve life's problems	——	——	——
Physical health	——	——	——
General self confidence	——	——	——
Ability to concentrate on complex tasks	——	——	——
Work performance (studies)	——	——	——
Ability to communicate	——	——	——
Relations with employers / seniors	——	——	——
Memory	——	——	——
General coordination	——	——	——
General level of energy	——	——	——
Excitement and enthusiasm for life	——	——	——

3. Why do you like to smoke marijuana?
4. What do you dislike about marijuana?
5. Have you ever made a conscious decision to stop smoking? If so, for what reasons, and how long did you give up for? Why did you start again?

CASST (Hannifin, 1987)

1. Have people close to you complained about your cannabis use?   Y / N
2. Do you have problems with short-term memory?   Y / N
3. Have you ever experienced paranoid episodes following cannabis use?   Y / N
4. Do you find it difficult to get through a day without a joint?   Y / N
5. Do you lack the energy to get things done in the way you used to?   Y / N
6. Do you ever worry about the effects of your cannabis use?   Y / N
7. Do you have more difficulty in understanding new information?   Y / N
   (e.g. difficulty in studying)
8. Have you ever unsuccessfully attempted to cut down or stop your cannabis use?   Y / N
9. Do you like to get stoned in the morning?   Y / N
10. Are you spending more and more time stoned?   Y / N
11. Do you experience cravings, headaches, irritability or difficulty in concentration when you cut down or cease cannabis use?   Y / N

References

Abbott, A. (1990). The switch that turns the brain on to cannabis. *New Scientist*, **127**, 19.

Abel, E.L. (1971a). Retrieval of information after use of marihuana. *Nature*, **231**, 58.

Abel, E.L. (1971b). Marihuana and memory: acquisition or retrieval? *Science*, **173**, 1038–40.

Abel, E.L. (1980). *Marijuana: The First Twelve Thousand Years*. New York: Plenum Press.

Abood, M.E. & Martin, B.R. (1992). Neurobiology of marijuana abuse. *Trends in Pharmacological Science*, **13**, 201–6.

Abood, M.E., Sauss, C., Fan, F., Tilton, C.L. & Martin, B.R. (1993). Development of behavioral tolerance to Δ^9-THC without alteration of cannabinoid receptor binding or mRNA levels in whole brain. *Pharmacology Biochemistry and Behavior*, **46**, 575–9.

Adams, I.B. & Martin, B.R. (1996). Cannabis: pharmacology and toxicology in animals and humans. *Addiction*, **91**, 1585–614.

Adams, P.M. & Barratt, E.S. (1975). Effect of chronic marijuana administration on stages of primate sleep-wakefulness. *Biological Psychiatry*, **10**, 315–22.

Adler, L.E., Pachtman, E., Franks, R.D., Pecevich, M., Waldo, M.C. & Freedman, R. (1982). Neurophysiological evidence for a defect in neuronal mechanisms involved in sensory gating in schizophrenia. *Biological Psychiatry*, **17**, 639–54.

Agarwal, A.K., Sethi, B.B. & Gupta, S.C. (1975). Physical and cognitive effects of chronic bhang (cannabis) intake. *Indian Journal of Psychiatry*, **17**, 1–7.

Agurell, S., Halldin, M., Lindgren, J., Ohlsson, A., Widman, M., Gillespie, H. & Hollister, L. (1986). Pharmacokinetics and metabolism of Δ^1-Tetrahydrocannabinol and other cannabinoids with emphasis on man. *Pharmacological Reviews*, **38**, 21–43.

Akshoomoff, N.A. & Courchesne, E. (1992). A new role for the cerebellum in cognitive operations. *Behavioural Neuroscience*, **106**, 731–8.

Alho, K., Sams, M., Paavilainen, P., Reinikainen, K. & Näätänen, R. (1989). Event-related brain potentials reflecting processing of relevant and irrelevant stimuli during selective listening. *Psychophysiology*, **26**, 514–28.

Alho, K., Töttölä, K., Reinikainen, K., Sams, M. & Näätänen, R. (1987). Brain mechanisms of selective listening reflected by event-related potentials. *Electroencephalography and Clinical Neurophysiology*, **68**, 458–70.

References

Alho, K., Woods, D., Algazi, A. & Näätänen, R. (1992). Intermodal selective attention. II. Effects of attentional load on processing of auditory and visual stimuli in central space. *Electroencephalography and Clinical Neurophysiology*, **82**, 356–8.

Ali, S.F., Newport, G.D., Scallet, A.C., Gee, K.W., Paule, M.G., Brown, R.M. & Slikker, W., Jr (1989). Effects of chronic delta-9-tetrahydrocannabinol (THC) administration on neurotransmitter concentrations and receptor binding in the rat brain. *Neurotoxicology*, **10**, 491–500.

Ali, S.F., Newport, G.D., Scallet, A.C., Paule, M.G., Bailey, J.R. & Slikker, W., Jr (1991). Chronic marijuana smoke exposure in the rhesus monkey. IV. Neurochemical effects and comparison to acute and chronic exposure to delta-9-tetrahydrocannabinol (THC) in rats. *Pharmacology Biochemistry and Behavior*, **40**, 677–82.

Altman, H. & Evenson, R.C. (1973). Marijuana use and subsequent psychiatric symptoms. *Comprehensive Psychiatry*, **14**, 415–20.

American Psychiatric Association (1987). *Diagnostic and Statistical Manual of Mental Disorders (DSM-III-R)*, 3rd edn revised. Washington, DC: American Psychiatric Association.

American Psychiatric Association (1994). *Diagnostic and Statistical Manual of Mental Disorders (DSM-IV)*, 4th edn. Washington, DC: American Psychiatric Association.

Andreasson, S., Allebeck, P., Engstrom, A. & Rydberg, U. (1987). Cannabis and schizophrenia: a longitudinal study of Swedish conscripts. *Lancet*, **2**, 1483–6.

Anthony, J.C. & Helzer, J.E. (1991). Syndromes of drug abuse and dependence. In *Psychiatric Disorders in America*, ed. L.N. Robins & D.E. Regier, pp. 116–54. New York: The Free Press.

Arnsten, A.F.T., Neville, H.J., Hillyard, S.A., Janowsky, D.S. & Segal, D.S. (1984). Naloxone increases electrophysiological measures of selective information processing in humans. *Journal of Neuroscience*, **4**, 2912–19.

Arnsten, A.F.T., Segal, D.S., Neville, H.J., Hillyard, S.A., Janowsky, D.S., Judd, L.L. & Bloom, F.E. (1983). Naloxone augments electrophysiological signs of selective attention in man. *Nature*, **304**, 725–7.

Baddeley, A.D. (1986). *Working Memory*. Oxford: Oxford University Press.

Baddeley, A.D. & Hitch, G. (1974). Working memory. In *The Psychology of Learning and Motivation. Recent Advances in Learning and Motivation*, ed. G. Bower, vol. *VIII*, pp. 47–90. New York: Academic Press.

Barnett, G., Licko, V. & Thompson, T. (1985). Behavioral pharmacokinetics of marijuana. *Psychopharmacology*, **85**, 51–6.

Barnett, V. & Lewis, T. (1984). *Outliers in Statistical Data*, New York: John Wiley.

Barratt, E.S. & Adams, P.M. (1972). The effects of chronic marijuana administration on brain functioning in cats. *Clinical Toxicology*, **5**, 36.

Barratt, E.S. & Adams, P.M. (1973). Chronic marijuana usage and sleep-wakefulness cycles in cats. *Biological Psychiatry*, **6**, 207–14.

Beck, A.T. (1987). *Beck Depression Inventory*. San Antonio: The Psychological Corporation.

Belgrave, B.E., Bird, K.D., Chesher, G.B., Jackson, D.M., Lubbe, K.E., Starmer, G.A. & Teo, R.K.C. (1979). The effect of (-) trans-Δ^9-tetrahydrocannabinol, alone and in combination with ethanol, on human performance. *Psychopharmacology*, **62**, 53–60.

Belue, R.C., Howlett, A.C., Westlake, T.M. & Hutchings, D.E. (1995). The ontogeny of cannabinoid receptors in the brain of postnatal and aging rats. *Neurotoxicology and Teratology*, **17**, 25–30.

Bidaut-Russell, M., Devane, W.A. & Howlett, A.C. (1990). Cannabinoid receptors and modulation of cyclic AMP accumulation in the rat brain. *Journal of Neurochemistry*, **55**, 21–55.

Biegon, A. & Kerman, I. (1995). Quantitative autoradiography of cannabinoid receptors in the human brain post-mortem. In *Sites of Drug Action in the Human Brain*, ed. A. Biegon & N.D. Volkow, pp. 65–74. Boca Raton: CRC Press.

Black, S. & Casswell, S. (1993). *Drugs in New Zealand – A survey 1990*. Auckland, NZ: Alcohol and Public Health Research Unit, University of Auckland.

Block, R.I. (1996). Does heavy marijuana use impair human cognition and brain function? *Journal of the American Medical Association*, **275**, 560–1.

Block, R.I., Farinpour, R. & Braverman, K. (1992). Acute effects of marijuana on cognition: relationships to chronic effects and smoking techniques. *Pharmacology Biochemistry and Behavior*, **43**, 907–17.

Block, R.I., Farnham, S., Braverman, K., Noyes, R., Jr & Ghoneim, M.M. (1990). Long-term marijuana use and subsequent effects on learning and cognitive functions related to school achievement: preliminary study. In *Residual Effects of Abused Drugs on Behavior*, ed. J.W. Spencer & J.J. Boren, pp. 96–111. National Institute on Drug Abuse Research Monograph 101, Rockville, MD: U.S. Department of Health and Human Services.

Block, R.I. & Ghoneim, M.M. (1993). Effects of chronic marijuana use on human cognition. *Psychopharmacology*, **110**, 219–28.

Block, R.I. & Wittenborn, J.R. (1984). Marijuana effects on semantic memory: verification of common and uncommon category members. *Psychological Reports*, **55**, 503–12.

Block, R.I. & Wittenborn, J.R. (1986). Marijuana effects on the speed of memory retrieval in the letter-matching task. *International Journal of the Addictions*, **21**, 281–5.

Bloom, A.S. (1984). Effects of cannabinoids on neurotransmitter receptors in the brain. In *The Cannabinoids: Chemical, Pharmacological and Therapeutic Aspects*, ed. S., Agurell, W.L. Dewey & R.E. Willette, pp. 575–89. New York: Academic Press.

Blum, K. (1984). *Handbook of Abusable Drugs*. New York: Gardner Press.

Bowman, M. & Pihl, R.O. (1973). Cannabis: psychological effects of chronic heavy use. A controlled study of intellectual functioning in chronic users of high potency cannabis. *Psychopharmacologia*, **29**, 159–70.

Braden, W., Stillman, R.C. & Wyatt, R.J. (1974). Effects of marijuana on contingent negative variation and reaction time. *Archives of General Psychiatry*, **31**, 537–41.

Braff, D.L., Silverton, L., Saccuzzo, D.P. & Janowsky, D.S. (1981). Impaired speed of visual information processing in marijuana intoxication. *American Journal of Psychiatry*, **138**, 613–17.

Brill, N.Q. & Christie, R.L. (1974). Marijuana use and psychosocial adaptation: follow-up study of a collegiate population. *Archives of General Psychiatry*, **31**, 713–19.

Broadbent, D.E. (1958). *Perception and Communication*. New York: Pergamon Press.

Broadbent, D.E. (1971). *Decision and Stress*. London: Academic Press.

Broadbent, D.E. (1977). The hidden preattentive processes. *American Psychologist*, **32**, 109–18.

Broadbent, D.E. (1982). Task combination and selective intake of information. *Acta Psychologica*, **50**, 253–90.

Broadbent, D.E. (1985). A question of levels: comment on McClelland and Rumelhart. *Journal of Experimental Psychology: General*, **114**, 189–92.

Bull, J. (1971). Cerebral atrophy in young cannabis smokers. *Lancet*, **2**, 1420.

Campbell, A.M.G., Evans, M., Thomson, J.L.G. & Williams, M.J. (1971). Cerebral atrophy in young cannabis smokers. *Lancet*, **2**, 1219–24.

Campbell, D.R. (1971). The electroencephalogram in cannabis associated psychosis. *Canadian Psychiatric Association Journal*, **16**, 161–5.

Campbell, K.A., Foster, T.C., Hampson, R.E. & Deadwyler, S.A. (1986a). Δ^9-Tetrahydrocannabinol differentially affects sensory-evoked potentials in the rat dentate gyrus. *Journal of Pharmacology and Experimental Therapeutics*, **239**, 936–40.

Campbell, K.A., Foster, T.C., Hampson, R.E. & Deadwyler, S.A. (1986b). Effects of Δ^9-tetrahydrocannabinol on sensory-evoked discharges of granule cells in the dentate gyrus of behaving rats. *Journal of Pharmacology and Experimental Therapeutics*, **239**, 941–5.

Cappell, H.D. & Pliner, P.L. (1973). Volitional control of marijuana intoxication: a study of the ability to come down on command. *Journal of Abnormal Psychology*, **82**, 428–34.

Carlin, A.S. (1986). Neuropsychological consequences of drug abuse. In *Neuropsychological Assessment of Neuropsychiatric Disorders*, ed. I. Grant & K.M. Adams, pp. 478–97. New York: Oxford University Press.

Carlin, A.S., Bakker, C.B., Halpern, L. & Post, R.D. (1972). Social facilitation of marijuana intoxication: Impact of social set and pharmacological activity. *Journal of Abnormal Psychology*, **80**, 132–40.

Carlin, A.S. & Trupin, E.W. (1977). The effect of long-term chronic marijuana use on neuropsychological functioning. *International Journal of the Addictions*, **12**, 617–24.

Carter, W.E. (1980). *Cannabis in Costa Rica: a Study of Chronic Marihuana Use.* Philadelphia: Institute for the Study of Human Issues.

Casswell, S. & Marks, D. (1973a). Cannabis induced impairment of performance of a divided attention task. *Nature*, **241**, 60–1.

Casswell, S. & Marks, D. (1973b). Cannabis and temporal disintegration in experienced and naive subjects. *Science*, **179**, 803–5.

Catts, S., Shelley, A.M., Ward, P.B., Liebert, B., McConaghy, N., Andrews, S. & Michie, P.T. (1995). Brain potential evidence for an auditory sensory memory deficit in schizophrenia. *American Journal of Psychiatry*, **152**, 213–19.

Chait, L.D., Fischman, M.W. & Schuster, C.R. (1985). 'Hangover' effects the morning after marijuana smoking. *Drug and Alcohol Dependence*, **15**, 229–38.

Chait, L.D. & Pierri, J. (1992). Effects of smoked marijuana on human performance: a critical review. In *Marijuana/Cannabinoids: Neurobiology and Neurophysiology*, ed. L. Murphy & A.Bartke, pp. 387–423. Boca Raton: CRC Press.

Charalambous, A., Marciniak, G., Shiue, C.-Y., Dewey, S.L., Schlyer, D.J., Wolf, A.P. & Makriyannis, A. (1991). PET studies in the primate brain and biodistribution in mice using (-)- $5'$-^{18}F-Δ^8-THC. *Pharmacology Biochemistry and Behavior*, **40**, 503–7.

Chesher, G.B., Dauncey, H., Crawford, J.C. & Horn, K. (1986). *The interaction of alcohol and marijuana: a dose dependent study of effects on human moods and performance skills.* Canberra: Federal Office of Road Safety.

Chesher, G.B., Franks, H.M., Hensley, V.R., Hensley, W.J., Jackson, D.M., Starmer, G.A. & Teo, R.K.C. (1976). The interaction of ethanol and Δ^9-tetrahydrocannabinol in man: effects on perceptual, cognitive and motor functions. *Medical Journal of Australia*, **2**, 159–63.

Chesher, G.B., Franks, H.M., Jackson, D.M., Starmer, G.A. & Teo, R.K.C. (1977). Ethanol and Δ⁹-tetrahydrocannabinol: interactive effects on human perceptual, cognitive and motor functions. *Medical Journal of Australia*, 1, 478–81.

Chopra, G.S. (1971). Marijuana and adverse psychotic reactions: evaluation of different factors involved. *Bulletin on Narcotics*, 23, 15–22.

Chopra, G.S. (1973). Studies on psycho-clinical aspects of long-term marihuana use in 124 cases. *International Journal of the Addictions*, 8, 1015–26.

Chopra, G.S. & Smith, J.W. (1974). Psychotic reactions following cannabis use in East Indians. *Archives of General Psychiatry*, 30, 24–7.

Chopra, G.S. & Jandu, B.S. (1976). Psychoclinical effects of long-term marijuana use in 275 Indian chronic users: a comparative assessment of effects in Indian and USA users. *Annals of the New York Academy of Sciences*, 282 (Dornbush, R.L., Freedman, A.M. & Fink, M. (Eds) Chronic Cannabis Use), 95–108.

Co, B.T., Goodwin, D.W., Gado, M., Mikhael, M. & Hill, S.Y. (1977). Absence of cerebral atrophy in chronic cannabis users: evaluation by computerized transaxial tomography. *Journal of the American Medical Association*, 237, 1229–30.

Cohen, S. (1976). The 94-day cannabis study. *Annals of the New York Academy of Sciences*, 282 (Dornbush, R.L., Freedman, A.M. & Fink, M. (Eds) Chronic Cannabis Use), 211–20.

Cohen, S. (1982). Cannabis effects upon adolescent motivation. In *Marijuana and Youth: Clinical Observations on Motivation and Learning*, pp. 2–9. Rockville, MD: National Institute on Drug Abuse.

Cohen, S. (1986). Marijuana research: selected recent findings. *Drug Abuse and Alcoholism Newsletter*, 15, 1–3.

Collins, D.R., Pertwee, R.G. & Davies, S.N. (1995). Prevention by the cannabinoid antagonist, SR141716A, of cannabinoid-mediated blockade of long-term potentiation in the rat hippocampal slice. *British Journal of Pharmacology*, 115, 869–70.

Comitas, L. (1976). Cannabis and work in Jamaica: a refutation of the amotivational syndrome. *Annals of the New York Academy of Sciences*, 282 (Dornbush, R.L., Freedman, A.M. & Fink, M. (Eds) Chronic Cannabis Use), 24–32.

Cone, E.J. & Johnson, R.E. (1986). Contact highs and urinary cannabinoid excretion after passive exposure to marijuana smoke. *Clinical Pharmacology and Therapeutics*, 40, 247–56.

Cone, E.J., Johnson, R.E., Darwin, W.D., Yousefnajed, D., Mell, L.D., Paul, B.D. & Mitchell, J. (1987b). Passive inhalation of marijuana smoke: urinalysis and room air levels of delta-9-tetrahydrocannabinol. *Journal of Analytical Toxicology*, 11, 89–96.

Cone, E.J., Roache, J.D. & Johnson, R.E. (1987a). Effects of passive exposure to marijuana smoke. In *Problems of Drug Dependence 1986*, ed. L. Harris, National Institute on Drug Abuse Research Monograph 76, pp. 150–6. Rockville, MD: U.S. Department of Health and Human Services.

Consensus Report, C.D.P. Research Technology Branch, National Institute on Drug Abuse. (1985). Drug concentrations and driving impairment. *Journal of the American Medical Association*, 254, 2618–21.

Corbetta, M., Miezin, F.M., Dobmeyer, S., Shulman, G.L. & Petersen, S.E. (1991). Selective and divided attention during visual discriminations of shape, color, and speed: functional anatomy by positron emission tomography. *The Journal of Neuroscience*, 11, 2383–402.

References

Cowan, N. (1988). Evolving conceptions of memory storage, selective attention, and their mutual constraints within the human information processing system. *Psychological Bulletin*, **104**, 163–91.

Cox, B. (1990). Drug tolerance and physical dependence. In *Principles of Drug Action. The Basis of Pharmacology*, ed. W. Pratt & P. Taylor, pp. 639–90. New York: Churchill Livingstone.

Crawley, J., Corwin, R., Robinson, J., Felder, C., Devane, W. & Axelrod, J. (1993). Anandamide, an endogenous ligand of the cannabinoid receptor, induces hypomotility and hyperthermia *in vivo* in rodents. *Pharmacology Biochemistry and Behavior*, **46**, 967–72.

Culver, C.M. & King, F.W. (1974). Neuropsychological assessment of undergraduate marihuana and LSD users. *Archives of General Psychiatry*, **31**, 707–11.

Dackis, C.A., Pottash, A.L.C., Annitto, W. & Gold, M.S. (1982). Persistence of urinary marijuana levels after supervised abstinence. *American Journal of Psychiatry*, **139**, 1196–8.

Damasio, A.R. (1979). The frontal lobes. In *Clinical Neuropsychology*, ed. K.M. Heilman & E. Valenstein, pp. 360–412. New York: Oxford University Press.

Darke, S. (1988). Anxiety and working memory capacity. *Cognition and Emotion*, **2**, 145–54.

Darke, S., Wodak, A., Hall, W., Heather, N. & Ward, J. (1992). Prevalence and predictors of psychopathology among opioid users. *British Journal of Addiction*, **87**, 771–76.

Deadwyler, S.A., Bunn, T. & Hampson, R.E. (1996a). Hippocampal ensemble activity during spatial delayed-nonmatch-to-sample performance in rats. *Journal of Neuroscience*, **16**, 354–72.

Deadwyler, S.A., Byrd, D.R., Konstantopoulos, J.A., Evans, G.J.O., Rogers, G. & Hampson, R.E. (1996b). Enhancement of rat hippocampal ensemble activity by CX516 protects against errors in spatial DNMS. *Society of Neuroscience Abstracts*, **2**, 1131.

Deadwyler, S.A. & Hampson, R.E. (1995). Ensemble activity and behavior: what's the code? *Science*, **270**, 1316–18.

Deadwyler, S.A. & Hampson, R.E. (1997). The significance of neural ensemble codes during behavior and cognition. *Annual Review of Neuroscience*, **20**, 217–44.

Deadwyler, S.A., Heyser, C.J. & Hampson, R.E. (1995). Complete adaptation to the memory disruptive effects of delta-9-THC following 35 days of exposure. *Neuroscience Research Communications*, **17**, 9–18.

Deahl, M. (1991). Cannabis and memory loss. *British Journal of Addiction*, **86**, 249–52.

Deliyannakis, E., Panagopoulos, C. & Huott, A.D. (1970). The influence of hashish on human EEG. *Clinical Electroencephalography*, **1**, 128–40.

Derogatis, L.R. (1983). *SCL-90-R Administration, Scoring, and Procedures Manual – II*. Towson, MD.

Deutsch, D.G. & Chin, S.A. (1993). Enzymatic synthesis and degradation of anandamide, a cannabinoid receptor agonist. *Biochemical Pharmacology*, **46**, 791–6.

Deutsch, J.A. & Deutsch, D. (1963). Attention: some theoretical considerations. *Psychological Review*, **70**, 80–90.

Devane, W.A. & Axelrod, J. (1994). Enzymatic synthesis of anandamide, an endogenous ligand for the cannabinoid receptor, by brain membranes. *Proceedings of the National Academy of Sciences of the USA*, **91**, 6698–701.

Devane, W.A., Dysarz, F.A., Johnson, M.R., Melvin, L.S. & Howlett, A.C.

(1988). Determination and characterization of a cannabinoid receptor in rat brain. *Molecular Pharmacology*, **34**, 605–13.

Devane, W.A., Hanus, L., Breuer, A., Pertwee, R.G., Stevenson, L.A., Griffin, G., Gibson, D., Mandelbaum, A., Etinger, A. & Mechoulam, R. (1992). Isolation and structure of a brain constituent that binds to the cannabinoid receptor. *Science*, **258**, 1946–9.

Dewey, W.L. (1986). Cannabinoid pharmacology. *Pharmacological Reviews*, **38**, 151–78.

Di Marzo, V., Fontana, A., Cadas, H., Schinelli, S., Cimino, G., Schwartz, J-C. & Piomelli, D. (1994). Formation and inactivation of endogenous cannabinoid anandamide in central neurons. *Nature*, **372**, 686–91.

Di Tomaso, E., Beltramo, M. & Piomelli, D. (1996). Brain cannabinoids in chocolate. *Nature*, **382**, 677–8.

Dixon, L., Haas, G., Wedien, P.J., Sweeney, J. & Frances, A.J. (1990). Acute effects of drug abuse in schizophrenic patients: clinical observations and patient's self reports. *Schizophrenia Bulletin*, **16**, 69–79.

Domino, E.F. (1981). Cannabinoids and the cholinergic system. *Journal of Clinical Pharmacology*, **21**, 249s–55s.

Donchin, E. (1981). Surprise! . . . Surprise? *Psychophysiology*, **18**, 493–513.

Donchin, E. & Coles, M.G.H. (1988). Is the P300 component a manifestation of context updating? *Behavioral and Brain Sciences*, **11**, 355–72.

Donchin, E., Ritter, W. & McCallum, W.G. (1978). Cognitive psychophysiology: the endogenous components of the ERP. In *Event-Related Brain Potentials in Man*, ed. E., Callaway, P. Tueting & S.H. Koslow, pp. 349–412. New York: Academic Press.

Dornbush, R.L. (1974). Marijuana and memory: effects of smoking on storage. *Transactions of the New York Academy of Sciences*, **36**, 94–100.

Dornbush, R.L., Clare, G., Zaks, A., Crown, P., Volavka, J. & Fink, M. (1972). Twenty-one day administration of marijuana in male volunteers. In *Current Research in Marihuana*, ed. M.F. Lewis, pp. 115–27. New York: Academic Press.

Dornbush, R.L., Fink, M. & Freedman, A.M. (1971). Marijuana, memory, and perception. *American Journal of Psychiatry*, **128**, 194–7.

Dornbush, R.L. & Kokkevi, A. (1976). The acute effects of various cannabis substances on cognitive, perceptual, and motor performance in very long-term hashish users. In *Pharmacology of Marihuana*, ed. M.C. Braude & S. Szara, pp. 421–8. New York: Raven Press.

Douglas, R.J. (1967). The hippocampus and behavior. *Psychological Bulletin*, **67**, 416–42.

Drew, W.G., Weet, C.R., De Rossett, S.E. & Batt, J.R. (1980). Effects of hippocampal brain damage on auditory and visual recent memory: comparison with marijuana-intoxicated subjects. *Biological Psychiatry*, **15**, 841–58.

Edwards, G. (1982). Cannabis and the question of dependence. In *Advisory Council on the Misuse of Drugs. Report of the Expert Group on the Effects of Cannabis Use*. London: Home Office.

Edwards, G. (1983). Psychopathology of a drug experience. *British Journal of Psychiatry*, **143**, 509–12.

Eichenbaum, H. & Cohen, N.J. (1988). Representation in the hippocampus: what do hippocampal neurons encode? *Trends in Neuroscience*, **11**, 244–8.

Eldridge, J.C., Hu, H-Y., Extrom, P.C. & Landfield, P.W. (1992). Interactions between cannabinoids and steroids in the rat hippocampus. *Society of Neuroscience Abstracts*, **18**, 789.

Eldridge, J.C. & Landfield, P.W. (1990). Cannabinoid interactions with glucocorticoid receptors in rat hippocampus. *Brain Research*, **534**, 135–41.

Eldridge, J.C., Murphy, L.L. & Landfield, P.W. (1991). Cannabinoids and the hippocampal glucocorticoid receptor: recent findings and possible significance. *Steroids*, **56**, 226–31.

Ellis, G.M., Mann, M.A., Judson, B.A., Schramm, N.T. & Tashchian, A. (1985). Excretion patterns of cannabinoid metabolites after last use in a group of chronic users. *Clinical Pharmacology and Therapeutics*, **38**, 572–8.

ElSohly, M.A. & ElSohly, H.N. (1989). Marijuana: analysis and detection of use through urinalysis. In *Cocaine, Marijuana, Designer Drugs*, ed. K.K., Redda, C.A. Walker & G. Barnett, pp. 145–61. Boca Raton: CRC Press.

Emrich, H.M., Weber, M.M., Wendl, A., Zihl, J., Von Meyer, L. & Hanisch, W. (1991). Reduced binocular depth inversion as an indicator of cannabis induced censorship impairment. *Pharmacology Biochemistry and Behavior*, **40**, 689–90.

Entin, E.E. & Goldzung, P.J. (1973). Residual effects of marihuana use on learning and memory. *Psychological Record*, **23**, 169–78.

Eysenck, M.W. (ed) (1982). *Attention and Arousal (Cognition and Performance)*. Berlin: Springer Verlag.

Eysenck, M.W. (1988). Anxiety and attention. *Anxiety Research*, **1**, 9–15.

Feeney, D.M. (1979). Marihuana and epilepsy: paradoxical anticonvulsant and convulsant effects. In *Marihuana: Biological Effects. Analysis, Metabolism, Cellular Responses, Reproduction and Brain*, ed. G.G. Nahas & W.D.M. Paton, pp. 643–57. Oxford: Pergamon Press.

Fehr, K.O. & Kalant, H. (eds) (1983a).*Cannabis and Health Hazards. Proceedings of an ARF/WHO Scientific Meeting on Adverse Health and Behavioural Consequences of Cannabis Use*. Toronto: Addiction Research Foundation.

Fehr, K.O. & Kalant, H. (1983b). Long-term effects of cannabis on cerebral function: a review of the clinical and experimental literature. In *Cannabis and Health Hazards*, ed. K.O. Fehr & H. Kalant, pp. 501–76. Toronto: Addiction Research Foundation.

Feinberg, I., Jones, R., Walker, J., Cavness, C. & Floyd, T. (1976). Effects of marijuana extract and tetrahydrocannabinol on electroencephalographic sleep patterns. *Clinical Pharmacology and Therapeutics*, **19**, 782–94.

Felder, C.C., Briley, E.M., Axelrod, J., Simpson, J.T., Mackie, K. & Devane, W.A. (1993). Anandamide, an endogenous cannabimimetic eicosanoid, binds to the cloned human cannabinoid receptor and stimulates receptor-mediated signal transduction. *Proceedings of the National Academy of Sciences of the USA*, **90**, 7656–60.

Felder, C.C., Nielsen, A., Briley, E.M., Palkovits, M., Priller, J., Axelrod, J., Nguyen, D.N., Richardson, J.M., Riggin, R.M., Koppel, G.A., Paul, S.M., and Becker, G.W. (1996). Isolation and measurement of the endogenous cannabinoid receptor agonist, anandamide, in brain and peripheral tissues of human and rat. *Federation of European Biochemical Societies Letters*, **393**, 231–5.

Fergusson, D.M. & Horwood, L.J. (1997). Early onset cannabis use and psychosocial adjustment in young adults. *Addiction*, **92**, 279–96.

Fiez, J.A., Petersen, S.E., Cheney, M.K. & Raichle, M.E. (1992). Impaired non-motor learning and error detection associated with cerebellar damage. *Brain*, **115**, 155–78.

Fink, D.J., Ashworth, B. & Brewer, C. (1972). Cerebral atrophy in young cannabis smokers. *Lancet*, **1**, 143.

Fink, M. (1976a). Effects of acute and chronic inhalation of hashish, marijuana, and Δ⁹-tetrahydrocannabinol on brain electrical activity in man: evidence for tissue tolerance. *Annals of the New York Academy of Sciences*, **282** (Dornbush, R.L., Freedman, A.M. & Fink, M. (Eds) Chronic Cannabis Use), 387–98.

Fink, M. (1976b). Conference summary. *Annals of the New York Academy of Sciences*, **282** (Dornbush, R.L., Freedman, A.M. & Fink, M. (Eds) Chronic Cannabis Use), 427–30.

Fink, M., Volavka, J., Panayiotopoulos, C.P. & Stefanis, C. (1976). Quantitative EEG studies of marijuana, Δ⁹-tetrahydrocannabinol, and hashish in man. In *Pharmacology of Marihuana*, ed. M.C. Braude & S. Szara, vol. 1, pp. 383–91. New York: Raven Press.

Fletcher, J.M., Page, J.B., Francis, D.J., Copeland, K., Naus, M.J., Davis, C.M., Morris, R., Krauskopf, D. & Satz, P. (1996). Cognitive correlates of long-term cannabis use in Costa Rican men. *Archives of General Psychiatry*, **53**, 1051–7.

Fletcher, J.M. & Satz, P. (1977). A methodological commentary on the Egyptian study of chronic hashish use. *Bulletin on Narcotics*, **29**, 29–34.

Ford, J.M., White, P.M., Csernansky, J.G., Faustman, W.O., Roth, W.T. & Pfefferbaum, A. (1994). ERPs in schizophrenia: Effects of antipsychotic medication. *Biological Psychiatry*, **36**, 153–70.

Fox, A.M., Michie, P.T., Coltheart, M. & Solowij, N. (1995). Memory functioning in social drinkers: a study of event-related potentials. *Alcohol and Alcoholism*, **30**, 303–10.

Frank, I.M., Lessin, P.J., Tyrell, E.D., Hahn, P.M. & Szara, S. (1976). Acute and cumulative effects of marihuana smoking in hospitalized subjects: a 36 day study. In *Pharmacology of Marihuana*, ed. M.C. Braude & S. Szara, vol. 2, pp. 673–9. New York: Raven Press.

Fried, P. (1977). Behavioral and electroencephalographic correlates of the chronic use of marijuana: a review. *Behavioral Biology*, **21**, 163–96.

Fried, P. (1993). Prenatal exposure to tobacco and marijuana: effects during pregnancy, infancy, and early childhood. *Clinical Obstetrics and Gynaecology*, **36**, 319–37.

Fried, P. (1995). The Ottawa Prenatal Prospective Study (OPPS): methodological issues and findings – its easy to throw the baby out with the bath water. *Life Sciences*, **56**, 2159–68.

Fried, P. (1996). Behavioural outcomes in preschool and school-age children exposed prenatally to marijuana: a review and speculative interpretation. In *Behavioral Studies of Drug Exposed Offspring: Methodological Issues in Human and Animal Research*, ed. C.L. Wetherington, V.L. Smeriglio & L.P. Finnegan, National Institute on Drug Abuse Research Monograph 164, pp. 242–60. Washington DC: U.S. Government Printing Office.

Fried, P.A. & Charlebois, A.T. (1979). Cannabis administered during pregnancy: first and second generation effects in rats. *Physiological Psychology*, **7**, 307–10.

Friedman, D., Simpson, G. & Hamberger, M. (1993). Age-related changes in scalp topography to novel and target stimuli. *Psychophysiology*, **30**, 383–96.

Fuster, J.M. (1980). *The Prefrontal Cortex*. New York: Raven Press.

Gaoni, Y. & Mechoulam, R. (1964). Isolation, structure and partial synthesis of an active constituent of hashish. *Journal of the American Chemistry Society*, **86**, 1646–7.

Garmezy, N. (1977). The psychology of psychopathology of attention. *Schizophrenia Bulletin*, 3, 360–9.

Gatley, S.J., Gifford, A.N., Volkow, N.D., Lan, R. & Makriyannis, A. (1996).

Iodine-123 labeled AM251: a radioiodinated ligand which binds in vivo to the mouse brain CB1 cannabinoid receptor. *European Journal of Pharmacology*, **307**, 301–8.

Gerard, C.M., Mollereau, C., Vassart, G. & Parmentier, M. (1991). Molecular cloning of a human cannabinoid receptor which is also expressed in testis. *Biochemistry Journal*, **279**, 129–34.

Ghodse, A.H. (1986). Cannabis psychosis. *British Journal of Addiction*, **81**, 473–8.

Gianutsos, R. & Litwack, A.R. (1976). Chronic marijuana smokers show reduced coding into long-term storage. *Bulletin of the Psychonomic Society*, **7**, 277–9.

Gifford, A.N. & Ashby, C.R.J. (1996). Inhibition of acetylcholine release from hippocampal slices by the cannabimimetic aminoalkylindole WIN 55212-2, and evidence for the release of an endogenous cannabinoid inhibitor. *Journal of Pharmacology and Experimental Therapeutics*, **277**, 1431–6.

Gifford, A.N., Samiian, L., Gatley, S.J. & Ashby, C.R.J. (1997). Examination of the effect of the cannabinoid agonist, CP 55,940, on electrically-evoked transmitter release from rat brain slices. *European Journal of Pharmacology*, **324**, 187–92.

Goldstein, A. & Kalant, H. (1990). Drug policy: striking the right balance. *Science*, **249**, 1513–21.

Grant, I., Rochford, J., Fleming, T. & Stunkard, A. (1973). A neuropsychological assessment of the effects of moderate marihuana use. *Journal of Nervous and Mental Disease*, **156**, 278–80.

Grenyer, B.F.S., Luborsky, L. & Solowij, N. (1995). *Treatment Manual for Supportive-Expressive Dynamic Psychotherapy: Special Adaptation for Treatment of Cannabis (Marijuana) Dependence.* National Drug and Alcohol Research Centre Technical Report No. 26. Sydney: University of New South Wales.

Grenyer, B.F.S., Williams, G., Swift, W. & Neill, O. (1992). The prevalence of social-evaluative anxiety in opioid users seeking treatment. *International Journal of the Addictions*, **27**, 665–73.

Gross, S.J., Worthy, T.E., Nerder, L., Zimmermann, E.G., Soares, J.R. & Lomax, P. (1985). The detection of recent cannabis use by saliva delta-9-THC radioimmune quantitation. *Journal of Analytical Toxicology*, **2**, 98–100.

Grossberg, S. & Stone, G. (1986). Neural dynamics of word recognition and recall: attentional priming, learning and resonance. *Psychological Review*, **93**, 46–74.

Hall, W., Johnston, L. & Donnelly, N. (in press) Epidemiological evidence on patterns of cannabis use and their health consequences. World Health Organization Project on Health Implications of Cannabis Use.

Hall, W. & Solowij, N. (1996). Steering a course between the Charybdis of credulity and the Scylla of scepticism. Response to comments on Hall *et al.*'s Australian National Drug Strategy Monograph No. 25 "The Health and Psychological Consequences of Cannabis Use", *Addiction*, **91**, 770–3.

Hall, W. & Solowij, N. (1997). Long-term cannabis use and mental health. *British Journal of Psychiatry*, **171**, 107–8.

Hall, W., Solowij, N. & Lemon, J. (1994). *The Health and Psychological Consequences of Cannabis Use.* National Drug Strategy Monograph Series No. 25, Canberra: Australian Government Publishing Service.

Hampson, R.E., Byrd, D.R., Konstantopoulos, J.K., Bunn, T. & Deadwyler, S.A. (1996). Delta-9-Tetrahydrocannabinol influences sequential memory in rats performing a delayed-nonmatch-to-sample task. *Society of Neuroscience Abstracts*, **2**, 1131.

Hampson, R.E. & Deadwyler, S.A. (1996a). Ensemble codes involving hippocampal neurons are at risk during delayed performance tests. *Proceedings of the National Academy of Sciences of the USA*, **93**, 13487–93.

Hampson, R.E. & Deadwyler, S.A. (1996b). LTP and LTD and the encoding of memory in small ensembles of hippocampal neurons. In *Long-Term Potentiation*, ed. M. Baudry & J. Davis, vol. 3, pp. 199–214. Cambridge, MA: MIT Press.

Hannerz, J. & Hindmarsh, T. (1983). Neurological and neuroradiological examination of chronic cannabis smokers. *Annals of Neurology*, **13**, 207–10.

Hannifin, J. (1987). The ownership debate: cannabis and the concept of "cannabism". In *Marijuana: An International Research Report*, ed. G. Chesher, P. Consroe & R. Musty, National Campaign Against Drug Abuse Monograph Series No. 7, pp. 231–6. Canberra: Australian Government Printing Service.

Hansen, J.C. & Hillyard, S.A. (1980). Endogenous brain potentials associated with selective auditory attention. *Electroencephalography and Clinical Neurophysiology*, **49**, 277–90.

Hansen, J.C. & Hillyard, S.A. (1983). Selective attention to multidimensional auditory stimuli. *Journal of Experimental Psychology Human Perception*, **9**, 1–19.

Harper, J.W. & Heath, R.G. (1973). Anatomic connections of the fastigial nucleus to the rostral forebrain in the cat. *Experimental Neurology*, **39**, 285–92.

Harper, J.W., Heath, R.G. & Myers, W.A. (1977). Effects of cannabis sativa on ultrastructure of the synapse in monkey brain. *Journal of Neuroscience Research*, **3**, 87–93.

Harshman, R.A., Crawford, H.J. & Hecht, E. (1976). Marihuana, cognitive style, and lateralized hemisphere. In *The Therapeutic Potential of Marihuana*, ed. S. Cohen & R.C. Stillman, pp. 205–54. New York: Plenum Press.

Harter, M.R. & Aine, C.J. (1984). Brain mechanisms of visual selective attention. In *Varieties of Attention*, ed. R. Parasuraman & D.R. Davies, pp. 293–321. New York: Academic Press.

Hawks, R.L. (1982). The constituents of cannabis and the disposition and metabolism of cannabinoids. In *The Analysis of Cannabinoids in Biological Fluids*, ed. R.L. Hawks, National Institute on Drug Abuse Research Monograph 42, pp.125–37. Rockville, MD: U.S. Department of Health and Human Services.

Hawks, R.L. & Chiang, C.N. (eds) (1986). *Urine Testing for Drugs of Abuse*. National Institute on Drug Abuse Research Monograph 73. Rockville, MD: U.S. Department of Health and Human Services.

Hayden, J.W. (1991). Passive inhalation of marijuana smoke: a critical review. *Journal of Substance Abuse*, **3**, 85–90.

Heath, R.G. (1972). Marihuana – effects on deep and surface electroencephalograms in man. *Archives of General Psychiatry*, **26**, 577–84.

Heath, R.G., Fitzjarrell, A.T., Fontana, C.J. & Garey, R.E. (1980). Cannabis sativa: effects on brain function and ultrastructure in rhesus monkeys. *Biological Psychiatry*, **15**, 657–90.

Heath, R.G. & Harper, J.W. (1974). Ascending projections of the cerebellar fastigial nucleus to the hippocampus, amygdala and other temporal lobe sites: Evoked potential and histological studies in monkeys and cats. *Experimental Neurology*, **45**, 268–87.

Hegerl, U., Lipperheide, K., Juckel, G., Schmidt, L.G. & Rommelspacher, H. (1995). Antisocial tendencies and cortical sensory-evoked responses in alcoholism. *Alcoholism: Clinical and Experimental Research*, **19**, 31–6.

Heishman, S.J., Huestis, M.A., Henningfield, J.E. & Cone, E.J. (1990). Acute and residual effects of marijuana: profiles of plasma THC levels, physiological, subjective and performance measures. *Pharmacology Biochemistry and Behavior*, **37**, 561–5.

Heishman, S.J., Pickworth, W.B., Bunker, E.B. & Henningfield, J.E. (1993). Acute and residual effects of smoked marijuana on human performance. In *Problems of Drug Dependence 1992*, ed. L. Harris, National Institute on Drug Abuse Research Monograph 132, p. 270. Washington DC: U.S. Government Printing Office.

Heishman, S.J., Stitzer, M.L. & Bigelow, G.E. (1988). Alcohol and marijuana: Comparative dose effect profiles in humans. *Pharmacology Biochemistry and Behavior*, **31**, 649–55.

Heishman, S.J., Stitzer, M.L. & Yingling, J.E. (1989). Effects of tetrahydro-cannabinol content on marijuana smoking behavior, subjective reports, and performance. *Pharmacology Biochemistry and Behavior*, **34**, 173–9.

Herkenham, M. (1992). Cannabinoid receptor localization in brain: relationship to motor and reward systems. *Annals of the New York Academy of Sciences*, **654** (Kalivas, P.W. & Samson, H.H. (Eds) The Neurobiology of Drug and Alcohol Addiction), 19–32.

Herkenham, M., Lynn, A.B., de Costa, B.R. & Richfield, E.K. (1991a). Neuronal localization of cannabinoid receptors in the basal ganglia of the rat. *Brain Research*, **547**, 267–74.

Herkenham, M., Lynn, A.B., Johnson, M.R., Melvin, L.S., de Costa, B.R. & Rice, K.C. (1991b). Characterization and localization of cannabinoid receptors in rat brain: A quantitative in vitro autoradiographic study. *Journal of Neuroscience*, **11**, 563–83.

Herkenham, M., Lynn, A.B., Little, M.D., Johnson, M.R., Melvin, L.S., De Costa, B.R. & Rice, K.C. (1990). Cannabinoid receptor localization in brain. *Proceedings of the National Academy of Sciences of the USA*, **87**, 1932–6.

Hernández-Peón, R. (1966). Physiological mechanisms in attention. In *Frontiers in Physiological Psychology*, ed. R.W. Russell, pp. 121–47. New York: Academic Press.

Hernández-Peón, R., Scherrer, H. & Jouvet, M. (1956). Modification of electrical activity in the cochlear nucleus during attention in unanaesthetized cats. *Science*, **123**, 331–2.

Herning, R.I., Jones, R.T. & Peltzman, D.J. (1979). Changes in human event-related potentials with prolonged delta-9-tetrahydrocannabinol (THC) use. *Electroencephalography and Clinical Neurophysiology*, **47**, 556–70.

Heyser, C.J., Hampson, R.E. & Deadwyler, S.A. (1993). Effects of Δ^9-tetrahydrocannabinol on delayed match-to-sample performance in rats: Alterations in short-term memory associated with changes in task specific firing of hippocampal cells. *Journal of Pharmacology and Experimental Therapeutics*, **264**, 294–307.

Hillyard, S.A. & Hansen, J.C. (1986). Attention: Electrophysiological Approaches. In *Psychophysiology: Systems, Processes and Applications*, ed. M.G.H. Coles, E. Donchin & S.W. Porges, pp. 227–43. New York: The Guilford Press.

Hillyard, S.A., Hink, R.F., Schwent, V.L. & Picton, T.W. (1973). Electrical signs of selective attention in the human brain. *Science*, **182**, 177–80.

Hillyard, S.A. & Kutas, M. (1983). Electrophysiology of cognitive processing. *Annual Review of Psychology*, **34**, 33–61.

Hillyard, S.A. & Mangun, G.R. (1987). Commentary: sensory gating as a physiological mechanism for visual selective attention. In *Current Trends in Event-Related Potential Research*, ed. R. Johnson, J.W. Rohrbaugh & R. Parasuraman, pp. 61–7. Amsterdam: Elsevier Science Publishers.

Hirschhorn, T.N. & Michie, P.T. (1990). Brainstem auditory evoked potentials (BAEPs) and selective attention revisited. *Psychophysiology*, 27, 495–512.

Hochberg, J.E. (1978). *Perception*. Englewood Cliffs, NJ: Prentice Hall.

Hochman, J.S. & Brill, N.Q. (1973). Chronic marijuana use and psychosocial adaptation. *American Journal of Psychiatry*, 130, 132–40.

Hockman, C.H., Perrin, R.G. & Kalant, H. (1971). Electroencephalographic and behavioral alterations produced by Δ^1-tetrahydrocannabinol. *Science*, 172, 968–70.

Hollister, L.E. (1986). Health aspects of cannabis. *Pharmacological Reviews*, 38, 1–20.

Hollister, L.E., Gillespie, H.K., Ohlsson, A., Lindgren, J-E., Wahlen, A. & Agurell, S. (1981). Do plasma concentrations of Δ^9-tetrahydrocannabinol reflect the degree of intoxication? *Journal of Clinical Pharmacology*, 21, 171S–7S.

Hooker, W.D. & Jones, R.T. (1987). Increased susceptibility to memory intrusions and the Stroop interference effect during acute marijuana intoxication. *Psychopharmacology*, 91, 20–4.

Houghton, G. & Tipper, S.P. (1994). A model of inhibitory mechanisms in selective attention. In *Inhibitory Processes in Attention, Memory and Language*, ed. D. Dagenbach & T.H. Carr, pp. 53–112. San Diego: Academic Press.

Howlett, A.C. (1987). Cannabinoid inhibition of adenylate cyclase: relative activity of constituents and metabolites of marihuana. *Neuropharmacology*, 26, 507–12.

Howlett, A.C., Bidaut-Russell, M., Devane, W.A., Melvin, L.S., Johnson, M.R. & Herkenham, M. (1990). The cannabinoid receptor: biochemical, anatomical and behavioral characterization. *Trends in Neuroscience*, 13, 420–3.

Howlett, A.C., Evans, D.M. & Houston, D.B. (1992). The cannabinoid receptor. In *Marijuana / Cannabinoids: Neurobiology and Neurophysiology*, ed. L. Murphy & A. Bartke, pp. 35–72. Boca Raton: CRC Press.

Howlett, A.C., Johnson, M.R., Melvin, L.S. & Milne, G.M. (1988). Nonclassical cannabinoid analgetics inhibit adenylate cyclase: development of a cannabinoid receptor model. *Molecular Pharmacology*, 33, 297–302.

Howlett, A.C., Qualy, J.M. & Khatchatrian, L.L. (1986). Involvement of Gi in the inhibition of adenylate cyclase by cannabimimetic drugs. *Molecular Pharmacology*, 29, 307–13.

Huba, G.J., Bentler, P.M. & Newcomb, M.D. (1981). *Assessing Marijuana Consequences: Selected Questionnaire Items*, Research Issues No. 28, DHHS Publication No. ADM 81–1150, Washington, DC: U.S. Government Printing Office.

Huestis, M.A., Henningfield, J.E. & Cone, E.J. (1992a). Blood Cannabinoids: I. Absorption of THC and formation of 11-OH-THC and THCCOOH during and after smoking marijuana. *Journal of Analytical Toxicology*, 16, 276–82.

Huestis, M.A., Sampson, A.H., Holicky, B.J., Henningfield, J.E. & Cone, E.J. (1992b). Characterization of the absorption phase of marijuana smoking. *Clinical Pharmacology and Therapeutics*, 52, 31–41.

Huitema, B.E. (1980). *The Analysis of Covariance and Alternatives*. New York: Wiley.

Hunt, C.A. & Jones, R.T. (1980). Tolerance and disposition of tetrahydrocannabinol in man. *Journal of Pharmacology and Experimental Therapeutics*, 215, 35–44.

Institute of Medicine (1982). *Marijuana and Health*, Washington, DC: National Academy Press.

Iragui, V.J., Kutas, M., Mitchiner, M.R. & Hillyard, S.A. (1993). Effects of aging on event-related brain potentials and reaction times in an auditory oddball task. *Psychophysiology*, **30**, 10–22.

Isreal, J.B., Chesney, G.L., Wickens, C.D. & Donchin, E. (1980). P300 and tracking difficulty: Evidence for multiple resources in dual-task performance. *Psychophysiology*, **17**, 259–73.

Jaffe, J. (1990). Drug addiction and drug abuse: cannabinoids (Marihuana). In *The Pharmacological Basis of Therapeutics*, ed. A.G. Gilman, T.W. Rall, A.S. Nies & P. Taylor, 8th edn, pp. 549–53. New York: Pergamon Press.

James, W. (1890). *The Principles of Psychology*. New York: Dover.

Janowsky, D.S., Meacham, M.P., Blaine, J.D., Schoor, M. & Bozzetti, L.P. (1976). Marijuana effects on simulated flying ability. *American Journal of Psychiatry*, **133**, 384–8.

Johansson, E., Sjovall, J., Noren, K., Agurell, S., Hollister, L.E. & Halldin, M.M. (1987). Analysis of Δ^1-Tetrahydrocannabinol (Δ^1-THC) in human plasma and fat after smoking. In *Marijuana: An International Research Report*, ed. G. Chesher, P. Consroe & R. Musty, National Campaign Against Drug Abuse Monograph Series No. 7, pp. 291–6. Canberra: Australian Government Printing Service.

Johansson, E., Agurell, S., Hollister, L.E. & Halldin, M.M. (1988). Prolonged apparent half-life of Δ^1-tetrahydrocannabinol in plasma of chronic marijuana users. *Journal of Pharmacy and Pharmacology*, **40**, 374–5.

John, E.R., Prichep, L.S., Alper, K.R., Mas, F.G., Cancro, R., Easton, P. & Szerdlov, L. (1994). Quantitative electrophysiological characteristics and subtyping of schizophrenia. *Biological Psychiatry*, **36**, 801–26.

Johnson, R. Jr. (1993). On the neural generators of the P300 component of the event-related potential. *Psychophysiology*, **30**, 90–7.

Johnston, W.A. & Dark, V.J. (1982). In defense of intraperceptual theories of attention. *Journal of Experimental Psychology: Human Perception and Performance*, **8**, 407–21.

Jones, R.T. (1975). Effects of marijuana on the mind. In *Marijuana and Health Hazards*, ed. J.R. Tinklenberg, pp. 115–20. New York: Academic Press.

Jones, R.T. (1980). Human effects: an overview. In *Marijuana Research Findings: 1980*, ed. R.C. Petersen, National Institute on Drug Abuse Research Monograph 31, pp. 54–80. Rockville, MD: U.S. Department of Health and Human Services.

Jones, R.T. (1983). Cannabis tolerance and dependence. In *Cannabis and Health Hazards: Proceedings of an ARF/WHO Scientific Meeting on Adverse Health and Behavioral Consequences of Cannabis Use*, ed. K.O. Fehr & H. Kalant, pp. 617–89. Toronto: Addiction Research Foundation.

Jones, R.T. (1987). Drug of abuse profile: cannabis. *Clinical Chemistry*, **33**, 72B–81B.

Jones, R.T. & Stone, G.C. (1970). Psychological studies of marijuana and alcohol in man. *Psychopharmacologia*, **18**, 108–17.

Kahneman, D. (1973). *Attention and Effort*. New Jersey: Prentice Hall.

Kahneman, D. & Treisman, A. (1984). Changing views of attention and automaticity. In *Varieties of Attention*, ed. R. Parasuraman & D.R. Davies, pp. 29–61. New York: Academic Press.

Kalant, H. (1996). Good report but scanty research. Comments on Hall et al.'s Australian National Drug Strategy Monograph No. 25 "The Health and Psychological Consequences of Cannabis Use", *Addiction*, **91**, 759–73.

Kales, A., Hanley, J., Rickles, W., Kanas, N., Baker, M. & Goring, P. (1972). Effects of marijuana administration and withdrawal in chronic users and naive subjects. *Psychophysiology*, **9**, 92.

Kandel, D.B. (1984). Marijuana users in young adulthood. *Archives of General Psychiatry*, **41**, 200–9.

Kandel, D.B. and Davies, G.H. (1992). Progression to regular marijuana involvement: Phenomenology and risk factors for near daily use. In *Vulnerability to Drug Abuse*, ed. M. Glantz & R. Pickens, pp. 211–53. Washington, DC: American Psychological Association.

Kandel, D.B. & Logan, J.A. (1984). Patterns of drug use from adolescence to young adulthood. I. Periods of risk for initiation, continued use and discontinuation. *American Journal of Public Health*, **74**, 660–6.

Kandel, D.B. & Raveis, V.H. (1989). Cessation of illicit drug use in young adulthood. *Archives of General Psychiatry*, **46**, 109–16.

Karacan, I., Fernandez-Salas, A., Coggins, W.J., Carter, W.E., Williams, R.L., Thornby, J.I., Salis, P.J., Okawa, M. & Villaume, J.P. (1976). Sleep electroencephalographic-electrooculographic characteristics of chronic marijuana users. *Annals of the New York Academy of Sciences*, **282** (Dornbush, R.L., Freedman, A.M. & Fink, M. (Eds) Chronic Cannabis Use), 348–74.

Karayanidis, F., Andrews, S., Ward, P.B. & Michie, P.T. (1995). ERP indices of auditory selective attention in aging and Parkinson's disease. *Psychophysiology*, **32**, 335–50.

Kimble, D.P. (1968). Hippocampus and internal inhibition. *Psychological Bulletin*, **70**, 285–95.

Klonoff, H. (1974). Effects of marijuana on driving in a restricted area and on city streets: Driving performance and physiological changes. In *Marijuana: Effects on Human Behavior*, ed. L. Miller, pp. 359–97. New York: Academic Press.

Knight, R.T., Hillyard, S.A., Woods, D.L. & Neville, H.J. (1981). The effects of frontal cortex lesions on event-related potentials during auditory selective attention. *Electroencephalography and Clinical Neurophysiology*, **52**, 571–82.

Kokkevi, A. & Dornbush, R. (1977). Psychological test characteristics of long-term hashish users. In *Hashish: Studies of Long-Term Use*, ed. C. Stefanis, R. Dornbush & M. Fink, pp. 43–7. New York: Raven Press.

Kolansky, H. & Moore, R.T. (1971). Effects of marihuana on adolescents and young adults. *Journal of the American Medical Association*, **216**, 486–92.

Kolansky, H. & Moore, R.T. (1972). Toxic effects of chronic marihuana use. *Journal of the American Medical Association*, **222**, 35–41.

Kopell, B.S., Roth, W.T. & Tinklenberg, J.R. (1978). Time course effects of marihuana and ethanol on event-related potentials. *Psychopharmacology*, **56**, 15–20.

Kopell, B.S., Tinklenberg, J.R. & Hollister, L.E. (1972). Contingent negative variation amplitudes: marihuana and alcohol. *Archives of General Psychiatry*, **27**, 809–11.

Koukkou, M. & Lehmann, D. (1976). Human EEG spectra before and during cannabis hallucinations. *Biological Psychiatry*, **11**, 663–77.

Koukkou, M. & Lehmann, D. (1977). EEG spectra indicate predisposition to visual hallucinations under psilocybin, cannabis, hypnagogic and daydream conditions. *Electroencephalography and Clinical Neurophysiology*, **43**, 499–500.

Kouri, E., Pope, H.G., Yurgelun-Todd, D. & Gruber, S. (1995). Attributes of heavy vs occasional marijuana smokers in a college population. *Biological Psychiatry*, **38**, 475–81.

Kozel, N.J. & Adams, E.H. (1986). Epidemiology of drug abuse: an overview. *Science*, **234**, 970–4.

Kreuz, D.S. & Axelrod, J. (1973). Delta-9-tetrahydrocannabinol: Localization in body fat. *Science*, **179**, 391–3.

Kuehnle, J., Mendelson, J.H. & David, K.R. (1977). Computed tomographic examination of heavy marijuana users. *Journal of the American Medical Association*, **237**, 1231–2.

Kunert, H.J., Rinn, T., Moeller, M.R., Poser, W., Hoehe, M.R. & Ehrenreich, J. (1997). Early onset of cannabis use is associated with specific attentional dysfunctions in adult moderate users. In *1997 Symposium on the Cannabinoids*, p. 82. International Cannabinoid Research Society, Burlington, Vermont.

Lan, R., Gatley, S.J. & Makriyannis, A. (1996). Preparation of iodine-123 labelled AM251, a potential SPECT radioligand for the brain cannabinoid CB1 receptor. *Journal of Labelled Compounds and Radiopharmaceuticals*, **38**, 875–81.

Landfield, P.W., Cadwallader, L.B. & Vinsant, S. (1988). Quantitative changes in hippocampal structure following long-term exposure to Δ^9-tetrahydrocannabinol: possible mediation by glucocorticoid systems. *Brain Research*, **443**, 47–62.

Landfield, P.W. & Eldridge, J.C. (1993). Neurotoxicity and drugs of abuse: cannabinoid interaction with brain glucocorticoid receptors. In *Assessing Neurotoxicity of Drugs of Abuse*, ed. L. Erinoff, National Institute on Drug Abuse Research Monograph 136, pp. 242–56. Washington DC: U.S. Government Printing Office.

Law, B., Mason, P.A., Moffat, A.C., King. L.J. & Marks, V. (1984). Passive inhalation of cannabis smoke. *Journal of Pharmacy and Pharmacology*, **36**, 578–81.

Leavitt, J., Webb, P., Norris, G., Struve, F., Straumanis, J., Patrick, G., Fitz-Gerald, M.J. & Nixon, F. (1992). Differences in complex reaction time between THC users and non-user controls. In *Problems of Drug Dependence 1991*, ed. L. Harris, National Institute on Drug Abuse Research Monograph 119, p. 452. Washington DC: U.S. Government Printing Office.

Leavitt, J., Webb, P., Norris, G., Struve, F., Straumanis, J., Fitz-Gerald, M., Nixon, F., Patrick, G. & Manno, J. (1993). Performance of chronic daily marijuana users on neuropsychological tests. In *Problems of Drug Dependence 1992*, ed. L. Harris, National Institute on Drug Abuse Research Monograph 132, p. 179. Washington DC: U.S. Government Printing Office.

Leirer, V.O., Yesavage, J.A. & Morrow, D.G. (1989). Marijuana, aging, and task difficulty effects on pilot performance. *Aviation, Space and Environmental Medicine*, **60**, 1145–52.

Leirer, V.O., Yesavage, J.A. & Morrow, D.G. (1991). Marijuana carry-over effects on aircraft pilot performance. *Aviation, Space, and Environmental Medicine*, **62**, 221–7.

Lemberger, L. & Rubin, A. (1978). Cannabis: the role of metabolism in the development of tolerance. *Drug Metabolism Reviews*, **8**, 59–68.

Lemberger, L., Silberstein, S.D., Axelrod, J. & Kopin, I.J. (1970). Marihuana: Studies on the disposition and metabolism of delta-9-tetrahydrocannabinol in man. *Science*, **170**, 1320–1.

Leon-Carrion, J. (1990). Mental performance in long-term heavy cannabis use: A preliminary report. *Psychological Reports*, **67**, 947–52.

Leon-Carrion, J. & Vela-Bueno, A. (1991). Cannabis and cerebral hemispheres: A chrononeuropsychological study. *International Journal of Neuroscience*, **57**, 251–7.

Lewis, E.G., Dustman, R.E., Peters, B.A., Straight, R.C. & Beck, E.C. (1973). The effects of varying doses of Δ^9-tetrahydrocannabinol on the human visual and somatosensory evoked response. *Electroencephalography and Clinical Neurophysiology*, **35**, 347–54.

Lichtman, A.H., Dimen, K.R. & Martin, B.R. (1995). Systemic or intrahippocampal cannabinoid administration impairs spatial memory in rats. *Psychopharmacology*, **119**, 282–90.

Lichtman, A.H. & Martin, B.R. (1996). Delta-9-Tetrahydrocannabinol impairs spatial memory through a cannabinoid receptor mechanism. *Psychopharmacology*, **126**, 125–31.

Low, M.D., Klonoff, H. & Marcus, A. (1973). The neurophysiological basis of the marihuana experience. *Canadian Medical Association Journal*, **108**, 157–64.

Lukas, J.H. (1980). Human auditory attention: the olivocochlear bundle may function as a peripheral filter. *Psychophysiology*, **17**, 444–52.

Lukas, J.H. (1981). The role of efferent inhibition in human auditory attention. An examination of the auditory brainstem potentials. *International Journal of Neuroscience*, **12**, 137–45.

Lundqvist, T. (1995a). Specific thought patterns in chronic cannabis smokers observed during treatment. *Life Sciences*, **56**, 2141–4.

Lundqvist, T. (1995b). Chronic cannabis use and the sense of coherence. *Life Sciences*, **56**, 2145–50.

Lundqvist, T. (1995c). *Cognitive Dysfunctions in Chronic Cannabis Users Observed During Treatment: an Integrative Approach*. University of Lund and Stockholm: Almqvist and Wiksell International.

Luria, A.R. (1966). *Higher Cortical Functions in Man*. London: Tavistock.

Luthra, Y.K., Rosenkrantz, H. & Braude, M.C. (1976). Cerebral and cerebellar neurochemical changes and behavioral manifestations in rats chronically exposed to marijuana smoke. *Toxicology and Applied Pharmacology*, **35**, 455–65.

MacAvoy, M.G. & Marks, D.F. (1975). Divided attention performance of cannabis users and non-users following cannabis and alcohol. *Psychopharmacology*, **44**, 147–52.

Mackie, K., Hsieh, C. & Law, J. (1997). Rapid internalization of the CB1 cannabinoid receptor following agonist binding. In *1997 Symposium on the Cannabinoids*, p. 55. International Cannabinoid Research Society, Burlington, Vermont.

Mailleux, P. & Vanderhaeghen, J.J. (1992). Age-related loss of cannabinoid receptor binding sites and mRNA in the rat striatum. *Neuroscience Letters*, **147**, 179–81.

Mailleux, P. & Vanderhaeghen, J.J. (1994). Delta-9-Tetrahydrocannabinol regulates substance P and enkephalin mRNAs levels in the caudate-putamen. *European Journal of Pharmacology*, **267**, R1–R3.

Makriyannis, A. & Rapaka, R.S. (1990). The molecular basis of cannabinoid activity. *Life Sciences*, **47**, 2173–84.

Mallet, P.E. & Beninger, R.J. (1995). The endogenous cannabinoid receptor agonist anandamide impairs working memory but not reference memory in rats. *Society of Neuroscience Abstracts*, **21**, 167.

Mangun, G.R. & Hillyard, S.A. (1995). Mechanisms and models of selective attention. In *Electrophysiology of Mind: Event-Related Brain Potentials and Cognition*, ed. M.D. Rugg & M.G.H. Coles, pp. 40–85. Oxford: Oxford University Press.

Marciniak, G., Charalambous, A., Shiue, C-Y., Dewey, S.L., Schlyer, D.J.,

Makriyannis, A. & Wolf, A.P. (1991). ^{18}F-Labeled tetrahydrocannabinol: synthesis; and PET studies in a baboon. *Journal of Laboratory and Comparative Radiophysiology*, **XXX**, 413–15.

Marks, D.F. & MacAvoy, M.G. (1989). Divided attention performance in cannabis users and non-users following alcohol and cannabis separately and in combination. *Psychopharmacology*, **99**, 397–401.

Martin, B.R. (1986). Cellular effects of cannabinoids. *Pharmacological Reviews*, **38**, 45–74.

Mason, A.P. & McBay, A.J. (1985). Cannabis: pharmacology and interpretation of effects. *Journal of Forensic Sciences*, **30**, 615–31.

Mathew, R.J., Tant, S. & Berger, C. (1986). Regional cerebral blood flow in marijuana smokers. *British Journal of Addiction*, **81**, 567–71.

Mathew, R.J. & Wilson, W.H. (1992). The effects of marijuana on cerebral blood flow and metabolism. In *Marijuana/Cannabinoids: Neurobiology and Neurophysiology*, ed. L. Murphy & A. Bartke, pp. 337–86. Boca Raton: CRC Press.

Matsuda, L.A., Lolait, S.J., Brownstein, M., Young, A. & Bonner, T.I. (1990). Structure of a cannabinoid receptor and functional expression of the cloned cDNA. *Nature*, **346**, 561–4.

Matsuda, L.A., Bonner, T.I. & Lolait, S.J. (1992). Cannabinoid receptors: which cells, where, how, and why? In *Molecular Approaches to Drug Abuse Research, vol. II: Structure, Function and Expression*, ed. T.N.H. Lee, National Institute on Drug Abuse Research Monograph 126, pp. 48–56. Rockville: U.S. Department of Health and Human Services.

Matsuda, L.A., Bonner, T.I. & Lolait, S.J. (1993). Localization of cannabinoid receptor mRNA in rat brain. *The Journal of Comparative Neurology*, **327**, 535–50.

McBay, A.J. (1988). Interpretation of blood and urine cannabinoid concentrations. *Journal of Forensic Science*, **33**, 875–83.

McClelland, J.L. (1988). Connectionist models and psychological evidence. *Journal of Memory and Language*, **27**, 107–23.

McGahan, J.P., Dublin, A.B. & Sassenrath, E. (1984). Long-term Δ^9-tetrahydrocannabinol treatment: Computed tomography of the brains of rhesus monkeys. *American Journal of Diseases of Children*, **138**, 1109–12.

Mechoulam, R. (ed.) (1986). *Cannabinoids as Therapeutic Agents*. Boca Raton: CRC Press.

Mechoulam, R., Fride, E., Hanus, L., Sheskin, T., Bisogno, T., Di Marzo, V., Bayewitch, M. & Vogel, Z. (1997). Anandamide may mediate sleep induction. *Nature*, **389**, 25–6.

Mechoulam, R., Hanus, L. & Martin, B.R. (1994). Search for endogenous ligands of the cannabinoid receptor. *Biochemical Pharmacology*, **48**, 1537–44.

Melges, F.T., Tinklenberg, J.R., Hollister, L.E. & Gillespie, H.K. (1970). Marihuana and temporal disintegration. *Science*, **168**, 1118–20.

Mendelson, J.H., Rossi, M.A. & Meyer, R.E. (Eds) (1974). *The Use of Marihuana: a Psychological and Physiological Inquiry*. New York: Plenum Press.

Mendhiratta, S.S., Wig, N.N. & Verma, S.K. (1978). Some psychological correlates of long-term heavy cannabis users. *British Journal of Psychiatry*, **132**, 482–6.

Mendhiratta, S.S., Varma, V.K., Dang, R., Malhotra, A.K., Das, K. & Nehra, R. (1988). Cannabis and cognitive functions. *British Journal of Addiction*, **83**, 749–53.

Menkes, D.B., Howard, R.C., Spears, G.F.S. & Cairns, E.R. (1991). Salivary THC following cannabis smoking correlates with subjective intoxication and heart rate. *Psychopharmacology*, **103**, 277–9.

Mesulam, M.M. (1981). A cortical network for directed attention and unilateral neglect. *Annals of Neurology*, **10**, 309–25.

Mesulam, M.M. (1990). Large-scale neurocognitive networks and distributed processing for attention, language, and memory. *Annals of Neurology*, **28**, 597–613.

Meyer, R.E. (1986). How to understand the relationship between psychopathology and addictive disorders: Another example of the chicken and the egg. In *Psychopathology and Addictive Disorders*, ed. R.E. Meyer, pp. 3–16. New York: Guilford Press.

Michie, P.T., Bearpark, H.M., Crawford, J.M. & Glue, L.C. (1990a). The nature of selective attention effects on auditory event-related potentials. *Biological Psychology*, **30**, 219–50.

Michie, P.T., Fox, A.M., Ward, P.B., Catts, S.V. & McConaghy, N. (1990b). ERP indices of selective attention and cortical lateralization in schizophrenia. *Psychophysiology*, **27**, 209–27.

Michie, P.T., LePage, E.L., Solowij, N., Haller, M. & Terry, L. (1996). Evoked otoacoustic emissions and auditory selective attention. *Hearing Research*, **98**, 54–67.

Michie, P.T., Solowij, N., Crawford, J.M. & Glue, L.C. (1993). The effects of between-source discriminability on attended and unattended auditory ERPs. *Psychophysiology*, **30**, 205–20.

Middleton, F.A. and Strick, P.L. (1994). Anatomical evidence for cerebellar and basal ganglia involvement in higher cognitive function. *Science*, **266**, 458–61.

Mikuriya, T.H. & Aldrich, M.R. (1988). Cannabis 1988: old drug, new dangers – the potency question. *Journal of Psychoactive Drugs*, **20**, 47–55.

Miller, L.L. (1984). Marijuana: acute effects on human memory. In *The Cannabinoids: Chemical, Pharmacologic, and Therapeutic Aspects*, ed. S. Agurell, W.L. Dewey, & R.E. Willette, pp. 21–46. Orlando, FL: Academic Press.

Miller, L.L. & Branconnier, R.J. (1983). Cannabis: effects on memory and the cholinergic limbic system. *Psychological Bulletin*, **93**, 441–56.

Miller, L.L., Cornett, T. & MacFarland, D. (1978). Marijuana: an analysis of storage and retrieval deficits in memory with the technique of restricted reminding. *Pharmacology Biochemistry and Behavior*, **8**, 327–32.

Miller, L.L., Drew, W.G. & Kiplinger, G.F. (1972). Effects of marijuana on recall of narrative material and Stroop colour-word performance. *Nature*, **237**, 172–3.

Miller, L.L., McFarland, D., Cornett, T.L. & Brightwell, D.R. (1977a). Marijuana and memory impairment: Effect on free recall and recognition memory. *Pharmacology Biochemistry and Behavior*, **7**, 99–103.

Miller, L.L., McFarland, D., Cornett, T.L., Brightwell, D.R. & Wikler, A. (1977b). Marijuana: effects on free recall and subjective organization of pictures and words. *Psychopharmacology*, **55**, 257–62.

Millsaps, C.L., Azrin, R.L. & Mittenberg, W. (1994). Neuropsychological effects of chronic cannabis use on the memory and intelligence of adolescents. *Journal of Child and Adolescent Substance Abuse*, **3**, 47–55.

Moreau (de Tours), J.J. (1845). *Du Hachisch et de l'Alienation Mentale: Etudes Psychologiques*. Paris: Librairie de Fortin, Masson. (English edition: New York: Raven Press, 1972).

Morland, J., Bugge, A., Skuterud, B., Steen, A., Wethe, G.H. & Kjeldsen, T.

(1985). Cannabinoids in blood and urine after passive inhalation of cannabis smoke. *Journal of Forensic Sciences*, **30**, 997–1002.

Moskowitz, H., Hulbert, S. & McGlothlin, W.H. (1976). Marijuana: effects on simulated driving performance. *Accident Analysis and Prevention*, **8**, 45–50.

Moskowitz, H. & McGlothlin, W.H. (1974). Effects of marijuana on auditory signal detection. *Psychopharmacologia*, **40**, 137–45.

Moskowitz, H., Sharma, S. & McGlothlin, W. (1972). Effects of marijuana upon peripheral vision as a function of the information processing demands in central vision. *Perceptual and Motor Skills*, **35**, 875–82.

Moskowitz, H., Shea, R. & Burns, M. (1974). Effect of marihuana on the psychological refractory period. *Perceptual and Motor Skills*, **38**, 959–62.

Mugford, S. & Cohen, P. (1989). *Drug use, social relations and commodity consumption: A study of recreational cocaine users in Sydney, Canberra and Melbourne*. A Report to the Research Into Drug Abuse Advisory Committee. Canberra: National Campaign Against Drug Abuse.

Mule, S.J., Lomax, P. & Gross, S.J. (1988). Active and realistic passive marijuana exposure tested by three immunoassays and GC/MS in urine. *Journal of Analytical Toxicology*, **12**, 113–16.

Munro, S., Thomas, K.L. & Abu-Shaar, M. (1993). Molecular characterization of a peripheral receptor for cannabinoids. *Nature*, **365**, 61–5.

Musselman, D.L., Haden, C., Caudle, J. & Kalin, N.H. (1994). Cerebrospinal fluid study of cannabinoid users and normal controls. *Psychiatry Research*, **52**, 103–5.

Musty, R. (1988). Individual differences as predictors of marihuana phenomenology. In *Marijuana: An International Research Report*, ed. G. Chesher, P. Consroe & R. Musty, National Campaign Against Drug Abuse Monograph Series No. 7, pp. 201–6. Canberra: Australian Government Printing Service.

Musty, R.E. & Kaback, L. (1995). Relationships between motivation and depression in chronic marijuana users. *Life Sciences*, **56**, 2151–8.

Myers, W.A. & Heath, R.G. (1979). Cannabis sativa: ultrastructural changes in organelles of neurons in brain septal region of monkeys. *Journal of Neuroscience Research*, **4**, 9–17.

Näätänen, R. (1982). Processing negativity: An evoked-potential reflection of selective attention. *Psychological Bulletin*, **92**, 605–40.

Näätänen, R. (1985). Selective attention and stimulus processing: reflections in event-related potentials, magnetoencephalogram and regional cerebral blood flow. In *Attention and Performance, XI*, ed. M.I. Posner & O.S.M. Marin, pp. 355–73. Hillsdale, NJ: Erlbaum.

Näätänen, R. (1987). Regional cerebral blood flow: supplement to event-related potential studies of selective attention. In *Neurophysiology and Psychophysiology: Experimental and Clinical Applications*, ed. G.C. Galbraith, M.L. Kietzman & E. Donchin, pp. 144–56. Hillsdale, NJ: Lawrence Erlbaum.

Näätänen, R. (1988). Implications of ERP data for psychological theories of attention. *Biological Psychology*, **26**, 117–63.

Näätänen, R. (1990). The role of attention in auditory information processing as revealed by event-related potentials and other brain measures of cognitive function. *Behavioral and Brain Sciences*, **13**, 201–88.

Näätänen, R. (1992). *Attention and Brain Function*. Hillsdale, NJ: Erlbaum.

Näätänen, R. & Gaillard, A.W.K. (1983). The orienting reflex and the N2 deflection of the event-related potential (ERP). In *Tutorials in ERP Research: Endogenous Components*, ed. A.W.K. Gaillard & W. Ritter, pp. 119–41. Amsterdam: Elsevier Biomedical Press.

Näätänen, R. & Michie, P.T. (1979). Early selective attention effects on the evoked potential: a critical review and reinterpretation. *Biological Psychology*, 8, 81–136.

Näätänen, R. & Picton, T.W. (1986). N2 and automatic versus controlled processes. *Electroencephalography and Clinical Neurophysiology* (Suppl. 38 McCallum, W.C., Zappoli, R. & Denoth, I. (eds) *Cerebral Psychophysiology: Studies in Event-Related Potentials*), 169–86.

Näätänen, R. & Picton, T. (1987). The N1 wave of the human electric and magnetic response to sound: A review and an analysis of the component structure. *Psychophysiology*, 24, 375–425.

Nahas, G.G. (ed) (1984). *Marihuana in Science and Medicine*. New York: Raven Press.

Nakamura, E.M., da Silva, E.A., Concilio, G.V., Wilkinson, D.A. & Masur, J. (1991). Reversible effects of acute and long-term administration of Δ^9-tetrahydrocannabinol (THC) on memory in the rat. *Drug and Alcohol Dependence*, 28, 167–75.

National Health and Medical Research Council (NH&MRC) (1986). *Is there a safe level of daily consumption of alcohol for men and women? Recommendations regarding responsible drinking behaviour*. Canberra: Australian Government Publishing Service.

National Institute on Drug Abuse (1982). *Marijuana and Youth: Clinical Observations on Motivation and Learning*. Rockville: National Institute on Drug Abuse.

Negrete, J.C. (1983). Psychiatric effects of cannabis use. In *Cannabis and Health Hazards: Proceedings of an ARF/WHO Scientific Meeting on Adverse Health and Behavioral Consequences of Cannabis Use*, ed. K.O. Fehr & H. Kalant, pp. 577–616. Toronto: Addiction Research Foundation.

Negrete, J.C. (1988). What's happened to the cannabis debate? *British Journal of Addiction*, 83, 359–72.

Negrete, J.C., Knapp, W.P., Douglas, D.E. & Smith, W.B. (1986). Cannabis affects the severity of schizophrenic symptoms: results of a clinical survey. *Psychological Medicine*, 16, 515–20.

Neisser, U. (1976). *Cognition and Reality*. San Francisco: W.H. Freeman and Co.

Nelson, H.E. (1982). *The National Adult Reading Test: Test Manual*. Windsor, Berks: NFER-Nelson.

Newcomb, M.D. & Bentler, P. (1988). *Consequences of Adolescent Drug Use: Impact on the Lives of Young Adults*. Newbury Park, California: Sage Publications.

Norman, D.A. & Shallice, T. (1980). *Attention to Action: Willed and Automatic Control of Behavior*. Center for Human Information Processing Technical Report No. 99. (Reprinted in revised form in R.J. Davidson, G.E. Schwartz & D. Shapiro, (1986). *Consciousness and Self-Regulation: Advances in Research and Theory*, vol. 4, pp. 1–18. New York: Plenum Press.)

O'Brien, C.P. (1996). Drug addiction and drug abuse. In *Goodman and Gilman's The Pharmacological Basis of Therapeutics*, ed. J.G. Hardman, L.E. Limbird, P.B., Molinoff, R.W. Ruddon & A.G. Gilman, 9th edn, pp. 557–77. New York: McGraw-Hill.

O'Connor, S., Bauer, L. Tasman, A. & Hesselbrock, V. (1994). Reduced P3 amplitudes are associated with both a family history of alcoholism and antisocial personality disorder. *Progress in Neuro-Psychopharmacology and Biological Psychiatry*, **18**, 1307–21.

Ohlsson, A., Lindgren, J-E., Wahlen, A., Agurell, S., Hollister, L.E. & Gillespie, H.K. (1980). Plasma delta-9-tetrahydrocannabinol concentrations and clinical effects after oral and intravenous administration and smoking. *Clinical Pharmacology and Therapeutics*, **28**, 409–16.

Oviedo, A., Glowa, J. & Herkenham, M. (1993). Chronic cannabinoid administration alters cannabinoid receptor binding in rat brain: a quantitative autoradiographic study. *Brain Research*, **616**, 293–302.

Page, J.B., Fletcher, J. & True, W.R. (1988). Psychosociocultural perspectives on chronic cannabis use: the Costa Rican follow-up. *Journal of Psychoactive Drugs*, **20**, 57–65.

Paige, S.R., Fitzpatrick, D.F., Kline, J.P., Balogh, S.E. & Hendricks, S.E. (1994). Event-related potential amplitude/intensity slopes predict response to antidepressants. *Neuropsychobiology*, **30**, 197–201.

Pardo, J.V., Pardo, P.J., Janer, K.W. & Raichle, M.E. (1990). The anterior cingulate cortex mediates processing selection in the Stroop attentional conflict paradigm. *Proceedings of the National Academy of Sciences of the USA*, **87**, 256–9.

Parsons, O.A., Sinha, R. & Williams, H.L. (1990). Relationships between neuropsychological test performance and event-related potentials in alcoholic and nonalcoholic samples. *Alcoholism: Clinical and Experimental Research*, **14**, 746–55.

Patrick, G., Straumanis, J.J., Struve, F.A., Nixon, F., Fitz-Gerald, M.J., Manno, J.E. & Soucair, M. (1995). Auditory and visual P300 event-related potentials are not altered in medically and psychiatrically normal chronic marihuana users. *Life Sciences*, **56**, 2135–40.

Patrick, G. & Struve, F.A. (1994). Brainstem auditory responses (BAER) in polydrug abuse. *Clinical Electroencephalography*, **25**, 1–7.

Perez-Reyes, M. (1990). Marijuana smoking: Factors that influence the bioavailability of tetrahydrocannabinol. In *Research Findings on Smoking of Abused Substances*, ed. C.N. Chiang & R.L. Hawks, National Institute on Drug Abuse Research Monograph 99, pp. 42–62. Washington DC: U.S. Government Printing Office.

Perez-Reyes, M., Di Guiseppi, S., Davis, K.H., Schindler, V.H. & Cook, C.E. (1982). Comparison of effects of marihuana cigarettes of three different potencies. *Clinical Pharmacology and Therapeutics*, **31**, 617–24.

Perez-Reyes, M., Di Guiseppi, S., Mason, A.M. & Davis, K.H. (1983). Passive inhalation of marihuana smoke and urinary excretion of cannabinoids. *Clinical Pharmacology and Therapeutics*, **34**, 36–41.

Perez-Reyes, M., Hicks, R.E., Bumberry, J., Jeffcoat, A.R. & Cook, C.E. (1988). Interaction between marihuana and ethanol: effects on psychomotor performance. *Alcoholism: Clinical and Experimental Research*, **12**, 268–76.

Perez-Reyes, M., Timmons, M.C. & Wall, M.E. (1974). Long-term use of marijuana and the development of tolerance or sensitivity to Δ⁹Tetrahydrocannabinol. *Archives of General Psychiatry*, **31**, 89–91.

Pertwee, R.G. (1988). The central neuropharmacology of psychotropic cannabinoids. *Pharmacology and Therapeutics*, **36**, 189–261.

Pertwee, R.G. (1992). *In vivo* interactions between psychotropic cannabinoids and other drugs involving central and peripheral neurochemical mechanisms. In

Marijuana / Cannabinoids: Neurobiology and Neurophysiology, ed. L. Murphy & A. Bartke, pp. 165–218. Boca Raton: CRC Press.

Pertwee, R., Griffin, G., Fernando, S., Li, X., Hill, A. & Makriyannis, A. (1995). AM630, a competitive cannabinoid receptor antagonist. *Life Sciences*, **56**, 1949–55.

Petersen, S.E., Fox, P.T., Posner, M.I., Mintun, M. & Raichle, M.E. (1989). Positron emission tomographic studies of the processing of single words. *Journal of Cognitive Neuroscience*, **1**, 153–70.

Pfefferbaum, A., Ford, J.M., White, P.M. & Roth, W.T. (1989). P3 in schizophrenia is affected by stimulus modality, response requirements, medication status, and negative symptoms. *Archives of General Psychiatry*, **46**, 1035–44.

Pfefferbaum, A., Wenegrat, B.G., Ford, J.M., Roth, W.T. & Kopell, B.S. (1984). Clinical application of the P3 component of event-related potentials. II. Dementia, depression and schizophrenia. *Electroencephalography and Clinical Neurophysiology*, **59**, 104–24.

Picton, T.W. (1992). The P300 wave of the human event-related potential. *Journal of Clinical Neurophysiology*, **9**, 456–79.

Picton, T.W. & Stuss, D.T. (1980). The component structure of event-related potentials. *Progress in Brain Research*, **54**, 19–49.

Pomara, N., Block, R., Demetriou, S., Fucek, F., Stanley, M. & Gershon, S. (1983). Attenuation of pilocarpine-induced hypothermia in response to chronic administration of choline. *Psychopharmacology*, **80**, 129–30.

Pope, H.G., Gruber, A.J. & Yurgelun-Todd, D. (1995). The residual neuropsychological effects of cannabis: the current status of research. *Drug and Alcohol Dependence*, **38**, 25–34.

Pope, H.G. & Yurgelun-Todd, D. (1996). The residual cognitive effects of heavy marijuana use in college students. *Journal of the American Medical Association*, **275**, 521–7.

Porjesz, B. & Begleiter, H. (1987). Evoked brain potentials and alcoholism. In *Neuropsychology of Alcoholism: Implications for Diagnosis and Treatment*, ed. O.A. Parsons, N. Butters & P.E. Nathan, pp. 45–63. New York: The Guilford Press.

Posner, M. (1978). *Chronometric Explorations of Mind*. Hillsdale, NJ: Erlbaum.

Posner, M.I. & Petersen, S.E. (1990). The attention system of the human brain. *Annual Review of Neuroscience*, **13**, 25–42.

Posner, M.I., Petersen, S.E., Fox, P.T. & Raichle, M.E. (1988). Localization of cognitive operations in the human brain. *Science*, **240**, 1627–31.

Pritchard, W.S. (1981). Psychophysiology of P300. *Psychological Bulletin*, **89**, 506–40.

Pritchard, W.S. (1986). Cognitive event-related potential correlates of schizophrenia. *Psychological Bulletin*, **100**, 43–66.

Raichle, M.E. (1983). Positron emission tomography. *Annual Review of Neuroscience*, **6**, 249–67.

Ray, R., Prabhu, G.G., Mohan, D., Nath, L.M. & Neki, J.S. (1978). The association between chronic cannabis use and cognitive functions. *Drug and Alcohol Dependence*, **3**, 365–8.

Reed, H.B.C. Jr. (1974). Cognitive effects of marihuana. In *The Use of Marihuana: A Psychological and Physiological Inquiry*, ed. J.H., Mendelson, A.M. Rossi & R.E. Meyer, pp. 107–14. New York: Plenum Press.

Reitan, R.M. (1986). Theoretical and methodological bases of the Halstead-

Reitan Neuropsychological Test Battery. In *Neuropsychological Assessment of Neuropsychiatric Disorders*, ed. I. Grant & K.M. Adams, pp. 3–30. New York: Oxford University Press.

Richmon, J., Murawski, B., Matsumiya, Y., Duffy, F.H. & Lombroso, C.T. (1974). Long-term effects of chronic marihuana smoking. *Electroencephalography and Clinical Neurophysiology*, **36**, 223–4.

Rinaldi-Carmona, M., Barth, F., Héaulme, M., Alonso, R., Shire, D., Congy, C., Soubrié, P., Brelière, J.C. & Le Fur, G. (1995). Biochemical and pharmacological characterisation of SR141716A, the first potent and selective brain cannabinoid receptor antagonist. *Life Sciences*, **56**, 1941–7.

Rinaldi-Carmona, M., Barth, F., Héaulme, M., Shire, D., Calandra, B., Congy, C., Martinez, S., Maruani, J., Neliat, G., Caput, D., Ferrara, P., Soubrié, P., Brelière, J.C. & Le Fur, G. (1994). SR141716A, a potent and selective antagonist of the brain cannabinoid receptor, *Federation of European Biochemical Societies Letters*, **350**, 240–4.

Riskind, J.H., Beck, A.T., Brown, G. & Steer, R.A. (1987). Taking the measure of anxiety and depression: Validity of the reconstructed Hamilton Rating Scale. *Journal of Nervous and Mental Disease*, **175**, 474–9.

Rittenhouse, J.D. (1979). *Consequences of alcohol and marijuana use: survey items for perceived assessment*. DHEW Publication No. ADM 80–920, Washington, DC: U.S. Government Printing Office.

Ritter, W., Simson, R., Vaughan, H.G. & Friedman, D. (1979). A brain event related to the making of a sensory discrimination. *Science*, **203**, 1358–61.

Robbe, H.W.J. & O'Hanlon, J.F. (1993). Marijuana's effect on actual driving: Summary of a 3-year experimental program. In *Alcohol, Drugs and Traffic Safety -T92*, ed. H.-D. Utzelman, G. Berghaus & G. Kroj, vol. 2. Köln: Verlag TÜV Rheinland.

Robinson, T.E. & Berridge, K.C. (1993). The neural basis of drug craving: an incentive-sensitization theory of addiction. *Brain Research Reviews*, **18**, 247–91.

Rochford, J., Grant, I. & LaVigne, G. (1977). Medical students and drugs: further neuropsychological and use pattern considerations. *International Journal of the Addictions*, **12**, 1057–65.

Rodin, E.A., Domino, E.F. & Porzak, J.P. (1970). The marihuana-induced "social high": neurological and electroencephalographic concomitants. *Journal of the American Medical Association*, **213**, 1300–2.

Rodriguez de Fonseca, F. Gorriti, M., Fernandez-Ruiz, J.J., Palomo, T. & Ramos, J.A. (1994). Downregulation of rat brain cannabinoid binding sites after chronic Δ^9-tetrahydrocannabinol treatment. *Pharmacology Biochemistry and Behavior*, **47**, 33–40.

Roffman, R.A. & George, W.H. (1988). Cannabis abuse. In *Assessment of Addictive Behaviors*, ed. D.M. Donovan & G.A. Marlatt, pp. 325–63. New York: Guilford Press.

Romero, J., Garcia, L., Fernandez-Ruiz, J., Cebeira, M. & Ramos, J. (1995). Changes in rat brain cannabinoid binding sites after acute or chronic exposure to their endogenous agonist, anandamide, or to Δ^9-tetrahydrocannabinol. *Pharmacology Biochemistry and Behavior*, **51**, 731–7.

Rosenkrantz, H. (1983). Cannabis, marihuana, and cannabinoid toxicological manifestations in man and animals. In *Cannabis and Health Hazards: Proceedings of an ARF/WHO Scientific Meeting on Adverse Health and Behavioral Consequences of Cannabis Use*, ed. K.O. Fehr & H. Kalant, pp. 91–175. Toronto: Addiction Research Foundation.

Ross, H.E., Glaser, F.B. & Germanson, T. (1988). The prevalence of psychiatric disorders in patients with alcohol and other drug problems. *Archives of General Psychiatry*, **45**, 1023–31.

Rossi, A.M. & O'Brien, J. (1974). Memory and time estimation. In *The Use of Marihuana: a Psychological and Physiological Inquiry*, ed. J.H. Mendelson, A.M. Rossi & R.E. Meyer, pp. 89–106. New York: Plenum Press.

Roth, W.T., Galanter, M., Weingartner, H., Vaughn, T.B. & Wyatt, R.J. (1973). Marijuana and synthetic Δ^9-trans-tetrahydrocannabinol: some effects on the auditory evoked response and background EEG in humans. *Biological Psychiatry*, **6**, 221–33.

Roth, W.T., Tinklenberg, J.R. & Kopell, B.S. (1977). Ethanol and marihuana effects on event-related potentials in a memory retrieval paradigm. *Electroencephalography and Clinical Neurophysiology*, **42**, 381–8.

Rounsaville, B.J. (1989). Clinical assessment of drug abusers. In *Treatment of Substance Use Disorders (Non-Alcohol)*, ed. H.D. Leber, pp. 1183–91. Washington, DC: American Psychiatric Association Press.

Rounsaville, B.J., Kosten, T.R., Weissman, M.M., Prusoff, B., Pauls, D., Foley Anton, S. & Merikangas, K. (1991). Psychiatric disorders in relatives of probands with opiate addiction. *Archives of General Psychiatry*, **48**, 33–42.

Rubin, V. & Comitas, L. (1975). *Ganja in Jamaica: a Medical Anthropological Study of Chronic Marihuana Use*. The Hague: Mouton Publishers.

Rugg, M.D. & Coles, M.G.H. (eds) (1995). *Electrophysiology of Mind: Event-Related Brain Potentials and Cognition*. Oxford: Oxford University Press.

Rumbaugh, C.L., Fang, H.C.H., Wilson, G.H., Higgins, R.E. & Mestek, M.F. (1980). Cerebral CT findings in drug abuse: Clinical and experimental observations. *Journal of Computer Assisted Tomography*, **4**, 330–4.

Rydlander, G. (1939). Personality changes after operations on the frontal lobes. *Acta Psychiatrica Neurologica*, Suppl. 30.

Salisbury, D.F., O'Donnell, B.F., McCarley, R.W., Shenton, M.E. & Benavage, A. (1994). The N2 event-related potential reflects attention deficit in schizophrenia. *Biological Psychology*, **39**, 1–13.

Santucci, V., Storme, J.J., Soubrie, P. & Le Fur, G. (1996). Arousal-enhancing properties of the CB1 cannabinoid receptor antagonist SR 141716A in rats as assessed by electroencephalographic spectral and sleep–waking cycle analysis. *Life Sciences*, **58**, 103–10.

Satz, P., Fletcher, J.M. & Sutker, L.S. (1976). Neuropsychologic, intellectual and personality correlates of chronic marijuana use in native Costa Ricans. *Annals of the New York Academy of Sciences*, **282** (Dornbush, R.L., Freedman, A.M. & Fink, M. (Eds) Chronic Cannabis Use), 266–306.

Scallett, A.C., Uemura, E., Andrews, A., Ali, S.F., McMillan, D.E., Paule, M.G., Brown, R.M. & Slikker, W., Jr (1987). Morphometric studies of the rat hippocampus following chronic delta-9-tetrahydrocannabinol (THC). *Brain Research*, **436**, 193–8.

Schaeffer, J., Andrysiak, T. & Ungerleider, J.T. (1981). Cognition and long-term use of Ganja (cannabis). *Science*, **213**, 465–6.

Schmahmann, J.D. (1996). From movement to thought: anatomic substrates of the cerebellar contribution to cognitive processing. *Human Brain Mapping*, **4**, 174–98.

Schneider, W. & Shiffrin, R.M. (1977). Controlled and automatic human information processing. I. Detection, search and attention. *Psychological Review*, **84**, 1–66.

Schwartz, R.H., Gruenewald, P.J., Klitzner, M. & Fedio, P. (1989). Short-term memory impairment in cannabis-dependent adolescents. *American Journal of Diseases of Children*, **143**, 1214–19.

Shallice, T. (1982). Specific impairments of planning. *Philosophical Transactions of the Royal Society of London B*, **298**, 199–209.

Shallice, T. (1988). *From Neuropsychology to Mental Structure*, Cambridge: Cambridge University Press.

Shannon, M.E. & Fried, P.A. (1972). The macro- and microdistribution and polymorphic electroencephalographic effects of Δ^9-tetrahydrocannabinol in the rat. *Psychopharmacologia*, **27**, 141–56.

Sharma, S. & Moskowitz, H. (1974). Effects of two levels of attention demand on vigilance performance under marihuana. *Perceptual and Motor Skills*, **38**, 967–70.

Shelley, A.M., Ward, P.B., Michie, P.T., Andrews, S., Mitchell, P.F., Catts, S.V. & McConaghy, N. (1991). The effect of repeated testing on ERP components during auditory selective attention. *Psychophysiology*, **28**, 496–510.

Shenton, M.E., Faux, S.F., McCarley, R.W., Ballinger, R., Coleman, M., Torello, M. & Duffy, F.H. (1989). Correlations between abnormal auditory P300 topography and positive symptoms in schizophrenia: a preliminary report. *Biological Psychiatry*, **25**, 710–16.

Shiffrin, R.M. & Schneider, W. (1977). Controlled and automatic human information processing. II. Perceptual learning, automatic attending and a general theory. *Psychological Review*, **84**, 127–90.

Sim, L.J., Hampson, R.E., Deadwyler, S.A. & Childers, S.R. (1996). Effects of chronic treatment with delta(9)-tetrahydrocannabinol on cannabinoid-stimulated [S-35] GTP-gamma-S autoradiography in rat brain. *Journal of Neuroscience*, **16**, 8057–66.

Skinner, J.E. & Yingling, C.D. (1977). Central gating mechanisms that regulate event-related potentials and behaviour – a neural model for attention. In *Progress in Clinical Neurophysiology: vol. 1. Attention, Voluntary Contraction and Event-Related Potentials*, ed. J.E. Desmedt, pp. 30–69. Basel: Karger.

Slikker, W., Jr, Paule, M.G., Ali, S.F., Scallet, A.C. & Bailey, J.R. (1992). Behavioral, neurochemical, and neurohistological effects of chronic marijuana smoke exposure in the nonhuman primate. In *Marijuana / Cannabinoids: Neurobiology and Neurophysiology*, ed. L. Murphy & A. Bartke, pp. 219–73. Boca Raton: CRC Press.

Smiley, A. (1986). Marijuana: on-road and driving simulator studies. *Alcohol, Drugs and Driving*, **2**, 121–34.

Smiley, A. (in press) Marijuana: on road and driving simulator studies. World Health Organisation Project on Health Implications of Cannabis Use.

Smith, D.E. (1968). Acute and chronic toxicity of marijuana. *Journal of Psychedelic Drugs*, **2**, 37–47.

Smith, P.B., Compton, D.R., Welch, S.P., Razdan, R.K., Mechoulam, R. & Martin, B.R. (1994). The pharmacological activity of anandamide, a putative endogenous cannabinoid, in mice. *The Journal of Pharmacology and Therapeutics*, **270**, 219–27.

Snyder, S. (1990). Planning for serendipity. *Nature*, **346**, 508.

Snyder, E. & Hillyard, S.A. (1976). Long latency evoked potentials to irrelevant deviant stimuli. *Behavioral Biology*, **16**, 319–31.

Sohlberg, M.M. & Mateer, C.A. (1989). *Introduction to Cognitive Rehabilitation. Theory and Practice*. New York: The Guilford Press.

Solowij, N. (1995). Do cognitive impairments recover following cessation of cannabis use? *Life Sciences*, **56**, 2119–26.

Solowij, N., Grenyer, B.F.S, Chesher, G. & Lewis, J. (1995a). Biopsychosocial changes associated with cessation of cannabis use: a single case study of acute and chronic cognitive effects, withdrawal and treatment. *Life Sciences*, **56**, 2127–34.

Solowij, N., Grenyer, B.F.S., Peters, R. & Chesher, G. (1997). Long-term cannabis use impairs memory processes and frontal lobe function. In *1997 Symposium on the Cannabinoids*, p. 84. International Cannabinoid Research Society, Burlington, Vermont.

Solowij, N., Michie, P.T. & Fox, A.M. (1991). Effects of long-term cannabis use on selective attention: an event-related potential study. *Pharmacology Biochemistry and Behavior*, **40**, 683–8.

Solowij, N., Michie, P.T. & Fox, A.M. (1995b). Differential impairments of selective attention due to frequency and duration of cannabis use. *Biological Psychiatry*, **37**, 731–9.

Solowij, N., Michie, P.T. & Fox, A.M. (1995c). ERP indices of selective attention in ex-cannabis users. *Biological Psychology*, **39**, 201.

Soueif, M.I. (1971). The use of cannabis in Egypt: A behavioural study. *Bulletin on Narcotics*, **23**, 17–28.

Soueif, M.I. (1975). Chronic cannabis users: further analysis of objective test results. *Bulletin on Narcotics*, **27**, 1–26.

Soueif, M.I. (1976a). Differential association between chronic cannabis use and brain function deficits. *Annals of the New York Academy of Sciences*, **282** (Dornbush, R.L., Freedman, A.M. & Fink, M. (eds) Chronic Cannabis Use), 323–43.

Soueif, M.I. (1976b). Some determinants of psychological deficits associated with chronic cannabis consumption. *Bulletin on Narcotics*, **28**, 25–42.

Soueif, M.I. (1977). The Egyptian study of chronic cannabis use: a reply to Fletcher and Satz. *Bulletin on Narcotics*, **29**, 35–43.

Souza, V.B.N., Muir, W.J., Walker, M.T., Glabus, M.F., Roxborough, H.M., Sharp, C.W., Dunan, J.R. & Blackwood, D.H.R. (1995). Auditory P300 event-related potentials and neuropsychological performance in schizophrenia and bipolar affective disorder. *Biological Psychiatry*, **37**, 300–10.

Spielberger, C.D., Gorsuch, R.L. & Lushene, R.E. (1970). *STAI Manual for the State-Trait Anxiety Inventory*. Palo Alto, California: Consulting Psychologists Press.

Squires, K.C., Donchin, E., Herning, R.I. & McCarthy, G. (1977). On the influence of task relevance and stimulus probability on event-related potential components. *Electroencephalography and Clinical Neurophysiology*, **42**, 1–14.

Squires, N.K., Squires, K.C. & Hillyard, S.A. (1975). Two varieties of long-latency positive waves evoked by unpredictable auditory stimuli in man. *Electroencephalography and Clinical Neurophysiology*, **38**, 387–401.

Stadnicki, S.W., Schaeppi, U., Rosenkrantz, H. & Braude, M.C. (1974). Crude marihuana extract: EEG and behavioral effects of chronic oral administration in rhesus monkeys. *Psychopharmacologia*, **37**, 225–33.

Stefanis, C. (1976). Biological aspects of cannabis use. In *The International Challenge of Drug Abuse*, ed. R.C. Petersen, pp. 149–78. Rockville: National Institute on Drug Abuse.

Stefanis, C., Dornbush, R. & Fink, M. (1977). *Hashish: Studies of Long-Term Use*. New York: Raven Press.

Stephens, R.S., Roffman, R.A. & Simpson, E.E. (1993). Adult marijuana users seeking treatment. *Journal of Consulting and Clinical Psychology*, **61**, 1100–4.

Stiglick, A. & Kalant, H. (1982a). Learning impairment in the radial-arm maze following prolonged cannabis treatment in rats. *Psychopharmacology*, **77**, 117–23.

Stiglick, A. & Kalant, H. (1982b). Residual effects of prolonged cannabis administration on exploration and DRL performance in rats. *Psychopharmacology*, **77**, 124–8.

Stillman, R.C., Weingartner, H., Wyatt, R.J., Gillin, C. & Eich, J. (1974). State-dependent (dissociative) effects of marihuana on human memory. *Archives of General Psychiatry*, **31**, 81–5.

Straumanis, J., Struve, F. & Patrick, G. (1993). Cerebral evoked potentials in chronic marijuana users. In *Problems of Drug Dependence 1992*, ed. L. Harris, National Institute on Drug Abuse Research Monograph 132, p. 351. Washington DC: U.S. Government Printing Office.

Straumanis, J., Struve, F., Patrick, G. & Raz, Y. (1991). Cognitive and sensory evoked potentials in chronic marihuana users. In *Biological Psychiatry*, ed. G. Racagni, N. Brunello, & T. Fakuda, vol. 2, pp. 21–4. New York: Elsevier Science Publishers.

Struve, F., Patrick, G. & Leavitt, J. (1995). Development of a "composite" measure of alpha hyperfrontality for use in THC research. In *Problems of Drug Dependence 1994*, ed. L.S. Harris, National Institute on Drug Abuse Research Monograph 153, p. 505. Washington DC: U.S. Government Printing Office.

Struve, F.A. & Straumanis, J.J. (1990). Electroencephalographic and evoked potential methods in human marihuana research: Historical review and future trends. *Drug Development Research*, **20**, 369–88.

Struve, F., Straumanis, J.J. & Patrick, G. (1994). Persistent topographic quantitative EEG sequelae of chronic marihuana use: a replication study and initial discriminant function analysis. *Clinical Electroencephalography*, **25**, 63–75.

Struve, F., Straumanis, J., Patrick, G., Norris, G., Leavitt, J. & Webb, P. (1992). Topographic quantitative EEG findings in subjects with 15+ years of cumulative daily THC exposure. In *Problems of Drug Dependence 1991*, ed. L. Harris, National Institute on Drug Abuse Research Monograph 119, p. 451. Washington DC: U.S. Government Printing Office.

Struve, F., Straumanis, J., Patrick, G., Norris, G., Nixon, F., Fitz-Gerald, M., Manno, J., Leavitt, J. & Webb, P. (1993). Altered quantitative EEG topography as sequelae of chronic THC exposure: a replication using screened normal Ss. In *Problems of Drug Dependence 1992*, ed. L. Harris, National Institute on Drug Abuse Research Monograph 132, p. 178. Washington DC: U.S. Government Printing Office.

Stuss, D.T. (1991). Interference effects on memory function in postleukotomy patients: an attentional perspective. In *Frontal Lobe Function and Dysfunction*, ed. H.S., Levin, H.M. Eisenberg & A.L. Benton, pp. 157–72. New York: Oxford University Press.

Stuss, D.T. & Benson, D.F. (eds) (1986). *The Frontal Lobes*. New York: Raven Press.

Substance Abuse and Mental Health Services Administration (1993). *National Household Survey on Drug Abuse: Population Estimates 1992*. Rockville, Maryland.

Susser, M. (1972). Cerebral atrophy in young cannabis smokers. *Lancet*, **1**, 41–2.

Swift, W., Williams, G., Neill, O. & Grenyer, B.F.S. (1990). The prevalence of minor psychopathology in opioid users seeking treatment. *British Journal of Addiction*, **85**, 629–34.

Tart, C. (1970). Marijuana intoxication: common experiences. *Nature*, **226**, 701–4.
Tashkin, D.P. (1993). Is frequent marijuana smoking harmful to health? *Western Journal of Medicine*, **158**, 635–7.
Tassinari, C.A., Peraita-Adrados, M.R., Ambrosetto, H.G. & Gastact, H. (1974). Effects of marihuana and Δ^9- THC at high doses in man: a polygraphic study. *Electroencephalography and Clinical Neurophysiology*, **36**, 94.
Tecce, J.J. (1972). Contingent negative variation (CNV) and psychological processes in man. *Psychological Bulletin*, **77**, 73–108.
Tecce, J.J. & Cole, J.O. (1974). Amphetamine effects in man: paradoxical drowsiness and lowered electrical brain activity (CNV). *Science*, **185**, 451–3.
Tennant, F.S. & Groesbeck, C.J. (1972). Psychiatric effects of hashish. *Archives of General Psychiatry*, **27**, 133–6.
Terranova, J.P., Storme, J.J., Lafon, N., Pério, A., Rinaldi-Carmona, M., Le Fur, G. & Soubrié, P. (1996). Improvement of memory in rodents by the selective CB1 cannabinoid receptor antagonist, SR 141716. *Psychopharmacology*, **126**, 165–72.
Thomas, H. (1993). Psychiatric symptoms in cannabis users. *British Journal of Psychiatry*, **163**, 141–9.
Thompson, L.K. & Cone, E.J. (1987). Determination of delta-9-tetrahydrocannabinol in human blood and saliva by high-performance liquid chromatography with amperometric detection. *Journal of Chromatography*, **421**, 91–7.
Thornicroft, G. (1990). Cannabis and psychosis: is there epidemiological evidence for association? *British Journal of Psychiatry*, **157**, 25–33.
Timsit-Berthier, M., Gerono, A., Rousseau, J.C., Mantanus, H., Abraham, P., Verhey, F.M.H., Lamers, T. & Edmonds, P. (1984). An international pilot study of CNV in mental illness: second report. *Annals of the New York Academy of Sciences*, **425**, 629–37.
Tinklenberg, J.R. (1972). Marihuana and alcohol. *Psychopharmacology Bulletin*, **8**, 9–10.
Tinklenberg, J.R., Kopell, B.S., Melges, F.T. & Hollister, L.E. (1972). Marihuana and alcohol: time production and memory functions. *Archives of General Psychiatry*, **27**, 812–15.
Tinklenberg, J.R., Melges, F.T., Hollister, L.E. & Gillespie, H.K. (1970). Marijuana and immediate memory. *Nature*, **226**, 1171–2.
Tipper, S.P. & Cranston, M. (1985). Selective attention and priming: inhibitory and facilitatory effects of ignored primes. *Quarterly Journal of Experimental Psychology*, **37A**, 591–611.
Towey, J.G., Bruder, G., Hollander, G., Friedman, D. & Erhan, H. (1990). Endogenous event-related potentials in obsessive-compulsive disorder. *Biological Psychiatry*, **28**, 92–8.
Towey, J.P., Tenke, C.E., Bruder, G.E., Leite, P., Friedman, D., Liebowitz, M. & Hollander, E. (1994). Brain event-related potential correlates of overfocused attention in obsessive compulsive disorder. *Psychophysiology*, **31**, 535–43.
Treisman, A.M. (1964a). Monitoring and storage of irrelevant messages in selective attention. *Journal of Verbal Learning and Verbal Behavior*, **3**, 449–54.
Treisman, A.M. (1964b). Verbal cues, language and meaning in selective attention. *American Journal of Psychology*, **77**, 206–19.
Treisman, A.M. & Gelade, G. (1980). A feature integration theory of attention. *Cognitive Psychology*, **12**, 97–136.
Tunving, K., Lundqvist, T. & Eriksson, D. (1988). "A way out of the fog": an outpatient program for cannabis users. In *Marijuana: An International*

Research Report, ed. G., Chesher, P. Consroe & R.Musty, National Campaign Against Drug Abuse Monograph Series No. 7, pp. 207–12. Canberra: Australian Government Printing Service.

Tunving, K., Thulin, O., Risberg, J. & Warkentin, S. (1986). Regional cerebral blood flow in long-term heavy cannabis use. *Psychiatry Research*, **17**, 15–21.

Vachon, L., Sulkowski, A. & Rich, E. (1974). Marihuana effects on learning, attention and time estimation. *Psychopharmacologia*, **39**, 1–11.

Vanderstelt, O., Gunning, W.B., Snel, J., Zeef, E. & Kok, A. (1994). Children of alcoholics – attention, information processing and event-related brain potentials. *Acta Paediatrica*, **83** (Suppl. 404), 4–6.

Varma, V.J., Malhotra, A.K., Dang, R., Das, K. & Nehra, R. (1988). Cannabis and cognitive functions: a prospective study. *Drug and Alcohol Dependence*, **21**, 147–52.

Vasey, M.W. & Thayer, J.F. (1987). The continuing problem of false positives in repeated measures ANOVA in psychophysiology: a multivariate solution. *Psychophysiology*, **24**, 479–86.

Vogel, Z., Barg, J., Levy, R., Saya, D., Heldman, E. & Mechoulam, R. (1993). Anandamide, a brain endogenous compound, interacts specifically with cannabinoid receptors and inhibits adenylate cyclase. *Journal of Neurochemistry*, **61**, 352–5.

Volavka, J., Fink, M., Stefanis, C., Panayiotopoulos, C. & Dornbush, R. (1977). EEG effects of cannabis in chronic hashish users. *Electroencephalography and Clinical Neurophysiology*, **42**, 730.

Volkow, N.D., Gillespie, H., Mullani, N., Tancredi, L., Grant, C., Ivanovic, M. & Hollister, L. (1991a). Cerebellar metabolic activation by delta-9-tetrahydrocannabinol in human brain: A study with positron emission tomography and ^{18}F-2-fluoro-2-deoxyglucose. *Psychiatry Research: Neuroimaging*, **40**, 69–78.

Volkow, N.D., Gillespie, H., Mullani, N., Tancredi, L., Grant, C., Valentine, A. & Hollister, L. (1996). Brain glucose-metabolism in chronic marijuana users at baseline and during marijuana intoxication. *Psychiatry Research: Neuroimaging*, **67**, 29–38.

Volkow, N.D., Gillespie, H., Mullani, N., Tancredi, L., Hollister, L., Ivanovic, M., and Grant, C. (1991b). Use of positron emission tomography to investigate the action of marihuana in the human brain. In *Physiopathology of Illicit Drugs: Cannabis, Cocaine, Opiates*, ed. G. Nahas & C. Latour, pp. 3–11. Oxford: Pergamon Press.

Volkow, N.D., Gillespie, H., Tancredi, L. & Hollister, L. (1995). The effects of marijuana in the human brain measured with regional brain glucose metabolism. In *Sites of Drug Action in the Human Brain*, ed. A. Biegon & N.D. Volkow, pp. 75–86. Boca Raton: CRC Press.

Waldo, M., Gerhardt, G.A., Baker, N., Drebing, C., Adler, L., and Freedman, R. (1992). Auditory sensory gating and catecholamine metabolism in schizophrenic and normal subjects. *Psychiatry Research*, **44**, 21–32.

Wall, M.E., Sadler, B.M., Brine, D., Taylor, H. & Perez-Reyes, M. (1983). Metabolism, disposition, and kinetics of Δ9-tetrahydrocannabinol in men and women. *Clinical Pharmacology and Therapeutics*, **34**, 352–63.

Walter, W.G., Cooper, R., Aldridge, V.J., McCallum, W.C. & Winter, A.L. (1964). Contingent negative variation: An electrical sign of sensorimotor association and expectancy in the human brain. *Nature*, **203**, 380–4.

Ward, P.B., Catts, S.V., Fox, A.M., Michie, P.T. & McConaghy, N. (1991).

Auditory selective attention and event-related potentials in schizophrenia. *British Journal of Psychiatry*, **158**, 534–9.

Webb, P., Struve, F., Leavitt, J., Norris, G., Fitz-Gerald, M., Nixon, F. & Straumanis, J. (1993). Time distortion as a persistent sequelae of chronic THC use. In *Problems of Drug Dependence 1992*, ed. L. Harris, National Institute on Drug Abuse Research Monograph 132, p. 177. Washington DC: U.S. Government Printing Office.

Weckowicz, T.E., Collier, G. & Spreng, L. (1977). Field dependence, cognitive functions, personality traits, and social values in heavy cannabis users and nonuser controls. *Psychological Reports*, **41**, 291–302.

Weckowicz, T.E. & Janssen, D.V. (1973). Cognitive functions, personality traits, and social values in heavy marijuana smokers and nonsmoker controls. *Journal of Abnormal Psychology*, **81**, 264–9.

Weil, A. (1970). Adverse reactions to marihuana. *New England Journal of Medicine*, **282**, 997–1000.

Wert, R.C. & Raulin, M.L. (1986a). The chronic cerebral effects of cannabis use. I. Methodological issues and neurological findings. *International Journal of the Addictions*, **21**, 605–28.

Wert, R.C. & Raulin, M.L. (1986b). The chronic cerebral effects of cannabis use. II. Psychological findings and conclusions. *International Journal of the Addictions*, **21**, 629–42.

Westlake, T.M., Howlett, A.C., Ali, S.F., Paule, M.G. & Scallett, W. Jr. (1991). Chronic exposure to delta-9-tetrahydrocannabinol fails to irreversibly alter brain cannabinoid receptors. *Brain Research*, **544**, 145–9.

Westlake, T.M., Howlett, A.C., Bonner, T.I., Matsuda, L.A., Herkenham, M. (1994). Cannabinoid receptor binding and messenger RNA expression in human brain: An in vitro receptor autoradiography and in situ hybridization histochemistry study of normal aged and Alzheimer's brains. *Neuroscience*, **63**, 637–52.

Wig, N.N. & Varma, V.K. (1977). Patterns of long-term heavy cannabis use in North India and its effects on cognitive functions: a preliminary report. *Drug and Alcohol Dependence*, **2**, 211–19.

Williams, H.L. (1987). Evoked brain potentials and alcoholism: questions, hypotheses, new approaches. In *Neuropsychology of Alcoholism: Implications for Diagnosis and Treatment*, ed. O.A., Parsons, N. Butters & P.E. Nathan, pp. 103–28. New York: The Guilford Press.

Woldorff, M.G., Gallen, C.C., Hampson, S.R., Hillyard, S.A., Pantev, C., Sobel, D. & Bloom, F.E. (1993). Modulations of early sensory processing in human auditory cortex during auditory selective attention. *Proceedings of the National Academy of Sciences of the USA*, **90**, 8722–6.

Woldorff, M.G., Hackley, S.A. & Hillyard, S.A. (1991). The effects of channel-selective attention on the mismatch negativity wave elicited by deviant tones. *Psychophysiology*, **28**, 30–42.

Woldorff, M.G. & Hillyard, S.A. (1991). Modulation of early auditory processing during selective listening to rapidly presented tones. *Electroencephalography and Clinical Neurophysiology*, **79**, 170–91.

Woods, D.L. (1989). The physiological basis of selective attention: implications of event-related potential studies. In *Event-Related Brain Potentials: Basic Issues and Applications*, ed. J.W., Rohrbaugh, R. Parasuraman & R. Johnson, pp. 178–207. New York: Oxford Press.

Woods, D.L., Alho, K. & Algazi, A. (1994). Stages of auditory feature conjunction: an event-related brain potential study. *Journal of Experimental Psychology: Human Perception and Performance*, **20**, 81–94.

Woods, D.L. & Knight, R.T. (1986). Electrophysiologic evidence of increased distractibility after dorsolateral prefrontal lesions. *Neurology*, **36**, 212–16.

Yesavage, J.A., Leirer, V.O., Denari, M. & Hollister, L.E. (1985). Carry-over effects of marijuana intoxication on aircraft pilot performance: a preliminary report. *American Journal of Psychiatry*, **142**, 1325–9.

Zablocki, B., Aidala, A., Hansell, S. & White, H. R. (1991). Marijuana use, introspectiveness, and mental health. *Journal of Health and Social Behavior*, **32**, 65–79.

Zeef, E.J. & Kok A. (1993). Age-related differences in the timing of stimulus and response processes during visual selective attention: performance and psychophysiological analyses. *Psychophysiology*, **30**, 138–51.

Index

Lightning Source UK Ltd.
Milton Keynes UK

171569UK00002B/12/A